THE DISEASE OF VIRGINS

THE DISEASE OF VIRGINS

Green sickness, chlorosis and the problems of puberty

Helen King

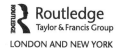

LONDON AND NEW YORK

First published 2004
by Routledge
2 Park Square, Milton Park, Abingdon, Oxon, OX14 4RN

Simultaneously published in the USA and Canada
by Routledge
270 Madison Ave, New York NY 10016

Routledge is an imprint of the Taylor & Francis Group

Transferred to Digital Printing 2009

Typeset in Garamond by Taylor & Francis Books Ltd

British Library Cataloguing in Publication Data
A catalogue record for this book is available from the British Library

Library of Congress Cataloging in Publication Data
A catalog record for this book has been requested

ISBN10: 0–415–22662–7 (hbk)
ISBN10: 0–415–55499–3 (pbk)

ISBN13: 978–0–415–22662–2 (hbk)
ISBN13: 978–0–415–55499–2 (pbk)

CONTENTS

Preface   vii
List of abbreviations   ix

Introduction   1

1 The nature of green sickness   18
   The humoral body 22
   From green jaundice to green sickness 24
   Green sickness and the disease of virgins 29
   How green was green sickness? 30
   Green sickness and love sickness 36

2 A new disease? The classical sources for the disease of virgins   43
   Lange's letter 45
   Hippocratic virginity 49
   The transmission of On the disease of virgins *51*
   What is a virgin? 53
   Other possible Hippocratic sources 59
   'Some unknown monster': the challenge of 'new' diseases 61

3 The menstruating virgin   67
   The Galenic physiology of menstruation 68
   Alternative theories of menstruation 71
   Letting blood in the Hippocratic and Galenic bodies 73
   'Marriage is a sovereign cure' 79
   The problem of puberty 83
   The philosophy of puberty 88
   Town and country 90

4 **Dietary factors**   94
Food and the growth of the body 98
Pica 103
Green sickness as a liver disorder 107
Constipation 112

5 **'The laboratory came to the rescue': technology and chlorosis** 116
The pulse 118
The stethoscope 120
Blood testing 121
Treatments 124
Shall we dance? 129
Rest 130
Alternatives to orthodoxy 131
Women physicians and chlorosis 134

Conclusion   139

Appendix   142
Notes   144
Bibliography   162
Index   188

PREFACE

When the late Roy Porter and George Rousseau published their history of gout, they began by attempting to disarm potential critics of this enterprise by stating that 'No apology is needed for writing the history of a malady and its cultural representation' (Porter and Rousseau 1998: 1). Roy enthusiastically supported my project but, unlike him, I feel I do need to apologise. First, because writing a history of 'a disease' seems a methodologically dubious pursuit, particularly when it is not clear to what extent this was a diverse collection of acute and chronic conditions which went under a single name – a point picked up in the title of Irvine Loudon's article of 1984, 'The diseases called chlorosis' – or, as I am suggesting here, a collection of symptoms which went under several different names but retained its core identity through the turmoil of medical change. Second, I would like to state now that, in following this disease from its Renaissance origins to its twentieth-century decline, I am all too aware that, as a historian of pre-modern medicine, I am entering the territory of those whose right to comment on it is far greater than mine. But sometimes it is worth taking the long view. I have been working on the disease of virgins for many years, and have been struck by the echoes across the centuries, although, as a scholar whose main interest hitherto has been in locating medical texts within very specific social and cultural contexts of production, I am aware that I could have done far more to tease out the subtle shifts beneath apparent continuities.

A preliminary attempt to understand the condition was supported by a British Academy Leave Award in 1995, and appeared as 'Hippocrates, Galen and the origins of the "disease of virgins"', *International Journal of the Classical Tradition* 2 (1996): 372–87, reprinted as chapter 10 of *Hippocrates' Woman: Reading the Female Body in Ancient Greece* (London: Routledge, 1998). Some of the material from that essay is revisited here in parts of chapters 1 and 2. The scope of this book expanded as a result of holding a University Award from the Wellcome Trust. Early versions of chapters were presented to the University of Birmingham Gender Seminar; the Leeds Historical Association; the London and Oxford Wellcome Units; KNHG

Voorjaarscongres, Den Haag; the Reading University Early Modern Research Centre; the American Association for the History of Medicine; and at the University of Victoria, British Columbia, as a Landsdowne Visiting Lecturer. The bulk of the manuscript was completed in the perfect conditions provided by the Netherlands Institute for Advanced Studies, during a fellowship held there in early 2001 as part of the project on medical history organised by Manfred Horstmanshoff and Marten Stol. The final stages have been much assisted by practical help from Janette Allottey, Leigh Hankin, Polly Harte, Edward James, Gordon Moger, Clare O'Sullivan and John Symons. My thanks to all who have shared my enthusiasm for this condition over the last ten years, including Ann Hanson, Cathy Crawford, Monica Green, Lucinda McCray Beier, Ursula Potter and Vivian Nutton, but above all to Irvine Loudon and Elaine Hobby, for reading the complete manuscript. All errors of fact or interpretation which remain are, of course, my own.

ABBREVIATIONS

AWP	[Hippocrates], *Airs Waters Places*
BL	British Library
BN	Bibliothèque Nationale
CMG	Corpus Medicorum Graecorum
CML	Corpus Medicorum Latinorum
CUL	Cambridge University Library
DNB	Dictionary of National Biography
DW	[Hippocrates], *Diseases of women*
GA	Aristotle, *De generatione animalium*
Gen.	[Hippocrates], *On generation*
Gyn.	Soranos, *Gynaecology*; Temkin 1956
K	Carl Gottlob Kühn (1821–33) *Claudii Galeni opera omnia*, 20 vols, Leipzig
L	Emile Littré (1839–61) *Oeuvres complètes d'Hippocrate*, 10 vols, Paris: Baillière
Loc. Aff.	Galen, *On the Affected Parts*
Loeb	Loeb Classical Library (Cambridge, MA and London)
MRCS	Member of the Royal College of Surgeons
NC	[Hippocrates], *On the nature of the child*
NW	[Hippocrates], *Nature of woman*
PA	Aristotle, *De partibus animalium*
QC	Plutarch, *Quaestiones convivales*
WMS	Wellcome manuscript

INTRODUCTION

What is the 'disease of virgins'? The simple answer to this question is that it was a historical condition involving lack of menstruation, dietary disturbances, altered skin colour and general weakness once thought to affect, almost exclusively, young girls at puberty. This answer may seem to side-step other questions which should come first: for example, what do we mean by 'a' disease? Were all the girls diagnosed as suffering from this disease really ill with the same condition? Were they ill at all? When trying to understand a disease which gripped the imaginations of people in the past, is the investigation over if we can match up the symptoms listed in our sources to a single named disease recognised today? Or is this when the role of the historian really begins? As Irvine Loudon has made admirably clear, the problem of retrospective diagnosis 'consists of attempting to reconcile conflicting evidence for the sake of a single disease hypothesis: the attempt is misguided and doomed to failure' (1984: 32).[1]

This is not, therefore, a book which seeks to diagnose – to identify in twenty-first-century terms – the 'disease of virgins'. Like Joan Jacobs Brumberg (1982: 1469; cf. Green 2001: 65–6), I do not believe that there is any simple 'one-to-one equivalent' between modern Western biomedical categories and those of the past. Instead, my interest lies in discovering the origins and uses of the idea of a 'disease of virgins', and the reasons for its popularity, not only in medical handbooks and treatises but also in popular literature, such as ballads and plays, and recipe collections, including those kept by women. Particularly important are physicians' case notes, in which a university-trained physician's understanding of disease came into negotiation with a patient's ideas about illness. Above all, I am interested in the roles served by the 'disease of virgins' in thinking about the body, and in regulating the sexuality of young women. As Ian Maclean (1980: 46) noted in his important study of Renaissance ideas about women, medical writings 'produce a "natural" justification for women's relegation to the home and exclusion from public office'; within the larger category of gynaecology, what was the message of discussions of the 'disease of virgins'?

1

In an important essay on the nature of disease, Charles Rosenberg (1992: xiii) noted that 'a disease does not exist as a social phenomenon until we agree that it does – until it is named'. For the disease of virgins, this focuses our attention on the period when it was first given its name, and on the alternative names it attracted; changes in the labelling of the condition, and in the explanations provided for its symptoms, can then provide a window on to wider shifts in medicine. The 'disease of virgins', or *morbus virgineus*, is just one of many names for a largely similar group of symptoms;[2] over a 400-year period, extending from 1554 to around 1930, other labels used included the white fever, the green sickness, chlorosis (a coined 'technical' word based on *chloros*, a Greek term for 'yellowish green') and, from the mid-nineteenth century, hypochromic anaemia.[3] French medicine included 'les pâles couleurs': German 'Bleichsucht' and Dutch 'geelzucht' also suggest 'the pale disease'.[4] These names suggest something of the richness of pre-modern diagnostic labels in their focus on colour. But different labels have always been available to apply to a young girl, 'pale, as if bloodless',[5] with disturbed eating patterns who failed to menstruate; and different stories can be told depending on whether food consumption is thought to affect menstrual cycles, or accumulated menstrual blood is assumed to depress the appetite for food, or another factor altogether is supposed to affect both appetite and the menstrual cycle. Today, I suspect that we would focus on the eating patterns, not worry unduly about the absence of menstrual periods, quiz the sufferer about her body image, and most probably diagnose anorexia nervosa. It has, indeed, been argued that the decline of chlorosis corresponds chronologically to the rise of anorexia nervosa as the culturally 'typical' ailment in young girls (Loudon 1980: 1674; 1984); Margaret Humphreys has gone further, calling anorexia nervosa 'a synonym for chlorosis' (1997: 163; cf. Theriot 1988: 121). In the early modern period, this label had not been created;[6] however, a young girl with the characteristic symptoms of the disease of virgins could also be thought to suffer from obstruction of the spleen,[7] consumption,[8] *cachexia virginea*,[9] love sickness, excess phlegm, or menstrual retention, due either to obstruction of the passages or to weakness of the expulsive faculty of the womb.[10] What factors influenced the decision to label her symptoms as 'the disease of virgins', 'green sickness' or 'chlorosis'? What were the implications of being labelled as a sufferer from the 'disease of virgins', and would they be identical for a girl 200 years later who was thought to have 'chlorosis'?

Over its history, the disease of virgins exhibits both similarity and difference, both stability and upheaval. Towards the end of the sixteenth century, Luis Mercado's *De mulierum affectionibus* (1579: 201) claimed that *morbus virgineus* was an alternative name for the white fever, 'because we observe that it occurs in a large number of virgins',[11] yet by the early nineteenth century, even its existence was being challenged. The Newcastle physician Andrew Fogo referred to it without hesitation as an 'imaginary disease', writing that

> The imaginary disease has had various names applied to it; such as amenorrhoea, chlorosis, green sickness, suppression of the menses, the want of *them*, *those*, the courses, the flowers, & c ...
>
> (Fogo 1803: 1)

Fogo combines what we would now consider to be 'symptoms' – absence of menses, expressed in formal classicising medical terminology or in the euphemisms of his day – with 'disease labels', such as chlorosis. This tendency is even more typical of pre-modern Western medicine, where our sources often classify as a 'disease' what we would regard only as 'symptoms'; for example, a headache, or lethargy, could be given the status of 'disease' (Wear 2000: 106–9). However, although there is generally some degree of difference here between early modern and modern medicine, we should not create too stark a dichotomy. In John Tanner's *The Hidden Treasures of the Art of Physick*, published in 1659, the chapter on green sickness follows that on 'pissing of blood', and immediately precedes that on 'stoppage of the terms'. Here, green sickness is a disease in its own right, placed logically after pathological loss of blood, but distinguished from the simple absence of menstruation, which is itself classified here as a 'disease'. In the early eighteenth century, John Maubray (1724: 42) noted that the virgins' disease was 'variously represented and taken, sometimes for a Disease, and sometimes for a Symptom'.

Beneath apparent shifts, the study of the disease of virgins thus reveals considerable continuity. Fogo's comment also gives a 200-year pedigree to the question of whether chlorosis ever existed: is it an imaginary disease, or a real disease? For the purposes of this book, the question is not central; endlessly transformed, it continued to be diagnosed. Later in the nineteenth century, Samuel Osborne Habershon (1863: 518) still considered that chlorosis was 'a state recognised with great facility', while Sir Andrew Clark (1887: 1003) stated that 'everyone acquainted with medical literature knows the great variety of names which has been given to this malady'; for these physicians, the existence of a single 'malady' behind the labels was not in doubt. Their certainty was increased by the medical technologies of the nineteenth century, which will be discussed in chapter 5; in particular, quantification of the pulse, and blood testing, were used to rescue chlorosis from any charge of being an imaginary disease, and to distinguish it from other conditions.

In his study of vernacular medical literature in Tudor England, Paul Slack (1979: 268) noted that a 'satisfactory' account of a disease at that time needed to include not just its name and its cure, but also its cause. Explanations of the cause of the disease of virgins varied as medical knowledge and theories changed; in different periods of its history, the symptoms were traced back to the womb, the intestines, the liver, the colon or the blood.[12] There is something circular about its aetiology, giving it almost a complete life-cycle; in the 1550s its symptoms were thought to be caused by abnormally thick and sticky blood becoming stuck in the internal channels of a virgin at menarche, while in its declining years at the beginning of the twentieth century it returned to being a blood disorder, but was now seen as the result of low specific gravity or inadequate blood manufacture by the body.

As for the ultimate cause, leading to the disturbance of the various body systems, this changed as ideas about virginity and puberty shifted. In the early eighteenth century, the surgeon Daniel Turner commented explicitly on the 'diverse Appellations' of the condition and noted that the name 'disease of virgins' marks the condition 'as more particular to young Women in the single State of life' (1714: 90). The French condition, 'les pâles couleurs', can have similar implications; an old French proverb, still being quoted in the nineteenth century, claims that 'A pale girl needs a male.'[13] 'The disease of virgins' seems to differ from the alternative labels, by including in the name of the disease its cure: ending the virgin state. If it is only virgins who can suffer in this way, then loss of virginity becomes a treatment, but one which can bring physicians into conflict with society; for must this loss of virginity necessarily take place within marriage? For example, Schurig (1730: 117) felt it necessary to stress that it is lawful intercourse, *coitus licitus*, which is needed.[14] As I shall show in chapter 1, the symptoms of the condition were close to those of love sickness; one way of understanding the disease of virgins is to see it as love sickness without a clear love-object. The label 'disease of virgins' also suggests that virginity is not always a healthy condition, which makes it problematic in Western society, where Christianity can present virginity as a valid life-style for women; it should come as no surprise that Protestant and Catholic authors, having different approaches to lifelong virginity, could hold somewhat different positions on the disease. It could be argued that the disease of virgins only became possible during the sixteenth century, with the rise of Protestantism favouring marriage even more as the goal for a faithful Christian girl.

This brings us to what may be an easier question to answer: namely, *when* was the 'disease of virgins'? It is an interesting condition for the history of medicine because it is one of very few diseases for which we can find a precise start date – in the mid-sixteenth century – and also one of the small number of diseases which seem subsequently to have vanished, in this case in the early twentieth century. But even these start and end dates are open to debate. In 1554, the physician Johannes Lange published what has subsequently been called 'the first medical description of this syndrome' (Crosby 1987: 2799). He left the diagnosis, in his own words, 'without a name, yet not without a treatment', but he headed the case *'De morbo virgineo'*, 'On the virgin disease'.[15] In using this heading, however, he was presenting it not as a new disease, but rather as something which had ancient antecedents. In creating a classical pedigree, he quoted from Galen, the extraordinarily prolific and influential medical writer who was born in Pergamum in Asia Minor in AD 129 and served as physician to the Roman emperor Marcus Aurelius and his family. He also referred to the works associated with the Greek 'Father of Medicine', Hippocrates, in the fifth and fourth centuries BC; in particular, Lange cited a short Hippocratic treatise known as *On the disease of virgins*.[16] For Lange, then, the disease was not new, but was already known in ancient Greece and Rome. As for the end date, although the rhetoric of Western biomedicine speaks of 'the conquest of disease', the notion of a 'disappearing disease' is not an easy one for medical writers to accept. Chlorosis disappeared from medical textbooks in the 1920s–30s; this disappearance, well documented over the last twenty-five years, has been linked to improved diet, changes in women's clothing, and a later age at first marriage.[17] However, there remains very little consensus either on what it was, or on why it is no longer found (Siddall 1982: 254), and it is still open to question whether it was ever 'conquered', or merely retired from the battlefield.[18]

Unease about a condition which vanishes for no clear reason may be particularly strong in the case of the 'disease of virgins' because of the symptom of altered skin colour which is implied in the alternate names. The idea of girls with green sickness turning green seems implausible to modern scholars from non-medical backgrounds, and has led to allegations that the symptom – and, by extension, the disease itself – never existed in the first place. As I shall show in chapter 1, there are other explanations for these names which do not require the sufferers to have been literally 'green', but these have not found favour with medical writers, who continue to maintain that the skin of a chlorotic is indeed green. For example, writing in the *Journal of the American Medical Association* in 1987, William H. Crosby insisted that,

> Based on my own experience, I am convinced that chlorosis did exist, for I have seen a chlorotic woman. It was about 1955 ... her face was green, its color accentuated by flaming red hair. The word was passed and doctors came from all over the hospital to gaze at her.
>
> (1987: 2799)

This recourse to first-hand observation – 'I have seen' – rather than to the technology of the laboratory, combined with the focus on the medical 'gaze', and the author's implied support for what earlier generations of physicians have also witnessed, is so frequent in medical sources that it suggests that, rather than being understood as part of the 'triumph' of medicine, the idea of a 'disappearing disease' is felt to be a threat to medical authority more generally.

Such resistance to the suggestion that the disease of virgins has disappeared, or that it never even existed, is symptomatic of the distinctive relationship it has with the medical men who have been called in to diagnose and treat it. Its 'creator', Johannes Lange, diagnosed it in a young girl, Anna, after her father – worried at the danger her appearance was posing to her marriage prospects – wrote to him outlining her symptoms. In 1554, Lange published what he presented as the letter giving his advice to her father, ending by saying that he hoped to be present at the girl's wedding; in this case, the caring physician appears as a sort of benign father-figure to the sick girl.[19] But other emotions besides pity could be aroused in the treatment of these young women. Here is the physician Frederick Hollick writing in the mid-nineteenth century:

> The subjects of chlorosis are the most interesting perhaps of all that come under the physician's care. Delicate and interesting, stricken by a disease from which they deeply suffer, but which often leaves their beauty untouched, or even heightens its attractions, they excite the liveliest emotions of pity and the most ardent desire to render them assistance.
>
> (1852: 193)

As I will discuss in chapter 3, in nineteenth-century medicine the onset of menstruation had itself become infused with male desire; and sufferers from the disease of virgins were commonly about to menstruate for the first time, or newly menstruant. Ambroise Rue described how menarche 'gives to this young beauty, no matter how sad or languid, the freshness and sparkle which mark the dawn of her life' (1819: 13–14). Half a century later, Armand Trousseau noted in a lecture on 'True and False Chlorosis' that 'The strange idea, after germinating in the heads of some physicians, has become popularised, that the erotic instincts are more developed in chlorotic than in other women' (1872: 112). Raciborski (1868: 332) was also keen to demolish this myth of the erotic chlorotic; he claimed to have asked chlorotic girls how they felt about it, and found that almost all of them expressed their disgust at the thought of sex.[20] However, physicians continued to find sufferers attractive: Lawson Tait (1889: 283) even wrote that chlorosis could be called 'the anaemia of good-looking girls', affecting those 'with a pretty pink and white complexion'. Although a new emphasis on the beauty of the chlorotic appears in nineteenth-century writing, the theme was already found in the sixteenth century in the work of Luis Mercado (1579: 201; cf. also Varandal 1619: 4; 1620: 2), while Rodrigues de Castro (1603: 129) explained that such girls were more inclined to use up only that venous blood which their bodies need for nourishment, and were thus more likely to be left with a surplus to make them prettily pink. This rationalisation depends on humoral theories of the body in Galenic medicine, which will be discussed in detail in the next chapter. However, Byrom Bramwell's description of the patient–doctor encounter deserves to be quoted at length:

> In blondes, the complexion often has a beautiful rosy-red tint when the patient first comes under the notice of the physician; patients suffering from chlorosis flush readily; their skin is usually thin and delicate; the temporary tinting of the skin which results from the flushing is very becoming, for many of the girls who are affected with chlorosis are very pretty. ... After the temporary excitement subsides, the face becomes pale ... almost entirely bloodless.
>
> (1899: 32)[21]

Chlorosis thus feeds into contemporary discussions about physician–patient relationships: it shows how such relationships can be sympathetic, but can easily become heavily eroticised. In Bramwell's description, the blushing patient appears to be responding to the physician as eagerly as he does to her.

Here, studying the disease of virgins both complements and challenges work on what has been seen as the disease of women, *par excellence*: hysteria. Entirely coincidentally, for both the disease of virgins and hysteria, the patient who has come to be seen as the origin of Lange's diagnosis is known to us as Anna, but the 'diagnosis-at-a-distance' of the sixteenth-century Anna through letters was as far as one can travel from the one-to-one 'talking cure' given to 'Anna O.' in the last decades of the nineteenth century.[22] At precisely the time when Freud colonised hysteria, updating it and making it into a twentieth-century condition, chlorosis started to fade away, disappearing from medical textbooks in the first decades of the twentieth century. Both chlorosis and hysteria have names coined on the basis of Greek roots, but which did not exist as discrete disease categories in the ancient world (King 1993; 1998: ch. 11); hysteria was named for the organ believed to dominate the female body, the womb (Greek *hystera*). But, in contrast to the hysterical woman, who is often presented as difficult and manipulative, with the label 'hysteria' being 'a sneer or an insult' (Duncan 1889: 973), the pubertal sufferer from the disease of virgins is usually seen as the ideal patient, entirely passive, controlled – like Anna – by her parents[23] and by the father-substitute of the physician.

The annoyance felt by those treating hysteria patients – in this case, a girl of fourteen – comes across clearly from the words of a Kentucky physician, Ap Morgan Vance, writing in 1908, a time when the contracture or 'drawing up' of a limb was a common symptom:

> I then, while alone, started to cut the plaster dressing off. After a section had been made the full length and I was pressing it open in

order to remove it, the girl cried, 'It is going to draw up; it is going to draw up;' at which I very sternly said, at the same time shaking my fist in her face, 'If it does draw up, I will break your d_____d little neck.' The limb did not draw up, and the child was cured.

(Vance 1908: 763, cited in Shorter 1986: 578 n.51)

Vance's treatment method, for hysteria patients of any age or gender, involved the removal of the patient from unhelpful influences, such as a mother who sent 'all the trashy French novels she could get' (Vance 1908: 763), cautery with a white-hot iron, or simply threats of burning. While 'a good "cussing"' was applied to all patients, on the grounds that 'Hysterics are all tyrants' (1908: 757), a 'good spanking' was reserved for the female patients. The most famous exponent of the assertion of mental and physical authority over hysteria patients was Lewis Yealland (1918), who combined what Elaine Showalter (1987: 176–7) has called his 'blatant use of power and authority' with electric shocks of increasing strength. Although, as we shall see in chapter 5, electricity was used in the treatment of chlorosis, girls of a similar age to Vance's young patient with 'the disease of virgins' or chlorosis tended to elicit much more sympathy from the medical profession.

Like hysteria, chlorosis was gendered as a female disease; and, in both cases, shifting the focus of the condition away from the womb raised the issue of whether men could suffer from it.[24] In the later nineteenth century, as the category of chlorosis grew, it expanded to embrace not only 'male chlorosis' (Siddall 1982: 255),[25] but also 'late chlorosis' or 'chlorosis tarda' (Stengel 1896: 351; Hudson 1977: 452). Because chlorosis was associated with the idea that women were 'less robust' than men (Ashwell 1836: 534), some men were thought sufficiently 'weak' or 'feeble' to be eligible as sufferers (Hamilton 1805: 94). Samuel Fox (1839), who regarded chlorosis not as a consequence of the menstrual function, but rather as a liver disorder,[26] claimed that it could also appear in 'young and delicate' men, while Samuel Ashwell (1836: 534) discussed the possibility of 'a kind of chlorosis' in 'Delicate and feeble' boys. It could, however, be argued that these new categories only show that the *typical* sufferer was still expected to be female and pubertal, chlorosis remaining 'essentially a disease of the female' (Bramwell 1899: 22).[27]

But the passive, weak, innocent, beautiful and suffering victim of the disease of virgins remained distant from the manipulative hysteric. In the seventeenth century Robert Pierce, who generally omitted the names of women patients in deference to the modesty of their sex, made an exception and named sufferers from green sickness because, he explained, the condition was not due to 'their faults' (1697: 188–9). Whereas a girl with hysteria could be regarded as having 'a kind of selfishness' (Duncan 1889: 973), appearing 'vainglorious', with a sense of 'selfimportance … the evident feeling that she was a curiosity or an interesting subject to the medical profession' (Vance 1908: 760), girls with chlorosis were considered 'For the most part gentle and inoffensive' (Clark 1887: 1004).

The 'most part' is, however, significant here; beneath the concern, even desire, for the sufferer from the disease of virgins, there remains a hint of caution and distance. Such girls could sometimes be 'odd in their behaviour' (Trousseau 1872: 106), 'snappy' and lacking respect (W. Johnson 1849: 44–5), or unduly fond of 'darkness and solitude' (Hamilton 1805: 90).[28] Other texts of the late nineteenth century suggest a more conscious manipulation of the viewer by the chlorotic; the doctor Frederick Taylor (1896: 720) described a developed colour sense in girls with chlorosis, so that 'chlorotics wear green ribbons and seem to object to pink' (Jones 1897: 28). Above all, physicians expressed the fear that their patients' behaviour may not be entirely honest. For example, when sufferers from chlorosis appeared to be taking very little food, there was some suspicion that they could in fact be eating rather more than their physicians realised; Ashwell warned that 'families and medical men are *occasionally* deceived on this point' (1836: 541; italics in original).

Throughout its history, for most medical writers, the prime symptom of the condition remained the absence of menstruation: an ambiguous symptom, because it could mean that this ideally passive young woman had in fact evaded paternal control and become pregnant. Astruc (1743: 83–4; 1761: 150–2) warned that women lie: maidens and widows who fall pregnant try to explain their paleness away as 'menstrual suppression'.[29] In early modern medicine, a missed period was not considered a certain sign of pregnancy; it could simply indicate that the blood had accumulated but had failed to come out due to some sort of blockage. This absence of menstruation did, however, initiate an interval of uncertainty which was only clarified by the eventual appearance of blood, or by 'quickening', the sensation which confirmed the presence of a viable infant (see, for example, Pollock 1989: 59; Duden 1991: 159–60; Wiesner 1993: 64). During this interval, practitioners were aware that treatment carried risks. In a list of remedies for menstrual suppression, Jacques Dubois gave a special recipe which he claimed could safely be used if conception was suspected; if the woman was indeed pregnant, then it would warm and strengthen the foetus, but if she had not conceived, then it would move the menses (1559: 182). The seventeenth-century midwife Jane Sharp warned, after listing treatments for suppressed menstruation, 'But do none of these things to women with Child, for that will be Murder' (1671: 296; Hobby 1999: 221).

One may expect that the girl who had never menstruated at all would be treated with sympathy and become the object of concerned care, while one who had already menstruated, but stopped, would perhaps be treated with suspicion. In the eighteenth-century move towards the classification of diseases on the model of Linnaeus and the natural sciences some writers, including William Cullen, labelled the former as menstrual 'retention', and the latter as menstrual 'suppression' (1786: 33). By the nineteenth century, the first was 'primary amenorrhoea', and the second 'secondary amenorrhoea' (Strange 2000: 611). The distinction between the two situations was not, however, as great as we may expect, because both categories of girl were thought capable of pregnancy. Early modern medicine held that women could not normally become pregnant without menstruation, because it provided the blood on which the male seed would then impose its form. However, if the blood had collected in the womb ready to flow out, and intercourse occurred at this precise moment, then conception could occur in the apparent absence of menstruation.[30] Over a period in which the role of the ovaries was much debated (see chapter 3 of this volume), eighteenth- and nineteenth-century medical writers had no difficulty in accepting that a girl who had never menstruated could become pregnant; the arguments and evidence were summarised by Raciborski (1868: 4–5), who himself believed that ovulation occurred immediately prior to menstruation, and that menstruation served to expel any unfertilised ripe eggs. For us, with our current understanding of ovulation, pregnancy without menstruation is no longer a conundrum;[31] but in previous centuries, when writers held different views on the timing of ovulation, and accumulated menstrual blood was thought to be necessary to form the foetus, late menarche could very easily be interpreted as possible pregnancy. Both chlorosis and pregnancy were thought to cause paleness, but the areas of potential overlap between them were reinforced by a further, and striking, symptom they had in common: pica, the consumption of non-food substances such as earth, coal, chalk and ashes.[32] The belief that pica was possible in women who were not pregnant had the authority of Galen; it was thought to be a feature of menstrual suppression (e.g. Green 2001: 73) and, in the eighteenth century, pica came to be seen as a major symptom of chlorosis.

A further question may be: *why* the disease of virgins? My interest in the condition grew after I realised that the ancient texts cited by Lange to 'prove' this was not something new and strange, but a perfectly respectable condition with a classical pedigree, do not in fact say what he claims (King 1996a; 1998: ch. 10). It became increasingly clear that the condition was a construct: but why would a writer of the mid-sixteenth century want to construct such a disease, and in this specific way? Why was the construct so powerful that it survived into the early twentieth century, in very different social and medical contexts? This led me in two directions. First, it made me think about the sources of medical authority in the sixteenth century. I would argue that, at a time when 'truth' could not be established by pathology, but could only be supported by other texts, the citation of Greek and Latin sources acted as a substitute for laboratory results.[33]

Studying the diagnosis of chlorosis enables us to enter into the key period of the mid-sixteenth century when the long-dominant Galenic medical theories began to be challenged by the rediscovery of the works of Galen's self-proclaimed 'master', Hippocrates. The ancient Greek texts transmitted under the name of Hippocrates date from the late fifth century to the first century BC, but for most of their history they have been read through the filter of Galenic medicine, dominant through the Middle Ages and into the early modern period both within university-based medical training and in popular knowledge of the body. Galen comprehensively imposed his own image of the Hippocratic texts on subsequent readers. Those texts which most resonated with his own medical views were hailed as the 'genuine works' of the great Hippocrates: those which did not were rejected as spurious. For Galen, 'Hippocrates was God, and Galen was his prophet' (Harris 1973: 267), but Galen also created this God in his own image (Smith 1979).

Largely lost to the Middle Ages, Hippocratic gynaecology only became available in the Latin which the learned community could read in 1525, when Marco Fabio Calvi's translation of the entire Hippocratic corpus was printed in Rome; in the following year it was reprinted by Cratender in Basle (Nutton 1989: 426), and the four main texts on gynaecology were also reprinted in Paris in a smaller, cheaper format.[34] Hippocratic gynaecology was opposed to Galenic gynaecology in several ways. In contrast with another text included in the Hippocratic corpus, *On generation/Nature of the child* (Lonie 1981), the three volumes of the fifth-century BC Hippocratic *Diseases of women* denied the existence of an active female 'seed', seeing women only as providers of the raw material for the foetus: blood. They assumed that the womb was free to wander around the body in search of moisture, a belief which should have been destroyed for good by the human dissections performed by Herophilos in third-century BC Alexandria, but which instead lingered on for many centuries. They put enormous emphasis on regular and heavy menstruation, regarding menstrual blood as a substance produced of necessity by all women except those too young, too old or with child (Clologe 1905: 63). Ideally, blood flowed 'like that of a sacrificial victim' (*DW* 1.6; L 8.30; King 1998: 88–98), a Hippocratic image still being used as the opening words of Edward Tilt's chapter on menstruation in a mid-nineteenth century textbook on women's diseases (1853: 108, cf. 116). Retained menstrual blood was seen as something so serious that it could lead to masculinisation of the body; the Hippocratic text *Epidemics* 6.8.32 (Loeb VII, 289–91) describes the patient Phaethousa of Abdera who, after her periods stopped, developed body hair – including a beard – and a harsh voice, dying shortly after the onset of the condition. Soranos, who wrote in the second century AD, challenged such ideas; he argued that, apart from its contribution to conception, menstruation is actually bad for women's health (*Gyn.* 1.27–32; Temkin 1956: 23–30).[35] But his views were eclipsed by the development of the Hippocratic/Galenic tradition,[36] and the belief that menstruation was essential to maintain women's health was still unanimously accepted in the seventeenth century (Crawford

1981: 53); the specific suggestion that failure to menstruate could make a woman's body become masculine was repeated as late as 1836, when Samuel Ashwell claimed that persistent chlorosis would lead to 'approximation to the male sex. Instances are not wanting, where the sexual distinctions seem to have passed away' (1836: 531). According to the French physician Victor Burq (1852: 19), one of the signs that treatment for chlorosis is working is that the girl has her heaviest period ever.

As these examples of nineteenth-century medicine show, the Hippocratic insistence on the importance of a regular, heavy menstrual flow survived virtually unchallenged; when the physician Emile Littré published his edition and translation of the Hippocratic corpus between 1839 and 1861, this was no antiquarian gesture, his explicit intention being to improve the medical practice of his own day (Jouanna 1983: 293–5).[37] In Hippocratic medicine, menarche was seen as a time of serious danger, as blood began to flow through channels only barely wide enough to allow its passage; in the short treatise *On the disease of virgins*, cited by Lange as the origin of his 'disease of virgins', a graphic picture was given of the mental and physical symptoms which could be caused by menstrual retention in girls at menarche. The text, and Lange's use of it, will be discussed in detail in chapter 2.

In contrast, Galen never wrote a gynaecological text; his early treatise *On the dissection of the uterus* is purely anatomical, and says nothing at all about physiology (CMG V. 2.1; Goss 1962). Israel Spach (1591: 130) includes 'Galeni liber spurius' in his listing of works on the diseases of women known in the sixteenth century; this may be the pseudo-Galenic work *On the secrets of women* which circulated in the Arab world, dating from before the ninth century (Levey and Souryal 1968), but there is no other evidence that this text was known in the West. It is therefore more likely that the 'spurious book of Galen' refers to a medieval treatise called *De passionibus mulierum* or *De gynaeceis*, printed under Galen's name for the first time in 1490.[38] In the absence of a dedicated volume on the diseases of women from Galen, a 'Galenic gynaecology' has to be pieced together from scattered sections in other works (Flemming 2000). Galen's medical system is far more closely tied to the theory of the four humours (discussed on pp. 22–3); the Hippocratic gynaecological texts mention these, but for them the overriding importance of blood in the female body makes the other three humours virtually redundant. Galen shares a concern with blood – for example, he states that suppressed menses make a woman 'certain to fall into every sort of illness' (*On bloodletting against Erasistratos* 5, K 11.166; Brain 1986: 27) – but, whereas *Diseases of women* is entirely focused on menstrual blood, the Galenic woman also has to contend with female seed, the retention of which causes even more serious problems for her health.[39] Moreover, although Galen believed *Diseases of women* to be a 'genuine work' of Hippocrates, he never wrote a commentary on it (Green 1987: 303 n. 15). This made the

Hippocratic text more difficult to read for medieval and Renaissance physicians who were trained by studying Galenic commentaries on Hippocratic treatises.

As we have already seen, the direct evidence of the senses was considered very important when the sick girl was observed by her physician and found to be 'green'. But the textual component of the early history of the disease of virgins raises serious questions about the relationship between theory and observation in the origin of the diagnosis. Lange never saw Anna; he carried out her diagnosis by letter, and it is even possible that she never existed except as a cipher to give his Hippocratic story a human dimension.[40] Lange was writing his letter in the decades immediately after the publication of Calvi's Latin translation of the complete works of 'Hippocrates'. Indeed, from echoes in the text, to be discussed in chapter 2, it is clear that he had Calvi's work open in front of him as he was writing. But Calvi did not always have access to the best Greek manuscripts, and the choices he made in translating from Greek to Latin are significant. The 'Hippocrates' available to Lange was one seen through Calvi's translation. In addition, as I have already noted, Lange himself also had a particular agenda in approaching Anna's symptoms. For subsequent writers, Anna is the Ur-patient of chlorosis: for Lange, the central point of his letter is that she is nothing of the kind. Writing within a contemporary debate, stimulated in particular by syphilis and the English Sweat, as to whether new diseases were possible in a creation finalised in the seven days of *Genesis*, Lange wanted to use Anna's symptoms to argue that there are no truly 'new' diseases. Immediately before the 'disease of virgins', Lange discussed the English Sweat; elsewhere he argued that syphilis is not new, and what appears to be a 'new disease' may really be a medley of many diseases, while one disease can easily change into others.[41] For him, precursors can be found for all apparently novel diseases by reading the work of the ancient writers, and the newly available Hippocratic text *On the disease of virgins* is the ancestor of the condition affecting Anna.

In addition to its value as a way into sixteenth-century uses of classical medical texts, the disease of virgins took me in a second direction. It raised questions about the study of female puberty over time; how far did views of what was normal and abnormal change? How did medicine try to account for the processes of puberty? The presence of chlorosis among young girls at puberty led some writers, especially in the nineteenth century, to stress the dramatic changes in the female body at this time, and to magnify these so that they became an explanation for the symptoms; puberty was thought to require a large amount of 'constitutional or vital power' (Ashwell 1836: 532), putting an enormous strain on the 'blood-forming' organs (Bramwell 1899: 25). But was chlorosis found in adolescent girls because of the physiology of puberty, or did social and cultural concerns about puberty lead to the invention of chlorosis as a way of controlling the behaviour of adolescent girls?

Here, the disease of virgins also becomes a test case for one of the questions which opened this investigation, and which itself has a considerable history: what do we mean by 'a' disease or condition? How far are diseases 'dynamic conceptions that change constantly in response to cultural and social forces' (Hudson 1977: 448)? For pre-modern Western medicine, is it a legitimate strategy for us to focus exclusively on descriptive labels like 'the disease of virgins' or 'green sickness', or should we be investigating all discussions of one of the symptoms? In the latter case, do we then privilege cases of changed skin colour, menstrual suppression, or dietary disturbance? So far, I have been using the various labels largely interchangeably, but with a stress on different terms in different historical periods: the issue of whether the disease of virgins, green sickness, chlorosis and the white fever were 'the same thing' in any useful sense will be revisited in the Conclusion.

But the problems continue to multiply. In addition to the question of whether the different labels favoured in different periods cover 'the same' condition, we could consider whether different individual physicians working in the same country in the same period would have used a single label in an identical way. In 1923, when J.M.H. Campbell studied the admissions records for a range of English hospitals between 1888 and 1922, he noted the problem of whether the word 'chlorosis' 'has been used in exactly the same sense during the period under review' (1923: 253) and suggested that, even within a single hospital, 'the exact meaning of chlorosis may have varied from time to time under the influence of different teachers' (1923: 248). If this is the case within a forty-year time frame in a single country, then the variation over four centuries could be enormous.

Part of the uncertainty derives from the variety and the vagueness of the symptoms. In the late seventeenth century, the posthumously published *Processus Integri* of Thomas Sydenham, known as 'the English Hippocrates' because of his insistence on close observation of symptoms, listed eleven which would have been recognised to varying degrees throughout the history of chlorosis, although – as I shall show in this book – the relative emphasis on different aspects of this symptom picture could, and did, shift over time.[42] In a mid-eighteenth century English translation this list reads as follows:

> This indisposition is attended with (1.) a bad colour of the face, and whole body; (2.) a swelling of the face, eyelids and ankles; (3.) heaviness of the whole body; (4.) a tension and lassitude of the legs and feet; (5.) difficult respiration; (6.) palpitation of the heart; (7.) pain in the head; (8.) feverish pulse; (9.) drowsiness; (10.) an unnatural longing for such things as are noxious, and unfit for food; and (11.) a suppression of the menstrual discharge.
>
> (1753: 658)[43]

From the range of symptoms given in lists such as this it is possible to argue that, at certain historical points, 'any sickly but normal girl in an irritable mood was in danger of being so labelled' (Loudon 1984: 32); indeed, Campbell's comparative study concluded that chlorosis was 'an exaggeration of a physiological change occurring in all girls rather than a disease *sui generis*' (1923: 267). Brumberg (1988: 173) suggests that, in the Victorian era, 'all adolescent girls were potentially chlorotic', while, for the period 1870–1920, chlorosis 'represented an entire conception of the female adolescent', being an expected crisis necessary to the attainment of womanhood, a pattern of behaviour learned 'from family, friends, and the popular press as well as from their doctors' (Brumberg 1982: 1468, 1475; cf. Loudon 1984: 34).

The range of symptoms also made the 'disease of virgins' or chlorosis into umbrellas under which other diseases could hide. At the end of the nineteenth century, Byrom Bramwell (1899: 44–8) listed the most likely areas of overlap as being with dyspepsia and ulceration of the stomach, tuberculosis, Bright's disease, lead poisoning, organic mitral disease, ulcerative endocarditis, and pernicious anaemia. Ward's list (1914: 318) included neurasthenia, and 'unsuspected pregnancy'. Campbell (1923: 256) noted that some sufferers labelled as chlorotics fifty years earlier would, in his day, have been diagnosed as having gastric ulcer and secondary anaemia. There have been some modern attempts to link hysteria and the disease of virgins, for example by the nutritionist Karl Guggenheim, who has tried to bring the disease of virgins into a Freudian arena by claiming that 'The idea that suppressed sexuality caused disease was expressed by Lange more than 300 years before Freud' (1995: 1822). However, in the sixteenth century Mercado (1579: 202–3) categorically separated hysteria from the disease of virgins: in the former, he says, the womb itself is disturbed, while in the latter the obstruction occurs *outside* the womb. In the nineteenth century, however, some believed that a girl could suffer from both chlorosis and hysteria at the same time (e.g. Burq 1852: 5), and in the early twentieth century Ward (1914: 312) regarded hysteria as a *symptom* of chlorosis; the categories shifted, as concepts of causation and models of the body changed.

It is sometimes claimed that, in the nineteenth century, chlorosis 'became' hypochromic anaemia, finally moving from being an ill-defined condition to the haven of diagnostic certainty as a result of increasingly sophisticated blood testing (Wailoo 1997: 27–8); for example, surveying the history of the condition, Guggenheim stated that 'The once-prevalent disease known as chlorosis is now generally believed to be hypochromic anemia' (1995: 1822). However, it must be noted that, at the time when the diagnosis of anaemia was becoming more common, writers often denied outright that chlorosis was related to any form of anaemia:[44] in a popular health manual, which ran into many editions, Frederick Hollick wrote that 'The peculiar state of decay and weakness, called *Anemia*, or decline, has also

15

been taken for Chlorosis by inattentive persons' (1852: 194), while Trousseau stated 'I am far from looking on anaemia and chlorosis as the same disease' (1872: 95). Trousseau pointed out that the symptoms of chlorosis could disappear at the return of menstruation, whereas one would expect the menstrual blood loss to exacerbate, rather than cure, anaemia (1872: 108).

ₐ This book therefore concerns the interplay in medicine between theory and observation, and between appeals to the authority of the ancients and claims to innovation. It concerns the construction of 'a disease' from symptoms, and the roles of age and gender in assigning diagnoses. Very different disorders could have been given a label such as 'disease of virgins' or 'chlorosis', not because of the lack of clinical tests to distinguish between them but simply because they appeared in girls of the right age (Humphreys 1997: 164). Brumberg (1982: 1472) pointed out that, in the nineteenth century, similar symptoms would receive very different diagnoses depending on the age and gender of the patient; thus medical labelling 'reinforced the gender and age categories that were the basis of the Victorian social order'. Lawson Tait, for example, insisted that the condition was 'absolutely limited to the first ten or twelve years of menstrual life' (1889: 282). Throughout its history, the target population of the diseases being investigated here remained young girls; for example, in the late nineteenth century chlorosis was known as 'the special anaemia of young women', the subtitle chosen for Ernest Lloyd Jones' discussion of the condition, published in 1897 (cf. Rosin 1907: 187). But Brumberg's analysis could apply equally well to earlier centuries; in the seventeenth century, for example, John Tanner (1659: 317) regarded menstrual suppression as something affecting 'a woman of ripe Age', while a young girl with menstrual suppression would be diagnosed as having 'green sickness'.[45] Jane Sharp (1671: 292) listed the differences between the effects of menstrual suppression in maids and in women: 'Maids, they presently fall into the Green sickness by it', whereas women vomit, do not want to eat, or crave unnatural foods.[46] John Maubray (1724: 48) regarded 'the Virgin-Disease, commonly called the Green-Sickness' as the only one of the 'Indispositions of Life, which can properly be accounted peculiar to Virgins'.

In demonstrating the extent to which the Western gynaecological tradition continued to be based on a set of ancient texts, I also want to keep in mind changes within medicine and its place in society. In the first chapter I will look at the solidification of the category of the disease of virgins, discussing the sixteenth-century diseases from which it emerged and with which it remained in closest dialogue: green jaundice, green sickness, and love sickness. Chapter 2 investigates the issue of the possibility of new diseases, situating Lange's letter within an established debate on this topic and probing further his relationship to his classical sources; in particular, his use of the Hippocratic *On the disease of virgins*. Chapter 3 concentrates on menstruation and bloodletting, looking at the anatomy and physiology of the virgin's body in Hippocratic and Galenic medicine, and examining changes in the medical perception of puberty up to the nineteenth century. Chapter 4 turns to the role of diet in chlorosis, exploring the function of the liver and colon in the condition. In chapter 5 I consider the changing role of technology in diagnosis and treatment; case books, recipe collections and medical advertisements also demonstrate the extent to which women believed themselves to be suffering from this textually constructed condition, and I investigate the responses of women healers to it. I will be examining how the different disease labels applied to young girls have themselves influenced expectations of symptoms and treatments. Throughout their history, the disease of virgins, green sickness and chlorosis remained tied, above all, to virgins at menarche, so that marriage – provided with ever-changing medical rationales – continued to be seen as the ultimate cure.

1

THE NATURE OF
GREEN SICKNESS

In sixteenth-century England, there was a disease known as 'green sickness'. In this chapter I will be discussing how ideas about this condition developed during the sixteenth century, examining in particular the relationship between lay ideas of disease and 'official' medical versions of the female body. Although I have already mentioned the role of Johannes Lange as the 'creator' of the precise symptom picture of the disease of virgins, I have deliberately chosen to start, not with him, but with green sickness in English vernacular sources. There are two reasons for this strategy.

First, there are chronological considerations. Lange's letter, in which he describes the disease of virgins, was published in 1554 but, as I will show here, green sickness was described both before and after this date. In this and the following chapter, I will be arguing that Lange's 'disease of virgins' may have reinforced the transformation of the English green sickness from a digestive disorder affecting all ages and both sexes to a condition found only in young women.

Second, starting with green sickness means giving priority to popular, vernacular medicine rather than elite Latin medicine. Lange's contribution, although important, distorts the image we have of sixteenth-century medicine; when we accept his letter as the 'first medical description of this syndrome' (Crosby 1987: 2799), the tendency is to privilege technical literature written in Latin, and to regard vernacular works as being merely derivative from Latin texts. However, in early modern Europe, while some Latin medical texts were translated into several different languages, vernacular medical texts were also translated into Latin in order to make them more easily accessible to the European medical elite; this two-way movement meant that early modern European medical knowledge was increasingly cross-cultural. I am also not convinced that medical ideas begin with a university-trained physician's reading – or, as I shall show in chapter 2, misreading – of the classical sources and are then imposed on a population to whom they were previously unknown. The connections which Lange drew between his 'disease of virgins' and the classical medical writers have been very influential, but they do not represent the whole story. The speed with which this condition gripped the imaginations of European medical writers, becoming, within a generation, something which 'occurs in a large number of virgins' (Mercado 1579: 201), and its appearance in case notes and in popular literature, suggest that it was embraced by patients as much as by physicians. Indeed, in his letter to Anna's father, Lange himself said that his 'disease of virgins' was already known under other names to ordinary people, being 'what the women of Brabant usually call "white fever", on account of the pale face, as well as "love fever" '.[1]

Which came first: the technical terms or the popular terms? Guggenheim (1995: 1822) states that 'chlorosis' 'led to the popular English term "green sickness" ', but this is simply an error: the vernacular term predated the coining of the technical label 'chlorosis'. It is one of the many peculiarities of the disease of virgins that its history, in many ways so opaque, nevertheless contains several events which can be clearly dated. The first use in print of the term 'chlorosis' is one of these events; it occurred in 1619, in the Latin edition of the work of Varandal of Montpellier published by his students two years after his death, where a list of alternative names for the condition is given, ending with 'the disease of virgins, which we, from Hippocrates, call Chlorosis' (Varandal 1619: 4–5; 1620: 1).[2] Varandal very consciously separated this allegedly 'Hippocratic' name from the other labels he gave, all of which were classified as the terms used by the 'common people' (Latin *vulgus*). One of the few women of the early modern period to write about the condition, the midwife Jane Sharp (1671: 256–70; Hobby 1999: 194–204), continued to prefer to use 'green sickness' over fifty years after Varandal, but the 'vulgar' label survived well beyond this date; for example, in the Glossary to Ruddock's homeopathic manual for ladies, first published in 1869, 'Chlorosis' is explained as 'Green sickness' as late as the tenth edition of 1892, while Stengel's 1896 encyclopaedic essay on diseases of the blood gave green sickness as 'the popular name' and chlorosis as 'the technical name' (1896: 343).

For Varandal to be 'the godfather' of the condition (Schwarz 1951: 14), he must have been using the word 'chlorosis' in his lectures some years earlier. This could push back the origin of the term to the 1590s, when he was teaching at Montpellier.[3] It is clear that the label 'green sickness' was already in use in English medicine at this time. In his study of the casebooks of Richard Napier, an English astrological priest-physician working in the south-east Midlands in the early seventeenth century, Ronald Sawyer suggested that one of the earliest uses of 'green sickness' to denote a condition specific to women aged between 17 and 22, with the absence of menstruation as a defining symptom, occurs in Napier's records for 1603 (see Sawyer 1986: 591 in conjunction with Loudon 1984: 29).[4] Work published subsequent to Sawyer's dissertation pushes back even further the earliest reference to this term in doctors' case notes; in her work on the physician Dr Barker of Shrewsbury, Lucinda McCray Beier found that green sickness was one of the gynaecological disorders named in his case notes, which date from 1595–1605 (Beier 1987: 120, 122); specifically, it appears in the notes from 1596.[5]

Outside doctors' case notes, where the label seems to have been established as uncontroversial, at least by the first years of the seventeenth century, 'green sickness' already appeared as a cause of death in the records of the London parish of St Botolph without Aldgate in the late sixteenth century (Forbes 1971: 100–1); as the 'searchers of the dead' were ordinary women, who decided on the cause of death in their neighbours (Munkhoff 1999), this suggests that the label was familiar outside medical texts. So does its use in Shakespeare's *Henry IV Part 2*, first performed in about 1597; there, Falstaff says

> There's never none of these demure boys come to any proof; for thin drink doth so over-cool their blood,[6] and making many fish-meals, that they fall into a kind of male green-sickness; and then, when they marry, they get wenches. They are generally fools and cowards.
>
> (*Henry IV Part 2*, IV.iii.90)[7]

But green sickness appeared in English writing, both medical and lay, considerably earlier than the 1590s. Timothie Bright mentioned green sickness so casually in a list of diseases that the reader gets the impression that it was the common cold of its day:

> Hath God so dispensed his blessings, that a medicine to cure iawndies, or the greene sicknes, or the rheume, or such like, should cost more oftentimes then one quarter of the substance that the patient is worth?
>
> (Bright 1580: 23)[8]

In Shakespeare, the joke depends on green sickness normally being a condition of young women: in Bright, there is no suggestion that it is gendered. However, if it was already known as an exclusively female disorder, then Bright would not need to spell out 'or the green sickness in women', just as we would not need to specify 'or period pains in women'. In a romance licensed in the Stationers' Register in the same year as Bright's book was published, and which appeared in print only three years later (Newcomb 2002: 42), Robert Greene's *Mamillia. A mirrour or looking-glasse for the ladies of Englande* (1583; Grosart 1881–3: II.36), green sickness was not only gendered as feminine, but also linked to virginity. Gonzaga realised that his daughter Mamillia was 'marriageable, knowing by skill and experience, that the grasse being ready for the sieth [scythe], would wither if it were not cut; and the apples being rype, for want of plucking would rotte on the tree; that his daughter beeing at the age of twentie yeeres, would either fall into the green sicknes for want of a husband, or els if she scaped that disease, incurre a farther inconvenience [i.e. illegitimate pregnancy]'. He therefore found her a suitor.

In 1583 Walter Cary also discussed green sickness in chapter 15 of his *A Brief Treatise called Caries Farewell to Physicke*. He continued to regard the condition as a digestive disorder, attributing it to a weakened liver, which led to water rather than blood being made, to the extent that 'if they chance to cut a finger, no bloud, but water will rather followe'. He noted that 'It is found most in maidens' and suggested that they bring it on themselves by an inadequate diet because they 'desire to abate their colour, and to be over fine'. He included headache, difficulty in breathing, faintness and absence of menses as symptoms (1583: 40–1).[9] For him, green skin colour was part of the absence of 'good blood', patients being 'verie pale and greenish'.

Letters from the early modern period demonstrate that green sickness was something experienced by women, and expected by men. In her late thirties Margaret, Countess of Cumberland, described how she had been affected by green sickness in the second seven-year period of her life; she was born in 1560, and appears to have been ill between the ages of about thirteen and sixteen, the condition ending with her marriage, at nearly seventeen years old, in 1577 (Williamson 1920: 11, 286). She attributed the affliction to 'unbrotherly dealing [which] pierced my thoughts' (Williamson 1920: 285).[10] Another case of the condition, this time occurring over twenty years before Bright, Greene and Cary, is described in a letter written in June 1558, in which Sir William Pagett describes his daughter Jane as 'still troubled as she was before her going thither with the greine sicknes'.[11] Jane was not, like Mamillia or Margaret, in 'want of a husband'; like other aristocratic women of the Tudor period, she married in her middle or late teens and, rather than setting up a new household, lived with her husband Thomas Kitson at the home of his mother, the countess of Bath (Harris 2001: 249). Her father was writing to her mother-in-law to explain why, having visited London to see her parents and to attend her sister's lying-in, she was unable to return; he announced that he was keeping her in London, 'where there is the best remedy to be had therfore, for which purpose I do use the advise of the best learned in Englande, not doubting but that she shall be remedied thereof'. At the time of her London green sickness, Jane had been married for a year, or even less. Her father suggests that she had suffered from green sickness before her move to Hengrave ('before her going thither'), and it is possible either that the marriage had not yet been consummated (Harris 2001: 248 n. 11), or that she had not yet reached menarche.[12] She was ill again in late 1559 – this time, her mother thought that she had consumption – and died before November 1560.

How can we combine the hint that Jane had green sickness before her marriage, the possibility that the marriage had not yet been consummated at the time of her green sickness in 1558, and her mother's fear of consumption in 1559? Both disorders were associated with weakness, difficult breathing, and paleness; in 1559, at least, we know that Jane's appearance was the subject of discussion, with her mother thinking her unwell, but her father considering that she had never looked better (Harris 2001: 249).[13] It may be valid here to compare the shift in label with one which occurred fifty years later, in the casebooks of Richard Napier. Here, case histories in which the diagnosis 'green sickness' was given were subsequently emended to 'obstruction of the spleen' if the patient menstruated (Sawyer 1986: 491 n. 41). For Napier, 'green sickness' was always a diagnosis dependent on the absence of menstruation. The evidence – flimsy as it is – could be read to suggest that Jane reached menarche later in 1558 or in 1559, making green sickness no longer a possible label for her weakness. Her father's claims that the learned physicians of London could provide the best remedy could indicate that he had been hoping that they could bring on her menstrual flow.

Returning to published medical texts, the earliest use of 'green sickness' for a distinct condition which I have been able to trace in English writing dates back ten years before Jane Kitson's illness, to 1547, when Andrew Boorde's *Breviary of Helthe* used 'grene sicknes' as the direct equivalent of 'grene Jawnes', one of three types of jaundice mentioned: yellow, black and green.[14] The green variant was seen as the result of the corruption of blood from a mixture of yellow bile and phlegm. Like Bright, however, Boorde did not state that this condition is specific to any age/sex group, nor did he regard it as in any way 'new' (1547: 75[r]; see Norri 1992: 336); on the contrary, he gave it an Arabic origin, saying that the 'grene sicknes' is 'named Agriaca' in Arabic texts (1547: 74[r]).[15]

The humoral body

The causation of green jaundice/green sickness was thus originally understood in the context of 'the seductive coherence of Galenic humoral theory' (Schoenfeldt 1999: 3). As Gail Kern Paster has argued, 'whenever the early modern subject became aware of her or his body ... the body in question was always a humoral entity' (Paster 1993: 10). To understand green sickness, it is necessary to appreciate some of the implications of such a body. Based on the work of the Hippocratic writers and Galen, and serving as the dominant model of the body through the middle ages up to at least the eighteenth century, the humoral system concentrated on what Galen made into the canonical four humours: blood, phlegm, yellow bile and black bile.[16] In its most complete form, the humoral body linked these constituent fluids to the four elements, the four qualities – hot, cold, wet and dry – and the four seasons, placing the human body within the wider cosmos and explaining its reactions to changes in the environment, while classifying people by their dominant humour, or 'temperament'.[17] Unlike a system in which the same pill – perhaps in different doses – is valid for the same condition, regardless of the individual in whom that condition is found, humoral medicine requires knowledge of the many individual features leading to illness in a specific person: this means that, ideally, the physician needs an extensive training, a detailed knowledge of the patient, and a lengthy – and expensive – consultation (Wear 2000: 42). Yet, in a diluted, over-the-counter form, humoral medicine could also be easily understood by lay people. In the absence of books or doctors, they could discuss their predominance of phlegm or blood with family and friends, attempt self-treatment or decide on the best sort of healer to consult (Wear 2000: 108–16).

The humoral body was, above all, a place of fluids, not of organs.[18] When studying the female patients of an eighteenth-century German physician, Johannes Pelagius Storch, Barbara Duden speculated on the impact of writing on perceptions of the body. In pre-literate cultures, such as that of ancient Greece before the Hippocratic corpus, knowledge too is 'fluid', and 'reality does not solidify' (Duden 1991: 33). But, even in the Western medical tradition of text-based medical education (Bates 1995), this less-than-solid body persisted in medical thinking and popular knowledge into the modern period alongside a body made of organs. The role of the organs in the humoral bodily economy was, however, secondary: to collect, transform and transmit the humours. The four humours could accumulate to cause blockages anywhere in the body or, as in 'green jaundice', could form inappropriate mixtures. But other fluids, too, because they derived from blood, needed to be taken into consideration by the patient and her physician. Blood, according to Aristotle, was cooked or 'concocted' into breast milk and, in men, whose greater innate heat allowed a greater level of concoction, into semen.[19] The transformative potential of the fluids into each other was accompanied by an interchangeability of the routes by which fluids travelled. When a fluid was present in excess, or trapped so that it rotted, noxious vapours could be produced which would rise up and affect other parts of the body; or, the superfluous fluid could move around the body before finding, and using, any available way out.

The transformation of the fluids and the range of their possible exits was valid for both male and female bodies (Schoenfeldt 1999: 36–7), but there was a particularly strong association between women and liquids. Paster (1993: 79) points out that, in humoral medicine, plethora is constructed as the natural state for a woman: women's blood is not only more plentiful, but also colder and thicker than that of a man, and the female body is also seen as more 'leaky' (Paster 1993: 44).[20] In the female humoral body, menstrual blood could erupt from any orifice, or through the skin. This belief was widespread and lasting; it had a particularly strong impact on the 'disease of virgins', which was often linked to the onset of menstruation. It had Hippocratic precedents; the treatise *Aphorisms*, widely used in Western medical education and in the Arab world, and one of the first Hippocratic texts to be printed, states that suppressed menstrual blood can come out of the body as a nosebleed, or as vomited blood (*Aphorisms*, 5.32, 33; Loeb IV, 166).[21] Another Hippocratic text, *On the use of liquids* 6 (L 6.130; Loeb VIII, 332), states that the menses can run back under the skin, and should be treated by cold topical applications.

By the eighteenth century, in women patients, bleeding from various orifices was still widely accepted as 'diverted menstruation'.[22] The authority of the Hippocratic texts was cited for such bodily redirection (e.g. Wiltshire 1885: 513). Routes listed typically included the ears, skin, gums, fingers, navel, little finger, ring finger, saliva glands and tear ducts (Sennert 1664: 90; Schurig 1729: 83–118; Duden 1991: 120–1); as recently as 1953, some of these routes were still included in an article on the topic in the *Nursing Mirror* – although the author commented on menstruation through tears and sweat, 'this is doubted' (Bender 1953: 159–60). Fleetwood Churchill's textbook *On the Diseases of Women*, first published in 1850, allowed for 'vicarious menstruation' from the nose, eyes, ears, gums, lungs, stomach, arms, bladder, nipples, the ends of fingers and toes, the joints, and so on (Churchill 1864: 204–5; cf. Wiltshire 1885: 517). He included the case of Mary Murphy, aged 21, whose missed period was resolved by the appearance of between fifteen and twenty ounces of blood from her ears, followed by vomiting blood (1864: 205–6). Vicarious bleeding from the stomach by vomiting continued to be seen as an encouraging symptom in Samuel Ashwell's discussion of chlorosis (1836: 539–40), because it demonstrated that there was sufficient blood present in the body to make menstruation possible. In his discussion of chlorosis, Ashwell mentioned one of Henry Oldham's chlorosis cases, a 24-year-old woman named as 'Eliza H.' who vomited blood at every period for six months, and a case of his own, the 17-year-old 'Sarah' who bled from a cyst on her breast whenever she menstruated (Ashwell 1836: 556 ff.). Not all writers of the eighteenth and nineteenth centuries accepted vicarious menstruation; for example, Thomas Denman (1788: 154–5; 1832: 102) believed that bleeding classified as such was more commonly due to disease, being independent of menstruation; and Walter Johnson (1849: 38) considered that some cases of vomiting blood in chlorosis were the result of ulceration of the stomach lining.

From green jaundice to green sickness

All forms of jaundice were thought to arise from inappropriate mixtures of humours corrupting the blood; in this sense, green sickness began as a blood condition. When nineteenth-century medicine explored ways of analysing the constituents of blood, attempts were made to find something in the blood itself which could cause the symptoms elsewhere in the body (see chapter 5); in sixteenth-century medicine, the blood could be altered in its consistency, or by the presence of other humours.

Somewhere between 1547 and Jane Kitson's illness in 1558, green sickness became a condition in its own right, rather than a form of jaundice, and – in the process – it became associated with young women. This dating can be supported by medical writing in English, where the recommended remedies suggest that it was seen as a condition exclusive to women some fifty years earlier than Sawyer (1986: 591) suggested, and that it involved digestive problems or blockages, menstrual suppression, and a bad facial colour. It was in the same year that Jane Kitson's father consulted London physicians for her green sickness that the Galenist physician William Bullein's *A Newe Booke Entituled the Government of Healthe* (1558)[23] explicitly called it 'a new disease', although he did not link it to menstrual suppression, nor restrict it only to virgins. Bullein recommended the remedy mithridatum – a compound drug with as many claimed virtues as it had ingredients – 'for women whiche have a newe disease peraccidentes[24] called the grene syckenes' (1558: 120^v; 1559: 228); he referred to onions helping 'the grene sickness' (1558: 64^r; 1559: 124); and, finally, he mentioned 'greene sicknes' as a possible consequence of eating too much pepper (1558: 115^r; 1559: 217). Bullein's aetiology for the condition will be discussed in detail shortly. Andrew Boorde had written of 'the grene sicknes or the grene Jawnes' (1547: 11^r): in 1547, green sickness was simply green jaundice. It was not new – it could be found in Arabic texts. It was not specific to any age/sex group. Yet by 1558 – that is, four years after the publication of Lange's letter on the 'disease of virgins' – green sickness seems to have broken away from jaundice to become not only a 'new' condition, but also one specific to women.

In the second half of the sixteenth century, however, green sickness remained very close to jaundice, and continued to be understood by many people as essentially a digestive disorder. For example, in a manuscript collection of medical recipes probably written in 1564 by Henry Dingley, who himself owned a copy of the 1558 edition of Bullein's *A Newe Booke Entituled the Gouernement of Healthe*, remedies for green sickness appear immediately after those for black jaundice, yellow jaundice and green jaundice, and before remedies for 'payne in the spleene' (WMS 244: 209).[25] 'Green jaundice' and 'green sickness' appear on the left and the right sides of the page, separated but adjacent, but still within the wider category of digestive disorders.[26] For many commentators on the exclusively female 'green sickness', too, it was understood mainly in terms of the digestive system.[27]

Bullein's *Government of Health* was a very popular health guide of the time, written after he returned from a period of travel on the continent in order to study medicine. This exposure to other ideas may be significant but, unfortunately, we know nothing about Bullein's precise movements at the time. The first edition of 1558–9 was followed by a second in 1595. After setting up a medical practice in London in 1561, Bullein was imprisoned for debt after successfully pleading his innocence on a far more serious charge of murdering a previous employer, Sir Thomas Hilton of Tynemouth; while in prison, he wrote a second book, the *Bulwark of Defence*, published in 1562–3, which entered a second edition in 1579. It may be possible to tease out some of the ideas lying behind Bullein's views on green sickness by examining the other circumstances in which he employed the therapies which he recommends for this condition.

When Bullein gave mithridatum as a cure for the new disease of green sickness, it was as a theriac, a cure for poisons, venomous stings and bites: it is also good for 'ye biting of a mad dogge'.[28] This could suggest that green sickness operated as a form of internal poisoning. This would be compatible with the Galenic view that the retention in the womb of menstrual blood and, to an even greater degree, 'female seed', can lead to the substance rotting, giving off noxious vapours which affect the rest of the body (*Loc. Aff.* 6.5; K 8.420, 424, 432–3). Based on the model of an apparently minor bite or sting from a poisonous creature causing possibly fatal symptoms, Galen argued that the effects of the retention of blood or seed could be dramatic (Debru 1996: 239). In other herbals of the mid-sixteenth century, however, such as Nicolaus Myrepsus' *Liber de compositione medicamentorum* of 1541, mithridatum is commonly recommended not only for all types of poisoning, but also to provoke the menstrual periods, cure 'all diseases of the womb', restore appetite and bring a good colour to the body (1541: ch. 466, followed by Fuchs 1555: 156). Any, or indeed all, of these aspects would make it appropriate to green sickness. However, Bullein's own uses of mithridatum could support a slightly different aetiology. He also states that it is 'veri good against the stone' (1558: 120ᵛ; 1559: 228). This would suggest that green sickness is due to a blockage, an explanation which will be examined in more detail below.

Bullein's section on the medical use of onions states that they 'bringe good couler to the face, and help the grene sickness' (1558: 64ʳ; 1559: 124). Like mithridatum, then, onions can restore a 'good couler'. So far, Bullein's brief references to green sickness suggest that it is new, female, involves a poor colour of the face – but not necessarily a 'green' colour – and, in terms of its cause, can be understood as the result of menstrual suppression or of blockage. Can the use of onions help us to define the likely cause of the symptoms, as he understood it? In Dioscorides' herbal (2.144 or 145, depending on the edition), a work dating from the first century AD and frequently reprinted and widely used in the sixteenth century, onions, like mithridatum in Myrepsus, are recommended both against the bites of mad dogs and to bring on a suppressed menstrual period.[29] The section on the onion in Fuchs' *De historia stirpium* (1542: 429) repeats Dioscorides' 'it moves suppressed menses', Galen's 'it thins thick humours' and Simeon Seth's 'it thins thick and sluggish humours'.[30] This group of writers represents the combined classical heritage of sixteenth-century botany available to Bullein: their consensus is that onions, considered hot and dry, can thin any abnormally thick humours in the body, including menstrual blood.

We know that Bullein owned a copy of Fuchs' *De medendi methodo* dated 1539, which is held by the Wellcome Institute for the History of Medicine. In this work, the section on menstrual suppression describes the situations in which menstruation is not to be expected: it does not occur in women who are very young or old, or who are hot, who take much exercise, or are particularly fat or thin. It is also scanty or absent in countrywomen. Otherwise, its absence is due to the blood being thick or sluggish, or coming out somewhere else; through the nose, in the stools, or as sweat or vomit. If none of these applies, it can be the result of too much or too little food. In some cases of menstrual suppression, then, where it is due to thick blood, onions are the answer. In the 1578 English edition of Rembert Dodoens' herbal, first published in French in 1557, onions not only 'scatter, and make thinne grosse and clammie humours' but also cure 'the white spottes of all the body', thus providing another possible reason for their recommendation for green sickness, as the symptoms also went under the name of the 'white fever' (e.g. Dodoens 1578: 640–1; Tanner 1659: 314). The link between green sickness and the white fever is clear in a manuscript recipe collection in which an early seventeenth-century hand has added to two recipes for green sickness a further one against the white fever, '*contra febrem album*' (WMS 244: 210).

In the first edition of Bullein's *Bulwark of Defence* (1562), the section on simple medicines from *Government of Health* appears in a slightly different form; cast as a dialogue, but with different characters. Here, any reference to green sickness, 'new' or otherwise, has been dropped from the description of the uses of mithridatum, although mithridatum is now explicitly described as a good remedy 'to provoke the menstruall terms' (Bullein 1562: xiv^v). Claims for the novelty of green sickness have been moved into the discussion of onions:

> They doe make thyn the Bloude … [they] bee hoat in the thyrd degree, but they warme and cleanse the Stomacke, brynge good Colour to the face, and then they muste be good for the neewe Greene Sycknesse.
>
> (Bullein 1562: vi^r)

There is nothing here to suggest whether this 'neewe Greene Sycknesse' is already seen as a condition only affecting young girls, but again it is associated with digestive problems, with a 'bad' colour of the face, and possibly with menstrual suppression due to thick blood; above all, it is significant that it continues to be seen as 'new'. William Langham's *The Garden of Health*, published in 1597, drew heavily on Bullein; Langham's account of onions repeated the wording of Bullein (1562), including the reference to 'the newe green sicknesse' (Langham 1597: 446). Langham also recommended for green sickness a remedy based on ash which used a number of red plants, perhaps suggesting a 'homoeopathic' association with menstruation:

> Greene sicknesse, seethe powder of the Keyes [i.e. ash] with Betonie, red Sage, red Mynts, and Magerom [i.e. marjoram] in running water from a pottell to a quart, and drinke thereof a good draught with sugar warme morning and evening.
>
> (Langham 1597: 40, no. 10)[31]

However, the presence of green sickness in the section on 'Blessed Thistle' suggests not only the idea of 'obstruction of the passages' but also a continued association with digestive disturbance:

> eat it against palsie, use powder for colic. Drink a decoction for green sickness, griping and pain of belly, to open obstructions, cause passage of urine.
>
> (Langham 1597: 82, no. 48)

The final herbal remedy for green sickness recommended by Langham employs rue, a traditional expulsive or abortifacient herb, with 'red' sage:

> Stamp 1 handful Rue, 2 Red Sage, strain juice, add to 1pt hot honey, spoonful Pepper. Stir. Give 1 spoonful and half, blood warm, morning and evening. Plus to eat, 4 or 5 times daily, 5 or 7 'Raisins of the Sunne'.
>
> (Langham 1597: 553, no. 210)

Langham's use of pepper as part of this remedy for green sickness forms an interesting contrast with the third reference to green sickness in Bullein's 1558 *Government of Health*. Bullein warned that women who would 'fayne be fayre' eat pepper and dried corn, and drink vinegar, 'with such like bagage', in order to dry up their blood. Bullein cautioned that most of these women 'fal into weaknes, greene sicknes, stinking breathes and oftentimes sodain death' (1558: 115ʳ; 1559: 217).

This suggests that, at an early stage of its history, green sickness could be seen as a self-inflicted condition. Varandal (1619: 5; 1620: 2) also believed that this was true of his 'chlorosis'. He suggested that, because it was thought that a pale complexion was more attractive, virgins and widows were using 'art and industry' to make themselves appear pale; on the side of 'industry', he included an aversion to food, and a poor diet. The theme of sufferers' attitude to food will be taken up in chapter 4.

Green sickness and the disease of virgins

The next step for green sickness was to move from being a digestive disorder most common in women, to become a disease characteristic of young girls, particularly virgins. In the Western medical tradition, symptoms and diseases ideally need classical names. *Proctalgia fugax* sounds far more impressive than 'a fleeting pain in the rectum', but it simply translates the words into Latin. In the next chapter, I will argue that the specific impetus to the focus on virgins came from Lange's letter of 1554, where the symptoms became *morbus virgineus*. Lange also located the cause not in digestive blockages, but as a consequence of the sufferer's virginity, understood as obstructing the normal motion of blood through her body. Later writers – maintaining the digestive theme – linked such obstructions to an inappropriate diet making the virgin's blood thick and sluggish. Its focal organ could be the liver – the traditional seat of blood production in Galenic medicine – the womb, or the stomach.

However, Lange would not have had such influence were it not for ideas about the importance of menstruation to the female body which were already present in the Hippocratic/Galenic medical tradition. As we have seen, the remedies associated with green sickness in sixteenth-century herbals easily elided the digestive and the menstrual: but the use of the label 'disease of virgins', despite its inclusion of digestive symptoms, moved the condition further towards the womb, and the menstrual function. Sydenham (see p. 14) gave absence of menstruation as the final item on his list of the symptoms of chlorosis, but it was fundamental to the diagnosis of green sickness in girls in the sixteenth and early seventeenth centuries. The concern with ensuring an adequate menstrual loss was very much a feature of medicine at this time; in the London practice of Simon Forman – memorably characterised by Michael MacDonald as having 'a mesmerizing personality and the sexual appetite of a goat' (MacDonald 1981: 25) – many female patients were found to have 'stopped menses' as a symptom (Traister 1991: 438). In taking a case history from a female patient in the first decades of the seventeenth century, Forman's friend Richard Napier would always ask for details of the menstrual cycle (Sawyer 1986: 484); his habit of crossing out 'green sickness' and writing in 'obstruction of the spleen' if menstruation subsequently took place shows that, if the patient menstruated, the initial diagnosis always had to be revised (Sawyer 1986: 491 n. 41; p. 22 of this volume). Although Napier's method of diagnosis was astrological, the remedies he gave were usually the standard purges and bleedings of the early modern period. The records we have of his cases are, however, fuller than those of 'standard' doctors because, for an astrological practitioner, it was important to have details of the time of consultation, and the date of birth of the patient. One in five of Napier's women patients 'complained to the doctor of a gynaecological or obstetrical problem in addition to her psychological distress' (MacDonald 1981: 38). Napier used the label 'green sickness' alongside that of 'the virgin's disease'

(Sawyer 1986: 491). It is not certain that he knew Lange's description of *morbus virgineus*, but it is possible; the relevant letter was mentioned by Mercado (1579: 201) and was also popularised at the end of the sixteenth century through the compilation of medical cases edited by Schenck von Grafenberg, where it was classified, significantly, not under digestive conditions, but under disorders of menstrual suppression.[32]

As the disease of virgins was overtaken in medical writing by the label of 'chlorosis', it broadened out in terms of suggested aetiologies. In the process, there was overlap; some physicians still believed that absence of menstruation was the fundamental symptom, while others argued that alternative disturbances to the menstrual function were equally common in sufferers. By the nineteenth century, some writers privileged the absence of menstruation as cause rather than effect, turning the categories around so that chlorosis was seen as a disease of menstruation, 'the most common derangement of the menstrual function' (Ashwell 1836: 529–30). But others disputed this centrality of amenorrhoea: Tilt (1853: 69) and Trousseau (1872: 107) considered that, although it was common, it was 'not always the accompaniment of chlorosis', some sufferers instead having a very heavy loss of blood; Edward Johnson claimed that 'The monthly periods are sometimes suppressed, sometimes profuse, sometimes irregular, sometimes as in perfect health' (1856: 155); Clark (1887: 1003) thought that most patients suffering from chlorosis had perfectly regular menstruation; and Cabot argued that amenorrhoea occurred only in 120 out of 387 cases studied (1908: 644). Yet, in the dying years of the condition, Campbell continued to see amenorrhoea as 'one of the cardinal symptoms' (1923: 272).

How green was green sickness?

While the absence of menstruation moved from being the defining characteristic of the disease of virgins to meet a series of challenges from the mid-nineteenth century onwards, another symptom – the skin colour of the sufferer, discussed briefly in the Introduction – remains a problem for historians of the disease of virgins, green sickness and chlorosis. The latter two disease labels, unlike 'the disease of virgins', place the focus of the disease on an external, visible sign, the green hue of the sufferer's skin.[33] Broadly speaking, in the early history of the condition, taking up Anna's cheeks and lips being described by Lange as pale 'as if bloodless',[34] a loss of colour was expected; in the later history, a green tint was thought to be more characteristic. However, beneath this general pattern lies considerable variation.[35] Although some of the earliest writers on the disease describe sufferers as green because of the watery nature of their blood (e.g. Cary 1583: 40–1; Sennert 1664: 101), sixteenth-century profiles of the sufferer usually prefer variations on paleness – 'leaden or whitish' (Mercado 1579: 201)[36] – rather than green. Bullein's discussion of onions claimed that they 'bring good couler to the face, and helpe the grene sickness' (1558: 64^r; 1559: 124). Sydenham too gave as the first symptom on his list 'a bad colour of the face, and whole body' (1753: 658); however, he did not specify *which* colour, merely *decoloratio*, loss of colour (Sydenham 1827: 557).

The interest in the colour of the sufferer increased after the introduction of the label 'chlorosis' in 1619; as I have already noted, although Varandal said that this word comes 'from Hippocrates', in fact it is a newly coined word based on a Greek term for a particular shade of green. By the late nineteenth century, some writers regarded as 'most characteristic of all' a 'greenish-yellow' skin colour (Stengel 1896: 343), while others disagreed emphatically; Cabot considered that it 'takes the eye of faith' to see green (1908: 644). But Stengel's symptom-picture also included paleness; he transferred it to the hair, suggesting that it may become 'light coloured in spots'. A similar shift in the 'pale' motif was used by Sir Andrew Clark, who suggested that 'now and then a finger, or a small tract of skin upon the body, will become suddenly blanched and remain in that condition for hours' (Clark 1887: 1004), and by Ralph Stockman (1895b: 1473), who stated that the patient's bodily products were also 'very pale', specifically the urine and faeces (cf. Ward 1914: 311).

As well as observing the long survival of the earlier expectation of paleness, sometimes shifted on to specific body parts or products, we can also challenge the idea that the green skin colour was ever agreed upon as fundamental to 'green sickness' or 'chlorosis' in young girls. When Varandal first used the term 'chlorosis' in 1619, he gave a list of alternative names for the condition, ending with 'the disease of virgins, which we, from Hippocrates, call Chlorosis, which is a type of cachexia accompanied by a certain bad colour from white, more or less to green'.[37] But the word translated here as 'green' (*virescente*) can also mean 'flourishing', so this does not by any means solve the problem of the green skin colour; were it not for his new label for the condition, Varandal could be read as saying that the colour range covers several degrees of paleness. In this case, why did he choose to base his new disease name on the Greek word *chloros*? In this section, I want to investigate the nuances of this word for a classically trained French physician such as Varandal, and also to consider the uses of 'green' by early modern English vernacular writers.

The analogies applied to the colour of the sufferer's skin by early modern writers tend, if anything, to complicate the picture rather than simplify it; for example, while John Pechey ([Pechey] 1694) used the relatively straightforward 'white as a Cloth', Astruc (1761–5, vol. 2: 4) said the skin is 'like wax or candle grease' but can be 'the yellow of a dead leaf, or a yellow tending towards green, or towards black'.[38] This is obviously a very wide colour range, in which 'green' is only one possibility. Nicholas Sudell's *Mulierum Amicus*, published in 1666 as a health guide aimed at women themselves, taught them:

1   What you are ... different from men, and that in the one particular in special, the womb.
2   What you are liable unto ... [the womb being] subject to innumerable company of diseases and calamities.
3   What assistance you have ... God having provided in his love ... very many supplies and remedies ... as well as laid punishment to shew his justice.

As the first sign of chlorosis, Sudell stated that 'the face and all the body is pale and white, and sometimes of a lead colour, blew [*sic*] and green' (1666: 7). This echoed John Tanner, who wrote that 'you may know the diseased, if you do but view their Faces, which are pale and white, sometimes of a Lead colour, blew or green' (1659: 315).

How could this protean confusion of colours come under some sort of intellectual control? Writing on 'les pâles couleurs', Liébault (1597: 12) suggested that the colour of the skin depended on the retained humoral materials: if the blood was serous or watery, the virgin would be pale; if yellow bile was retained, she would be yellow; and if black bile was retained, she would be bronzed. Varandal (1619: 5; 1620: 2) also took a similar line; *chloros* is relevant because the outer signs reveal the internal humoral imbalance. In the nineteenth century, Sir Andrew Clark tried to tie down the colour range in a different way, by suggesting that the colours could be associated with different parts of the face; the skin

> is of the colour of long-kept white wax, lighter or darker at different parts; on the forehead it is of a greenish-white tint; on the temples and neck it is of a yellowish hue; about the lips and nostrils it is of a very pale purple colour;[39] and about the eyelids it is like a withered autumn leaf.
>
> (1887: 1004)

Is this a supreme example of medical observation, or an imaginative attempt to retain all colour options in a single, ideal patient?

When the London surgeon Daniel Turner included green sickness alongside yellow jaundice in his 1714 treatise on 'diseases incident to the skin', he cast serious doubt on the green skin colour. In this work, he was asking that surgeons – whose sphere was restricted to externally manifest conditions – should be allowed to invade the territory of physicians, by administering internal medicines. His argument aimed at collapsing the categories of 'internal' and 'external'; although this shift in conceptions of the body had significant professional implications, it corresponded to patients' experiences of their own bodies.[40] Barbara Duden's study of the German physician Storch, a contemporary of Daniel Turner, discussed women's fears that matter which should be expelled had 'been driven back inside' and could then come out in a rash (Duden 1991: 133). This idea was also found in sixteenth-century medicine; Amatus Lusitanus (1556: 39) described how retained menstrual blood in an 18-year-old virgin could lead to 'very severe and disgusting symptoms', with skin eruptions occurring all over the body, but particularly on the face. The cure was to let blood at the ankle, in order to return the blood to the womb.[41] Turner classified both chlorosis and yellow jaundice under diseases of inward origin which presented themselves through external symptoms of the skin; because the pores allowed particles causing disease to be evacuated, they also provided a route into the interior of the body for remedies applied to the skin (Wilson 1999: 64–9). Turner's section on green sickness offered a direct challenge to the colour by calling it 'the Green-Sickness, *so called*', and then describing it as

> The Green (or rather give me leave to call it, the Pale or White) Sickness (since in its worst state the Complexion is rarely if ever a true Green, tho' bordering on that Hue).
>
> (Turner 1714: 90)

In *The Female Physician*, published ten years later, John Maubray (1724: 43) looked for 'a pallid greenish Tincture', but suggested that the complexion inclines only 'a little that way'.

As we have already seen (p. 5), the issue of whether or not sufferers were characteristically 'green' is not merely an antiquarian one; it is important for writers of the modern period who want to understand chlorosis as a condition which medicine is at last able to explain. Hudson (1977: 451, 460) notes that, after developments in haematology in the mid-nineteenth century placed many 'chlorotics' under the diagnostic label of hypochromic anaemia, the green skin colour was less frequently observed. Instead the focus lay on pallor: the extent of the pallor 'must be seen to be appreciated', according to Gordon Ward's *Bedside Haematology* (1914: 307). Writers of this later period who continued to list a green skin colour as one of the textbook signs of chlorosis admitted that they did not always observe it in the cases they themselves saw. Hudson does not, however, use this evidence to conclude that sufferers never had been, literally, green; instead, he proposes that

> unknown physiologic factors could have existed in certain chlorotics to explain the presence of a greenish caste in the skin, if, as is also possible, chlorosis was something more than a simple iron deficiency anaemia.
>
> (1977: 461)

When pushed, Hudson investigates the possibility of partial obstruction of the bile duct as one of these 'unknown physiologic factors', but admits that this is unlikely (1977: 462). Siddall too confesses that 'this green hue is very seldom observable', but still wishes to retain the symptom because a green or brown tint can both be linked to iron-deficiency anaemia (1982: 260; cf. Hudson 1977: 451). The wheel comes full circle: chlorosis may have been a type of anaemia, one sort of anaemia may involve green skin coloration, therefore the list of symptoms for chlorosis needs to include this coloration, even if the cases seen did not usually exhibit it. Neither Hudson nor Siddall wishes to abandon altogether the symptom of green skin; as Hudson puts it, 'one may not conclude that three centuries of careful clinical observers were reporting a striking physical finding that was not there' (1977: 461; cf. Hansen 1931: 176).

Or, perhaps, 'one may'. For sixteenth-century writers, a changed skin colour could indicate the underlying humoral imbalance. But green sickness was not always about turning green, and its long survival as an alternative name for the disease of virgins may owe more to its metaphorical uses. A comparable medical example may be the 'Black Death'; the label was not used by contemporaries, but was applied to the plague retrospectively because of its high mortality rate (e.g. D'Irsay 1926; Kjennerud 1948). Is something similar true of green sickness: just as sufferers from the Black Death did not turn black, so girls suffering from green sickness did not need to be, literally, green, although the expectation of some change in skin colour was part of the picture as early as 1547–58, when green sickness emerged from green jaundice?

I would suggest that, in the second half of the century, strengthened by the input from Lange's letter in 1554 associating the disorder predominantly with virgins, 'green' took on a less visual meaning. Loudon (1980) argued that the origin of the label lay instead in the use of 'green' to mean youthful, immature or inexperienced. Sixteenth-century texts would support this suggestion; for example, a cognate medical usage appears in the notes which Simon Forman (1552–1611) made of his medical practice from 1597 onwards, where he used the term 'grene' for 'newly delivered of a child' (Traister 1991: 441). Only when a metaphorical use invoking youth and immaturity began to fade was a physical interpretation of the colour again expected. English medical advertisements from the late seventeenth and early eighteenth centuries, by which practitioners publicised their services and their remedies, suggest that in this period the label of 'green sickness' remained the one to which potential patients would respond. However, while some handbills simply listed green sickness among the disorders they could cure, others specified the practitioner's ability to treat 'Green-sickness in Virgins (though never so weak)', or 'Green-sickness in Maids'.[42] This may suggest that, at this date, the label itself did not always suggest the youth of the patient sufficiently clearly for its audience. Metaphorical uses of 'green' continued to surface in medical literature; for example, in an inaugural dissertation presented to the Paris Medical Faculty on 1 May 1819, Olive claimed that the unsuitable foods eaten by the chlorotic girl include green – unripe – fruits (1819: 13), an assertion made as early as 1583 by Walter Cary (1583: 40–1). In the context of discussions of the disease of virgins, thought to affect girls like Anna or Mamillia who are 'ripe' for marriage, this suggests a disagreement between girls and their medical authorities as to what constitutes their own 'ripeness'.

However, there remain other possibilities which have not been explored by Loudon and which suggest further nuances to 'green sickness'; most importantly, the use of 'green' in early modern sexual imagery.[43] Ursula Potter (2002: 280–1) has discovered late sixteenth-century sources which link greenness in virgins to envy of their married sisters; for example, in *Romeo and Juliet* the virgin goddess Diana is described as 'sick and green' but also as 'envious' (II.ii.7–9). But green was also seen as the colour of sexuality and nature, hence the colour appropriate to the dress of a whore. Even more relevant to the disease of virgins, to have a 'green gown' or to be 'green-gowned' represents the loss of sexual innocence, the image suggesting an outdoor tumble (Williams 1994: 620–1). This is used in the ballad 'Enfield Common' (1705), where a girl with green sickness is offered 'ease in a green Gown' as a cure 'to stir the Blood'. The 'gallant' who offers to act as her physician observes that the cure is successful;

> Then with her leave there, a dose I gave her,
> She straight confes'd her Sickness I did nick it.[44]

This suggests that, for an early modern reader, the disease label 'green sickness' – like 'the disease of virgins' – could contain within itself the cure: sexual experience.

But this does not exhaust the rich potential of 'green sickness'. In addition to the youth of the sufferer, and the sexual cure, the name may also contain a suggestion as to how the label could move so readily from the realm of digestive disorders – green jaundice – into that of menstrual disturbance. Cressy (1997: 203–5) has argued that the use of 'green' for women who have just given birth, found from at least the 1580s, suggests that the post-partum period was linked to green sickness because in both cases menstruation was temporarily absent. In an important twelfth-century medical text, both green and 'the colour of grass' are presented as appropriate colours for sufferers from menstrual suppression. This text, known from its opening words as *Cum auctor*, is one of those associated with the name of Trotula.[45] Claiming its roots lie in the Hippocratic and Galenic texts (Green 2001: 70), it exists in many medieval manuscripts; indeed, before the 1520s, the Trotula texts were far better known than the Hippocratic gynaecological texts. The prologue to *Cum auctor*, first printed in the 1540s, and reprinted in the late sixteenth-century gynaecological compendium called the *Gynaeciorum*, ends with a list of symptoms of menstrual suppression; 'sometimes their face changes into a green or livid color or into a color like that of grass' (Lat. *gramen*).[46] The idea that green-ness can result from the absence of menstruation may be reinforced by the notion, found in the work of Hildegard of Bingen (1098–1179), that menstruation was itself a sign of the 'greenness and flowering' of a woman; 'As a tree, from its greenness, brings forth blossoms and leaves and bears fruit, so too woman, from the greenness of the rivulets of menstrual blood, brings forth blossoms and leaves in the fruit of her womb' (Berger 1999: 82).

Green sickness and love sickness

The phrasing of *Cum auctor* suggests that 'green' and 'grass' are not the same colour, but alternatives. However, bringing them into conjunction like this brought in other nuances for an early modern audience and for writers such as Varandal; these too derive from the classical tradition and draw green sickness alongside not only menstrual suppression, but also love sickness. The dividing line between green sickness and love sickness continued to be a thin one even into the nineteenth century: *The Edinburgh Practice of Physic, Surgery, and Midwifery*, based on the work of Cullen, stated in the 1803 edition that there was 'only one idiopathic species of this genus', namely '*chlorosis virginea*, or *chlorosis amatoria*' (Cullen 1803: 361), caused by 'love and other passions of the mind' (1803: 362). Emotion, particularly after the eighteenth century, was thought to play a key role in the development of chlorosis. As well as unrequited love (Johnson 1849: 50, 52–4), it could be caused by bereavement (Burq 1852: 16) or fright (Trousseau 1872: 108; Stengel 1896: 329; see Hudson 1977: 454–5). Pre-eighteenth century writers such as Dubois (1559: 148) had already listed anger and sorrow as factors leading to insufficient menstrual blood being produced. However, love was implicated as early as Lange, who claimed that the women of Brabant called his 'disease of virgins' not only white fever, but also love fever.

What was the appropriate complexion for a sufferer from love sickness? In medieval medicine, love sickness already existed as a recognised medical condition, derived from Constantine the African's *Viaticum*, a central text in the medical curricula of many European universities from the early thir-teenth century onwards. An adaptation of an Arabic text, al-Jazzār's *Kitab Zād al-Musāfir*, it included 'passionate love' as an autonomous disease cate-gory (Beecher 1988: 5; Wack 1990: xiii, 35). The chapter on love sickness, placing it after insomnia, frenzy and drunkenness, and before sneezing, epilepsy and apoplexy, provided a conceptual framework for the disease over the following four centuries. Its cause was thought to be humoral imbalance, but its seat was located in the brain. Mental and physical symptoms of the condition were traced back to the brain because, in Galenic theory, this organ was the seat of the passions (Wack 1990: 38–40). However, in the medieval and early modern periods, love sickness tended to be associated not with women, but with noble men; Mary Wack (1990: 46) argued that the association originated in word-play, with *eros*, 'erotic love', being associated with *heroicus*, that which belongs to a lord or nobleman. Appropriately for this class, it was then thought that excess wealth and leisure could encourage the condition, one of the symptoms of which was a yellow skin colour (Wack 1990: 40, 188).

In favour of paleness, however, was an important classical text for discussions both of love sickness and of chlorosis: Ovid's *Art of love* 1.729, which states that it is fitting that a lover becomes pale (*palleat*), because paleness is the colour most appropriate for a lover.[47] This text was among those cited by Lange in his description of Anna's condition. The definition of *pallens* given in the Oxford Latin Dictionary is 'Pale, wan', from illness, death or emotion; however, the entry goes on to suggest that, in Mediterranean populations, we should understand this as involving a yellowish or greenish tint, making the colour close to the Greek *chloros*. This denial that *palleat* simply means 'becomes pale' is also found in sixteenth- and seventeenth-century writers; in *Love's Labour's Lost* (c.1595) Shakespeare's 'fantastical Spaniard' Armado seems to have Ovid in mind when he remarks 'Green indeed is the colour of lovers' (I.ii.81), while in the early seventeenth century Ferrand called the colour of lovers one 'blended of white and yellow, or of white, yellow and green', and cited Galen as evidence that pale (Greek *ôchros*) and *chloros* are equivalent terms for a certain complexion.[48] Here he is using Giovan Battista della Porta's influential work, the four books of *De humana physiognomonia* (1601), which discussed the significance of different colours of the face and body; Ovid's comment on pale lovers is repeated here, and *chloros* is described as sometimes meaning 'pallid' (Porta 1601: 200, 201–5). This text further suggests that, in women, a white colour is associated with excessive sexual appetites (1601: 198).[49]

Like green sickness, therefore, love sickness can make its sufferer pale, yellow or green. Trotula's reference linking menstrual suppression with both a green complexion and a grass-like appearance would, for classically trained readers, recall the poetry of the sixth-century BC Greek lyric poet Sappho, who described turning 'more *chloros* [yellowish green?] than grass' while overcome with love. Nor was this exclusively an image for the educated elite: a ballad called 'A remedy for the green sickness' (c.1683) includes the verse:

A handsome buxom lass
lay panting on her bed.
She look't as green as grass
and mournfully she said
Unless I have some lusty lad to ease me of my pain
I cannot live
I sigh and grieve
My life I now disdain.[50]

Sappho's 'more *chloros* than grass' is the most influential use of *chloros* in Greek literature, and it is important to investigate its meaning if we are to understand the possible nuances of Varandal's label, 'chlorosis'. In the second century AD, Plutarch related a story set at the end of the fourth century BC; Antiochos fell in love with his stepmother Stratonike, a love presented as 'an incurable disease'. But the physician Erasistratos discovered the identity of Antiochos' love-object by his reactions in her presence: 'those tell-tale signs of which Sappho sings were all there in him', including pallor (*Life of Demetrios* 38). Jacques Ferrand, a practising physician whose treatise on love sickness was published in 1610, echoed this when he wrote that Sappho had already identified all the signs of love, leaving it to later physicians only to classify these; he also quoted from the Roman poets Catullus and Ovid.[51]

The phrase 'more *chloros* than grass' occurs in the partially preserved poem Sappho 31, known to medieval and Renaissance readers through its preservation in pseudo-Longinus, *On the sublime* 10.1–3, where it is used as an example of Sappho's excellence (*aretê*) in selecting the most important aspects of the symptoms of love's madness (*tais erôtikais maniais*).[52] Sappho describes the sensations she experiences in mind and body when seeing the woman she loves talking and laughing with a man. The man who hears the girl's sweet voice and lovely laughter seems to Sappho to be in a situation 'equal to the gods'. When Sappho looks at the girl 'even for a moment', her heart trembles in her breast, her senses are affected, and she is near death; unable to speak, she feels a fire beneath her flesh, her sight fails, her ears hum, she sweats and trembles and says, 'I am more *chloros* than grass' ('*chlorotera de poias emmi*', Sappho 31, lines 13–14).

Are these sensations the result of watching the beloved in animated conversation, or of having been supplanted in her affections by the man in the poem? The most common translation of the key phrase is 'greener than grass', a translation which has been used to support a reading of the poem which diagnoses what is affecting Sappho as jealousy, or as an 'anxiety attack'. Scholars – mainly male, and uncomfortable with the female homo-eroticism of the poem – who put forward this argument suggest that the girl Sappho loves is to be married; seeing the beloved relaxing in the company of the man who is to replace her causes Sappho to feel jealousy. The 'jealousy thesis' can be traced back to the 1850s, but the idea of an 'attack' of this kind was put forward by the psychiatrist George Devereux in 1970. In responding to Devereux, Marcovich pointed out that this is not a sudden 'attack', but a chronic problem; Sappho's use of the subjunctive *idô* in line 7 should be understood as '*each* time I look at you', while Sappho marvels at the nameless man who can 'keep sitting right opposite you and keep listening', implying that she can only see the beloved for a moment before being overwhelmed by her beauty (Marcovich 1972: 21, 25).

If being *chloros* is nothing to do with jealousy, then how should we understand it? The spectrum of meanings of *chloros* also associates it with paleness and moisture; Eleanor Irwin (1974: 33–56) argued that the core meaning was 'liquid'/'fresh', so that flowers or dew could be described as *chloros*. For her, the best translation of Sappho's words would be 'more grassy than grass', thus seeing becoming *chloros* 'not as a symptom of exhaustion, but of excitement' (Irwin 1974: 65–7). Snyder (1991: 13–14) followed up the idea that the main use of *chloros* was in connection with 'youth and life'; she therefore suggested that 'more *chloros* than grass' 'anchors the speaker's experience firmly in the natural world, a world of freshness, growth and moisture'. This recalls Hildegard's reference to greenness and flowering, and makes the expression contrast strongly with the next line, 'I seem to be little short of dying'. This reading of the poem is consistent with pseudo-Longinus' explanation of why he cited it in *On the sublime*; it is precisely Sappho's ability to capture the contradictory sensations central to the feeling of being in love which he praised.

As Irwin's study of Greek colour terminology demonstrates, words change their meanings over time. She traced a gradual shift in the meaning of *chloros* from 'green' in the eighth century BC to 'pale' or 'blanched' by the fourth century BC; in the Homeric poems, it was closest to 'green', and was seen as the colour appropriate to fear, because the frightened were thought to produce more bile from the liver, the organ in which fear was centred.[53] By the fourth century BC, those who were afraid were thought to become pale, because blood was believed to rush towards the heart, away from the surface of the body (Irwin 1974: 63–4; Aristotle fr. 243). The Roman poet Lucretius echoed Sappho's words in a description of the sensations of fear (*De rerum natura* 3.152–8), which included pallor; in the Roman world, then, Sappho 31 was certainly known. The poet Catullus produced a heterosexual 'creative translation' into Latin (Catullus 51; Gaisser 1993: 163), in which he stopped himself in mid-phrase, in order to end with a reminder to himself that these fantasies of another man with his beloved are only the result of too much leisure (*otium*). Catullus' version is cut short before he feels the sensation of being 'more *chloros* than grass'. But echoes of Sappho's poem also appear in Longus' novel *Daphnis and Chloe* (1.17.4).[54] This last work, from the late second or early third century AD, is an imitation rather than a translation; Longus develops 'more *chloros* than grass' into 'more *chloros* in the face than summer grass', which could suggest greenness but seems more likely to be based on an analogy with grass thoroughly bleached by the hot summer sun (Irwin 1974: 65–6). The main point of Gonzaga's analogy between his marriageable daughter Mamillia and the 'grasse being ready for the sieth' (Greene 1583: Grosart 1881–3: II.36) is to suggest the narrow window of opportunity between readiness and lost opportunity; but, as grass being harvested for winter storage needs to be pale, yellow, and dried out, otherwise it will not keep well, his fear of the green sickness does evoke the colour of summer grass.[55] Longus' interpretation of Sappho, which removes the sense of life/death contrast between this line and the following one, 'I seem to be little short of dying', was projected back on to the original poem by Monica Silveira Cyrino in her study of love sickness in early Greek poetry. Cyrino (1995: 153) suggested that Sappho is 'pale' because 'Eros has rendered her weak, bloodless, insensate, barely alive', making the image into a preparation for the 'near-death experience' of the final image of the poem, rather than a contrast to it.

Whatever its meaning for Sappho, 'greener than grass' therefore moved towards 'paleness', at least in Roman understandings of the poem. When would these classical texts have been available to writers of the Renaissance and beyond? Sappho, through pseudo-Longinus' *On the sublime*, was known in the fifteenth century, but *On the sublime* received little attention until the mid-sixteenth century, when Francesco Robortello published an edition in 1554. A few months later, in October of the same year, Marc-Antoine de Muret brought out his commentary on Catullus, where he was the first to identify in print Catullus 51 as a translation of Sappho 31 (Gaisser 1993: 163–4, 147; Muret 1554: 57). The materials needed to construct a connection between the colour *chloros* and love sickness were thus more easily available from the mid-sixteenth century onward; specifically, they became available in 1554, precisely the same year as Lange's letter on the disease of virgins. Varandal's 'chlorosis' may be a nod in the direction of Sappho and love sickness, masked as a reference back to a Hippocratic text which does not in fact exist.

While medieval writers on love sickness focused on men – a strategy which, Mary Wack has argued, was due to 'historical contradictions in aristocratic culture' (1990: 147, 150–1) – by the sixteenth century the seat of the condition had moved down from the brain to the genitals, and what had been the 'heroic disease' was also thought to affect women (Wack 1990: 121–5; Vandereycken and Van Deth 1994: 139). As love sickness moved to being a women's complaint, green sickness picked up the classical association of greenness or paleness with being in love (from Ovid and Sappho) and of both greenness and grassiness with menstrual suppression (from Trotula). On one reading of Sappho, the 'greenness' of green sickness could also suggest the fresh youthfulness of its now-typical sufferer: on another, it evoked a paleness more akin to love sickness. Jane Sharp suggested that puberty was a time when girls were likely to 'grow almost mad with love' (1671: 85; Hobby 1999: 69), and that green sickness is 'more common in maids of ripe years when they are in love and desirous to keep company with a man' (1671: 256; Hobby 1999: 194); but, for some girls, green sickness could be seen as a form of love sickness in which there is *no* specific love object.[56]

In the seventeenth and eighteenth centuries, another disorder – nymphomania – came to prominence, and was considered mainly to affect women (Groneman 1994: 343); young girls at puberty remained most vulnerable to this latter condition, particularly at the onset of the first menstrual period.

For example, the French doctor Bienville, whose treatise on nymphomania was published in 1771 and translated into English in 1775, wrote that

> This disorder frequently surprizes the younger part of the sex, at a marriageable age, when their hearts, premature in love, have warmly pleaded in favour of some youth, for whom they feel a desperate passion, the gratification of which is opposed by insurmountable obstacles.
>
> (1775: 29)[57]

Bienville (1775: 102; 107) believed that, like chlorosis and medieval love sickness, nymphomania could be detected from a 'pale, and even disfigured' face; again like these, it was best cured by marriage.

Another interesting feature of Bienville's treatise is that, despite its condemnation of novels and voluptuous pictures which can over-stimulate the emotions (1775: 76), long sections of the text consist of extended case histories which are themselves written as 'novels'. Novels were thought to contribute to chlorosis; one of Ashwell's chlorosis patients was a 34-year-old teacher 'devoted to reading ... but never called upon for any laborious exertion' (1836: 572), while Raciborski (1868: 317–18) recommended a total ban on novel-reading before the age of 20, with entry to public libraries being forbidden. Like many writers of the late nineteenth century, he regarded fiction as giving a deceptive image of the world, and encouraging immorality. Imagining the scenes of the novel was thought to have a direct physical effect on the sexual organs, leading to their premature development (Wood-Allen 1898: 122–3, 147).[58]

The case histories given by Bienville could be seen as forming precisely the sort of emotionally over-exciting stories which would lead to disease; they tell the stories of Lucilla of Lyons (1775: 91–102), Leonora (1775: 128–53) and Julia (1775: 164–84).[59] While George Rousseau (1982: 100) was correct to say that the book 'contains very little material of a disreputable nature', there is nevertheless a sense in which the reader is invited to be a voyeur here. The story of Leonora, for example, 'whose beauty had been the delight and admiration of the whole country' but 'was, now, become the terror of it' so that 'Several gentlemen of the neighbourhood had, with difficulty, escaped from her', involves a detailed description of how she is stripped, pinioned and tied to the bed so that 'she could not possibly apply her hands to the parts' (Bienville 1775: 130–1, 140–4). Julia, who began to suffer from the condition when she was 13, falls in love with a man and is taught by her maid to masturbate while she waits to satisfy her desires (Bienville 1775: 173–4). In the nineteenth century in particular, it was feared that 'Seclusion and solitary habits are frequently indulged' by the sufferer from chlorosis (Ashwell 1836: 541); masturbation (Hudson 1977: 457; Loudon 1984: 31), euphemistically described as 'secret impurities'

(Clark 1887: 60) or 'vices of personal hygiene' (Stengel 1896: 329; Brumberg 1982: 1471), was sometimes directly blamed for its onset. Mothers were encouraged to watch for signs of masturbation, and to act immediately, before the nervous system could be weakened (e.g. Raciborski 1868: 333; Ruddock 1892: 81). In Bienville on nymphomania, as in Lange on the disease of virgins, or Gonzaga on his daughter Mamillia, the most dangerous time of life is when a girl is 'at a marriageable age' or – in the words of the Hippocratic treatise *On the disease of virgins*, which will be discussed in the next chapter – 'ripe for marriage'. As Gonzaga knew, 'the apples being rype, for want of plucking would rotte on the tree' (Greene 1583).

A gendered green sickness thus existed in English vernacular medicine as early as 1558, when it was perceived as 'new'. It remained close to green jaundice, in its digestive components and its association with blockages but, as interest in its menstrual causes grew, it was narrowed down by the end of the sixteenth century to become a disorder of young girls. The green skin colour, adopted from green jaundice, was replaced by claims for the paleness of the sufferer's complexion, reinforced not only by medieval texts on menstruation and on the effects of menstrual suppression but also by classical images of love sickness. However, the 'green' label survived, picking up the intertwined imagery of youth, inexperience and the emergence of sexuality. At the same time, green sickness merged with a disease called the 'disease of virgins' which arose from Lange's reading of the newly available Hippocratic medical texts. Both conditions were as well known in popular literature as in medical texts, where one of their most characteristic features was the recommendation of marriage as one of the best therapies. In the next chapter, I will concentrate on the themes brought in by Lange's letter of 1554, investigating how academic medicine constructed the disease of virgins.

2

A NEW DISEASE?

The classical sources for the disease of virgins

In the previous chapter, I discussed claims for the novelty of green sickness in English vernacular medical writing, and the process by which the digestive disorder of green jaundice was repackaged and, drawing on imagery of 'green' as suggesting freshness, youth and sexuality, relaunched as the disease of virgins, and subsequently as chlorosis. In this chapter, I will return to Latin medical writing and to Johannes Lange, who made no such claims to novelty in his description of the disease of virgins in his *Medicinalium epistolarum miscellanea* 1.21 (1554). Although, as we have seen, he himself did not talk about being 'the first', historians of chlorosis have identified Lange's letter as 'doubtless the earliest account of chlorosis' (Ruhräh 1934: 393), 'the first distinct description of chlorosis' (Bird 1982: 134), the 'first medical description of this syndrome' (Crosby 1987: 2799) or, more cautiously, 'the account which all later commentators would agree upon as describing chlorosis' (Hudson 1977: 448–9). On the contrary, however, and in obvious contrast to Bullein's claims for the 'new' green sickness in 1558, Lange stressed that his 'disease of virgins' was far from being new. He referred to popular knowledge – among 'the women of Brabant' – of the condition which he described, but also gave it a 2,000-year past by naming classical precedents for this combination of symptoms. Modern discussions of the mysterious disappearance of chlorosis have also looked to classical precedents, but have identified different classical texts as the sources for the symptoms. Do any of these classical precedents exist and, more broadly, how did Lange use Greek medical texts to structure his 'disease of virgins'?

Lange cited 'the rich store of the medicine of Hippocrates' as the source of his advice to Anna's father. The most important ancient text for him was the Hippocratic treatise *On the disease of virgins*, and in this chapter I will investigate its content, and its transmission up to the sixteenth century. In the early seventeenth century, when the publication of his *De morbis et affectibus mulierum* (1619: 4–5; 1620: 1) relabelled the disease of virgins 'chlorosis', it is significant that Varandal gave authority to his new label by claiming it was 'from Hippocrates'. By the second half of the sixteenth century, 'Hippocrates' had become the buzz-word in gynaecology, the movement 'back to Hippocrates' being fuelled partly by the lack of material in Galen on women and children (Nutton 1989: 435). Giambattista da Monte, the humanist professor of medical practice at Padua known as the 'second Galen', died two years before Lange's letter was published; his *De uterinis affectibus*, first published posthumously in 1554, used an entirely Galenic model of menstruation, but still named Hippocrates, not Galen, as the expert guide to gynaecology.[1] In particular, he cited *Diseases of women* 1.62 as demonstrating Hippocrates' knowledge that disorders of the womb are difficult to treat due to inexperience and ignorance, shame and fear, on the part of both the patient and the doctor. It was Hippocrates, da Monte (1554: 63v; 1556: 3) wrote, who was the fullest authority and the most careful of all ancient doctors in addressing the problems raised by disorders of the womb. By the 1580s, it had become commonplace to praise Hippocrates for his gynaecological works; for example, Liébault's introduction to his French translation of his *De Sanitate, Fecunditate et Morbis Mulierum*, published in 1582, described the four separate books written by 'The divine Hippocrates, caring about the health and fertility of womankind, and stimulated by a charitable spirit to save her.'[2] Liébault went on to claim that few of Hippocrates' successors, ancient or modern, had been able to match his knowledge of gynaecology, because the subject is inherently shifting and unstable; the diseases of men are easier to treat because they remain constant over an individual's life, whereas women move between the categories of virgin, wife, pregnant woman and mother (cf. Maclean 1980: 46).

Taking up this enthusiasm for Hippocrates as gynaecological expert, historians of chlorosis have assumed that the Hippocratic texts must somewhere contain the earliest references to this disease, even if it was Lange who was the first to put forward an immediately recognisable description. For example, in a list of diseases for which the Greek names are preserved, Le Clerc (1699: 248) mentioned '(g) Virgins, the Diseases of Virgins' but added that 'This disease is described by *Hippocrates*, but he gave it no particular name' (cf. Astruc 1761–5, vol. 2: 5; 1762, vol. 1: 173). Even as recently as the 1930s, Fowler (1936: 168) was able to claim at least that 'it is probable that chlorosis was the disease in mind' in the Hippocratic treatise *On the disease of virgins*. This contrasts with Loudon's cautious 'Lange may well have based his description in part on Hippocrates' (1984: 35), and Figlio's even more measured assessment that 'the Hippocratic corpus refers to symptoms which were *later interpreted* as chlorosis' (1978: 174; my italics). However, despite the enormous confidence in its Hippocratic origins shown by medical writers from the early modern period onwards, neither the label 'chlorosis' nor the symptom picture characteristic of it can be found in the Hippocratic corpus. Furthermore, when Lange tells us what Hippocrates says, he adds material which is not found in the Greek text. Sometimes this is due simply to carelessness in specifying where a quotation ends, and Lange's own gloss on it begins, but on other occasions Lange's interpretation can help us to see how and why the version of the text he was using differs from the versions of the Greek text known today. The relationship between chlorosis and Hippocrates is thus far less direct than either Varandal's confident statement, 'from Hippocrates', or Lange's letter, with its claims for 'the rich store of the medicine of Hippocrates', may suggest. The evidence indicates that it is in the rediscovery and reinterpretation of ancient texts in the early sixteenth century, rather than in observed reality, that we can find the solutions to some of the problems which the disease of virgins poses.

Lange's letter

What did Lange say in his letter to Anna's father which was so significant that a new disease was created from it? Lange was born in Löwenburg in Silesia in 1485; he studied medicine at the universities of Leipzig, Ferrara and Pisa, receiving a master's degree in philosophy and natural sciences from Leipzig in 1514 and his medical qualification at Pisa in 1522. In his preface to the *Epistolae medicinales*, a work which he says is directed not only at doctors, but at all who are interested in natural history, he claims that his experiences in Italy showed him how outdated German medicine had become, with its excessive reliance on urine examination, and its inadequate knowledge of Hippocrates and Galen (Fossel 1914: 240). Lange served as Archiater to the Palatinate for forty years, travelling around Europe with the Kurfürst Friedrich II, and dying in Heidelberg in 1565. He was a highly knowledgeable writer, familiar with the medical debates of his day (Nutton 1984: 84; 1985: 94); he used the letter format, an Italian device which had become popular in medicine in this period (Fossel 1914: 238–40), and he was steeped in the classical tradition. His work may thus be set in the context of the transformation of science in the sixteenth and early seventeenth century by 'the systematic use of newly discovered classical texts and methods' (Grafton 1991: 4).

From close similarities of wording, it is clear that he owned a copy of the first printed edition of the complete Hippocratic corpus, the 1525 Latin translation made by Marco Fabio Calvi of Ravenna.[3] Calvi, who also translated Vitruvius' *De architectura* for Raphael, was probably in Rome from 1510 working on Hippocratic medicine; he tells us that he finished his transcription of the manuscripts on 24 July 1512, and completed the Latin translation on 14 August 1524. Captured during the sack of Rome in 1527, he was unable to pay the ransom demanded, and died in a hospital outside the city.

Although Lange preferred to cite Hippocratic treatises from Calvi's Latin translation rather than from the Aldine Greek text of the complete corpus published in 1526, he could read Greek when necessary; in the letter on the disease of virgins he cited Galen's commentary on *Regimen in acute diseases* in Greek, and in some of the sections in which he claimed to be giving

Hippocrates' words it may be possible to see him comparing the Greek and Latin texts before reaching his own version. This is consistent with what is known of the reading habits of other sixteenth-century humanists; Lisa Jardine and Anthony Grafton (1990) have shown that Gabriel Harvey read Livy by having several different books open in front of him at any one time. Also typical of the sixteenth century is the preference for Latin over Greek. The humanist enterprise stressed the importance of knowledge of Greek in order to purge medical texts of the errors caused by their complex transmission through Arabic and Syriac into the 'inelegant medieval Latin' versions used in medical education from the middle ages onwards (Nutton 1988: 113). However, as Grafton and Jardine (1986: 119) have shown, Greek nevertheless 'ended the Renaissance in the position in which it first entered Italy: as a new subject, something on the margins of the curriculum'.

The text of Lange's letter may be translated as follows.[4]

> You complain bitterly to me, as to your faithful Achates,[5] that your firstborn daughter Anna, who is now of marriageable age, is desired in marriage by many suitors of unblemished virtue, from families of distinction and with an abundance of wealth, so that the ancestry of your son-in-law would not be inferior to that of your ancestors. Yet, because of the infirmity of your daughter, you are forced to refuse them. But this is less worrying for you than the fact that, until now, not one of the doctors has been able to explain the internal cause and essence of the disease, or indeed to prescribe treatment. For one says that it is cardialgia, another palpitation of the heart; this one, that it is certainly dyspnoea, that one, suffocation of the womb; and there are also those who suppose that a defect of the liver has caused an aversion [towards food] in the stomach. The disagreement which they have expressed on your daughter's disease has, you say, made you wholly confused, and you cannot decide what to do.
>
> Because of this, by virtue of our long-standing friendship, you urgently request my opinion on your daughter's disease, and reliable advice on her marriage. In your letter, you accurately detail the symptoms of the disease which distresses her. You confirm that the character of her face, which during the past year blossomed in rosy cheeks and red lips, has lately turned pale, as if bloodless; her sad heart trembles severely at any bodily movement, and the arteries of her temples pulsate with feeling; she has an attack of dyspnoea when dancing or climbing stairs; her stomach turns away from food, above all from meat; her legs – especially near the ankles – swell with oedema at night. From these occurrences, and from the visible signs of the disease which betray its cause and its resources, and indicate its treatment, I am quite astounded that your family doctors did not recognise the cause and nature of the disease.

Indeed, they have not said its name, but as it contributes nothing to the treatment of the disease, this is of no importance. There are many illnesses in the catalogue of diseases, which although without a name are not without a treatment. This disease does not have its own name, but as it is peculiar to virgins it may be designated 'the disease of virgins'; which is what the women of Brabant usually call 'white fever', on account of the pale face, as well as 'love fever', since every lover is pale, and this colour is appropriate for a lover. However, a fever very seldom accompanies it.

But this disease often attacks virgins when, already ripe for a man, they have left behind their youth. For at this time, led by nature, the menstrual blood flows down from the liver to the pockets of the womb, and the veins.[6] This blood cannot break through because of the narrow mouths of the veins, which are not yet open and which are additionally obstructed by viscous and unconcocted humours and, finally, because of the thickness of the blood itself. Then it flows backwards through the branches of the vena cava and the greater artery, towards the heart, liver, diaphragm and the veins of the praecordia. A large amount is taken to the head, and causes severe symptoms around the viscera: dyspnoea, a trembling palpitation of the heart, swelling of the liver, aversion of the stomach towards food, cardialgia, and not uncommonly epilepsy with madness and delirium. Hippocrates vouches for this in his book *On the diseases of virgins*, in these words: Virgins, he says, for whom the time of marriage comes, and who are ripe for a man, are afflicted with fancied terrors of spectres, especially when the menstrual blood descends; for before this they are not much affected at all. Certainly afterwards the blood drops down and descends into the small spaces of the womb, as if it were going to flow out. But the mouths of exit[7] are blocked, while there remains very much blood collected there, its quantity increased due to food and the growth of the body. The blood does not flow out opening up the way out of the veins; because of its abundance it makes for the heart, the diaphragm and the belly. And when they are filled to overflowing, the heart does not remain stable, and it becomes numb, the numbness making the patient foolish and delirious. It is not at all surprising, as the liver is not purged of thick menstrual blood and the veins of the belly are crammed full of it, that the tissues of the hypochondria swell, and this compresses the diaphragm, as in dropsy, and causes difficulty in breathing. Galen bears witness to this at the end of his third book *On dyspnoea* where, as a general rule, he says: If an internal swelling or pain should exist around the hypochondria, then the breathing is shallow and frequent.[8] Next, then, the heart, stomach and liver – each of which is linked to each other, by the branches of the *vena chylis*[9] and the arteries, as if in a common bond – are of course crammed and blocked with coarse blood, with windy breath and vapour, so that the heart strives to drive these out and unstop them, and not to be stifled by the frequent motion of the arteries and the systole, and it trembles all over with palpitation. When it is exhausted by this, what prevents *asphixias, kai pneumatôn apolêpseis, kai apnoias*, an interruption of pulse, breath and respiration, from happening?[10] By which the patient is struck dumb, and lies there lamented. Whence, by Hercules, Galen cleverly says in *On diet in acute diseases*:[11] *dunatai de kai plêthos kai pachos haimatos, ou monon tas artêrias pneumatôsai pote kai diexodon ouk echein, alla kai autas idiôs onomazomenas phlebas*, that is, it is possible for blood, if both plentiful and thick, not only to inflate the arteries and block the way out, but also to block the veins in the strict sense of the term.

Finally, as to whether your daughter who is sick with this disease ought to marry, and what the treatment for it should be, see, I shall impart reliable advice from the rich store of the medicine of Hippocrates, who says in his little book on the diseases of virgins: the patient is cured of this disease by bloodletting, if there are no contraindications. But I myself – he says – order virgins suffering from this disease to live with men as soon as possible, and have intercourse. If they conceive, they recover. In fact, if they are not attacked by this disease during puberty, then it seizes them a little later, unless they have married a man. And of the married, it is certainly the barren who suffer this more. If to this most health-giving advice of the divine Hippocrates, you add medicines for provoking the menses and for opening up obstructions, to refine the coarse blood, then you will be able to discover and contrive nothing more effective than these. In using these for this disease of virgins, I have never been mistaken in treatment, or been disappointed in my hopes. So therefore, take courage, betroth your daughter: I myself will gladly be present at the wedding. Farewell.

Lange's claims for Hippocratic medicine are powerful ones. All doctors consulted so far have failed, leaving Anna's father confused. This is astonishing, Lange claims, because the diagnosis is obvious. It is a disorder already known in popular medicine, where the women of Brabant have more than one name for it. In learned medicine, it can be found in the Hippocratic *On the disease of virgins*, and supported from Galenic anatomy. The treatment given by Hippocrates never fails.

In the remainder of this chapter I will be investigating the sources for this text, and asking how Lange used Hippocratic and Galenic medicine. This will involve placing the Hippocratic text in its original context of production, before looking at how this letter can be situated within medical representations of virginity more generally.

Hippocratic virginity

In Lange's letter, the section commencing, 'Hippocrates vouches for this in his book *On the disease of virgins*, in these words' is a direct Latin translation, based on Calvi, of the Hippocratic text *Peri Partheniôn, On the disease(s) of virgins*. Interestingly, Calvi gave two different translations of *On the disease of virgins*, one headed 'Hippocrates' book on the nature of virgins',[12] the other 'Hippocrates' book on the diseases of virgins'.[13] In general, Lange's wording is closer to the first of these translations.

On the disease of virgins was written in the fifth or fourth century BC; Bonnet-Cadilhac (1993) argued for a late fourth-century date, on the grounds of supposed Aristotelian influence, but Flemming and Hanson (1998) could see no such influence and suggested a date in the late fifth or early fourth century. The text's location of the seat of intelligence at the heart and *phrenes* would also support an early date (Langholf 1990: 41, 45 n. 40). It is such a short text that many commentators have concluded that it is a fragment of a longer, lost, work on types of seizure (Flemming and Hanson 1998), or one on diseases in general (Jouanna 1992: 548). It was considered to be a fragment even in the sixteenth century; de la Corde (in Bauhin 1586–88, vol. 3: 67–8) and Mercuriale (in Bauhin 1586–88, vol. 2: 155; Mercuriale 1591: 186–7) described it as such, while in the eighteenth century Gruner (1772: 170) saw it as an extract from the main Hippocratic gynaecological compendia, *Diseases of women* Books 1 and 2.[14] On two occasions, the writers of *Diseases of women* may refer to a separate work on virgins' diseases; a discussion of alternative routes taken by suppressed menstruation notes that such blood may come out as vomit, or in the stools, 'as I have said concerning the diseases of virgins' (*DW* 1.2; L 8.22); while a further reference states that the mature woman patient 'will suffer all that has been said about the *parthenos* whose first menstrual period moves upwards' (*DW* 1.41; L 8.98). However, although this second reference could describe the extant *On the disease of virgins*, this little treatise does not mention blood appearing as vomit or in stools (Bonnet-Cadilhac 1993: 149 n. 11). Another possibility, therefore, is that our treatise is only part of a longer, lost, work on virgins' diseases.

On the disease of virgins describes the medical risks faced by young girls at menarche if they do not marry, despite being 'ripe for marriage' (Greek *hôrê gamou*). The treatise was neglected by classical scholarship and, until the rise of feminism in the Classics from the 1970s onwards, by Hippocratic studies,[15] although in the early modern period it enjoyed great popularity and influence. The number of editions published from the sixteenth century onwards (L 8.465; Celli 1984) gives only a hint of this; more significant are the large number of references to it, some direct quotations, others not acknowledging their source, in medical writing of the sixteenth and seventeenth centuries.

What does it say which was of such interest? The anonymous writer of *On the disease of virgins* begins by discussing 'the sacred disease', a condition usually identified with epilepsy which, he asserts, affects women more than men because the former are less courageous, and weaker. This 'natural' physical and mental difference between the sexes was a commonplace in both ancient and Renaissance medicine;[16] it would be self-evident to the reader, who would then be predisposed to agree with whatever the text claimed followed on from this difference. The ancient writer then describes a particular disorder affecting girls who, despite being 'ripe for marriage', remain unmarried. In the body of a girl of this age there is a greater quantity of blood than usual 'because of food and the growth of the body'. This blood, moving towards the womb ready to leave the body, is unable to escape because the 'mouth of exit' is not open. Instead of moving down, it is forced to move up the body, but it tends to become stuck around the area of the heart and diaphragm, where the channels along which it passes are 'at an angle'. Unable to move further, it exerts pressure on the heart, believed by some ancient writers to be the seat of consciousness. This causes mental disturbance, including a sensation of 'being strangled', seeing ghosts and 'desiring death as a lover'; in particular, trying to drown or hang oneself.[17] Some girls with this disorder are persuaded by diviners to make costly dedications to the goddess Artemis (traditionally associated with the process of maturation, and with women's diseases), but this is condemned by the writer as deception. With the exception of the treatise *On the sacred disease*, nowhere else in the Hippocratic corpus are the therapeutic recommendations of those to whom the Hippocratic medical practitioners oppose themselves so clearly outlined; here, rather than simply condemning all other brands of healer, the writer tells us their methods. He contrasts with these his own recommendation of marriage as a cure, because this will remove any obstacle preventing the blood from flowing out, and 'if they become pregnant, they will be cured'. However, the last lines of the text warn, even married women may suffer in this way if they do not have children.

The treatise could then be summarised as a description of the physical consequences for young girls of remaining unmarried, and an encouragement of marriage as close as possible to menarche. In this sense, it can be seen as an 'instrument of socialization' (Pinault 1992: 129), or as a form of 'medical terrorism' (Manuli 1980: 404). The symptoms occur at 'the descent of the menses, although previously they suffered no ill effect'. The Greek wording seems to imply the very first menstrual period (King 1998: 78); the first Renaissance commentator on the text, Maurice de la Corde, certainly understood the text in this way when he wrote, 'This fever is peculiar to virgins, who develop fever with numbness from the obstruction of the first issuing of the menses, just after the time of puberty' (Corde 1574: 54v). Lange's Anna seems to be at a slightly later age; over the past year she has 'blossomed in rosy cheeks and red lips', and there is no suggestion that she has not menstruated at all before her illness; for her, virginity, rather than menarche, is at the root of the problem.

Whatever the role of the Hippocratic treatise on *parthenoi* in the creation of the disease of virgins, however, a Greek *parthenos* is not precisely a 'virgin'. The presence of the hymen is not essential to the definition (Sissa 1990a), and Nicole Loraux (1993: 162) argued that *parthenos* is 'not so much the word for virgin as it is for a woman who is not yet married; it is less a physical state than a social status'. Loudon's comment that chlorosis 'was essentially a disease of young women and typically it was a disorder of virgins, or the unmarried, or occasionally the married but childless' (1980: 1670) replicates precisely the scope of the classical Greek term *parthenos*. Hippocratic gynaecology aimed to transform incomplete, immature girls into complete, reproductive women; in Greek terms, to make a *parthenos* into a *gynê*, a mature woman, a term covering both 'woman' and 'wife'. To be a *gynê* in the fullest sense it was also necessary to have given birth: the first menstrual period demonstrates the readiness of the body, in terms both of the availability of blood from which a foetus can be formed,[18] and the possibility of male semen gaining entry to the womb, while the lochial flow after birth completes the process, also 'breaking down' the woman's flesh so that excess blood can rest in the open spaces created (*NC* 30; L 7.538; *DW* 1.1; L 8.10–14). The classical Greeks tried to compress this process into the shortest possible amount of time, expecting menarche at age 13 and recommending marriage for girls at 14 (King 1985: 180–6; Hanson 1992: 49).

The transmission of *On the disease of virgins*

Western medicine was unfamiliar with *On the disease of virgins* before the early sixteenth century. Sections of *Diseases of women* – the first chapter and chapters 7–38 from Book 1, and extracts from Book 2 – had survived in the Western gynaecological tradition during the medieval period.[19] They were among the Hippocratic works translated from Greek into Latin in Ravenna between the fifth and seventh centuries AD, with the intention of creating short manuals of direct practical and instructional value; the early ninth-century manuscript Paris BN 11219, which includes *Diseases of women* 1.1 and 7–38, is one of several compilations including Hippocratic material which can be traced back to Ravenna. Another manuscript compilation – Leningrad Lat.F.v.VI.3, made in the eighth or ninth century AD – adds parts of three more chapters of *Diseases of women*, 1.10–12, with material from the second book; its practical intention can be seen from the way in which substitutions are made in the pharmacopoeia according to what was available in this period.[20] However, the short work *On the disease of virgins* did not survive in the West. As for the chapters which can be understood as referring the reader to a further book on virgins' diseases, even if *Diseases of women* 1.41 had been known, its mention of a *parthenos* whose menstrual period moved upwards could have been taken as a reference to another Hippocratic menstrual crisis, in *Epidemics* 7.123 (Loeb VII, 414): 'In the daughter of Leonidas her "natural things",[21] having made a start, turned aside; after it had turned aside, she bled at the nose. When she had bled at the nose, a change occurred. The doctor did not understand, and the young girl died' (King 1998: 54–74).

This contrasts with the fortunes of Hippocratic gynaecology in the Arabic tradition; in general, the 'Arabic Hippocrates' is fuller than the 'Latin Hippocrates', as the treatises translated included those of a more theoretical or speculative nature (Lippi and Arieti 1985: 401). While *Diseases of women* does not appear to have been translated as a complete treatise in the Arab world, two commentaries on its first eleven chapters, attributed respectively to Galen and to Asklepios, were known; the commentary attributed to Galen was spurious, no such work being mentioned in Galen's list of his own works, although he did mention that he intended eventually to write one.[22] Some of the ideas found in *Diseases of women* also survived in encyclopaedic works such as at-Tabart's *Paradise of wisdom*, completed in 850 AD (Meyerhof 1931: 13–15). In contrast, *On the disease of virgins* was translated from Greek in eighth- or ninth-century Baghdad, and was mentioned in about 900 AD by Rhazes (*Al-Hāwī* 9.67, 69), and in the thirteenth century by Ibn Abī Uṣaibi'a (1.32) (Ullmann 1970: 32). I have argued elsewhere that the availability of *On the disease of virgins* in the Arab world would account for the interest in diseases arising from the 'thick menstrual blood' of virgins in the writers Ibn al-Jazzār and al-Majūsī (King 1998: 239).

When Calvi's Latin Hippocrates was printed in 1525, it therefore brought the treatise *On the disease of virgins* before an entirely new audience in the West; Lange was only one of many writers inspired by it. Furthermore, the translation into Latin of the whole of *Diseases of women*, Books 1 and 2, with a further volume *On sterile women*, meant that Hippocratic gynaecology was now available in full. In the preface to his 1525 edition, Calvi declared Hippocrates 'of all physicians, without dispute, the prince', and it was this assessment of Hippocrates which dominated the period after the complete corpus became available. A further indication that, in the absence of any exclusively gynaecological texts by Galen, the particular Hippocratic contribution to this area was recognised, came with the publication in 1526 of Calvi's translations of the Hippocratic gynaecological texts in the cheaper sextodecimo format (see p. 11). The first commentary on Book 1 of *Diseases of women* did not follow until 1585, when Maurice de la Corde's *Hippocratis Coi, Medicorum Principis, liber prior de morbis mulierum* was published. De la Corde's commentary on *On the disease of virgins* had, however, been published a decade earlier, in 1574. Three further commentaries on this short text were produced, those of Giovanni Battista Donati (1582), Joannes Stephanus (1635), and Claude Tardy (1648).

Although Lange praised 'the rich store of the medicine of Hippocrates', and Liébault could describe the charity of the 'divine Hippocrates' in caring for women's health, such devotion to Hippocratic gynaecology should not blind us to what was going on behind the façade of enthusiasm. Most commonly, sixteenth-century readers understood the newly available Hippocratic texts in Galenic terms; the Galenic model of the body, dominant since the twelfth century, continued to guide the ways in which Hippocratic gynaecology could be interpreted. For example, Liébault stated that 'In the book on the sufferings of virgins, Hippocrates recognises no other origin for the virginal diseases than the difficult flow of menstrual blood, and the retention of the spermatic humour' (1597: 8). Since there is no mention of female sperm in the Hippocratic text, it is clear here that he is merging ideas from the theories of the Hippocratic writers (menstrual blood causes disease in women) and Galen (both blood and female seed cause disease in women). Liébault's suggested cure for menstrual retention was threefold: 'to release the menstrual flow, to moderate the ardour and to titillate the spermatic humour'.

In the seventeenth century, François Ranchin criticised the Hippocratic *On the disease of virgins* for not giving a complete list of the disorders to which virgins were most exposed. He gave a new classification, consisting of four classes of disorder (1627: 370–2). The first comprised diseases which were not exclusive to virgins, but which were more likely to afflict them than other women: this class included closure of the womb. In the second class, he placed conditions affecting younger virgins, before menarche: in this class he put chlorosis, glossed as 'white fever, or love fever' (1627: 371). His third class contained diseases affecting virgins after menarche but before defloration: here he included corruption of the seed, hysterical suffocation and uterine fury. His fourth and final class consisted of disorders associated with defloration, such as soreness of the vulva, and haemorrhage. However, although Ranchin's *Tractatus de morbis virginum* suggests that there are many 'diseases of virgins', the influence of Lange's letter meant that only one condition, chlorosis/green sickness, continued to bear the name.

What is a virgin?

Ranchin's treatise on the diseases of virgins opens with sections defining virginity (1627: 352–5); in the sixteenth century, too, published texts on women's diseases often started with definitions and questions related to virginity. For example, the *Harmonia Gynaeciorum* (Wolf 1566b; Fravega 1962) contains answers to questions concerning how long a girl should remain a virgin, how loss of virginity could be disguised, and what tests could demonstrate virginity.

Lange's choice of the title 'the disease of virgins' assumes that we know what a virgin is: he stated that, 'as it is peculiar to virgins it may be designated "the disease of virgins"'. But, as we have seen, the Greek *parthenos* is not identical to our current usage of 'virgin'. For Lange, then, what is a virgin? An unmarried woman? A woman with a hymen? A third gender, neither male nor female (Salih 1999: 100)? Or, regardless of the presence or absence of her hymen, a woman who has not had sexual intercourse with a man? Lange operated within the dual perspective of the authority of the classical world, and a millennium and a half of Christianity.

Several different models of virginity, *partheneia*, existed in classical cultures. In ancient Greek mythology, the virgin Hestia, goddess of the hearth, represented a fixed point of security devoted exclusively to the service of her father Zeus; she became the Roman Vesta, served by the Vestal Virgins (Beard 1980; 1995). Hestia/Vesta was a conservative figure, staying in her father's household, refusing to move to become a wife (Vernant 1983). Two other goddesses of the Olympic pantheon were also virgins, but their activity was focused on different aspects of virginity. For Athena, who was not only a virgin but was also born from her father, Zeus, after he swallowed her mother, Metis, virginity became a statement of autonomy but also of rejection of the procreative aspects of womanhood. Artemis, despite having been granted eternal *partheneia* by her father Zeus (Callimachos, *Hymn to Artemis* 5 ff.), acted to assist human girls across the boundary between childhood and adulthood (van Straten 1981: 90 n. 126; King 1998: 82); she insisted that they go where she did not. The virginity of Artemis is a fierce and wild virginity, but – for the girls and women who honour her – explicitly not a role model. On the model proposed by Halpern (1986: 93), the virginity of Hestia/Vesta can be seen as 'a passive virginity that suits a system of patriarchal control': that of Artemis, like that of the Amazons, may appear to represent an 'active virginity' which is a 'repudiation of the husband's ownership', but which is also used in the service of patriarchy to ensure that other women are still 'tamed' and 'yoked' by marriage.

What effect did the rise of Christianity have on these images of virginity? The uniqueness of the Virgin Mary has led to her deliberate exclusion from some recent studies of virginity (e.g. Cooper 1996: x; Kelly 2000: 2). In contrast to the work of Giulia Sissa (1990b: 361), which sees Christianity as introducing ideas about virginity as complete physical closure absent from pagan texts, Kate Cooper's examination of virginity in late antiquity shows how, in this period, the theological debates did not take place in a cultural vacuum, but still worked within the parameters set by traditional Greco-Roman views of sexuality. Replicating the Zeus/Hestia relationship, the only person an elite father in the Roman empire could fully trust may be his unmarried daughter, a person owing no political allegiance to another man, and able to nurture no political ambitions for herself (Cooper 1996: 76).

Cooper identifies Ambrose of Milan (consecrated Bishop in 374) as the man who 'catapulted the virginal ideal to prominence in the Latin church' by asserting the right of the Church to prevent families forcing consecrated virgins into marriage (1996: 78). Now virginity became a long-term option, rather than a valued but short-term role before the inevitable marriage. But, Cooper argues, the impetus towards such virginity did not only come from the early Church. The presence within a pious family of a consecrated virgin raised its social status (Cooper 1996: 74), parallel to the way in which Roman society had earlier used a man's conduct in marriage as an indicator of his fitness for public office (Cooper 1996: 3). Where selfhood was identified with family honour, self-mastery was equivalent to control of one's household, and showed one could be trusted to govern a larger body. Female virgins could thus be used in the service of male ambition; every upwardly mobile home should have one.

But, in Christian rhetoric, virginity could have another meaning, coming to represent resistance to the Roman ideal. While self-control was a social value, associated with equality and with serving the community, self-denial was antisocial, suggesting setting oneself up as superior to others. Cooper suggests that asceticism was 'a wild card in the game of social ranking' (1996: 85); but it became an acceptable way for a woman to publicise herself, and was open to upwardly mobile families, outside the senatorial aristocracy. Even married women could join in; if her husband was worthless in traditional terms, totally lacking self-control, a woman's asceticism could still raise the reputation of her family in the continence stakes.

Could there be 'virgins whose bodies were not virgin' (Sissa 1990b: 349)? In late antiquity, when the Church claimed for itself the right to define virginity, Basil of Ancyra argued that true virginity was the virginity of the soul, underlined by John Chrysostom in *On virginity* (c.380–90 AD): 'It is not enough to be unmarried to be a virgin. There must be spiritual chastity.'[23] Virginity developed different levels, with the virginity of the body not necessarily corresponding to the virginity of the soul; at her trial in 1431, Joan of Arc insisted on her 'virginity both of body and soul' (Edwards 1999: 140). However, for ordinary people, in the middle ages and Renaissance, it remained the physical sense of virginity which gripped their imaginations (Loughlin 1997: 28; Kelly 2000: 37–8).

The virginity of the body has long been considered particularly complex. Proverbially, virginity 'is a hard animal to keep watch over' (Joubert, in Rocher 1989: 209). Is the presence of a hymen the best evidence, 'the physiological mark *par excellence* of virginity' (Kelly 2000: 9)? Or, as a fourteenth-century commentator on Albertus Magnus' *De secretis mulierum* put it, was the hymen 'the guardian of virginity' (Lemay 1992: 127; Kelly 2000: 27) rather than being itself the locus of virginity? A recipe in an Arab text, possibly from the ninth century, and attributed to Galen, gives a way of softening the hymen so that it will rupture by itself, 'so that the girls become non-virgins without the contact of a man' (Levey and Souryal 1968: 213). Does the hymen even exist? In medicine up to the Renaissance, the membrane was not always recognised as a distinct structure (Joubert, in Rocher 1989: 214) and, even where it was, its meaning was open to challenge: it could be seen as a rare and pathological structure (Loughlin 1997: 29–31).[24] As Sarah Salih (1999: 107) has shown, St Augustine's vision of sex in Eden featured the entry of male seed into the female body 'without loss of maidenhead', as such entry was possible by the same passage through which menstrual blood came out (*City of God* 16.26). However, if there is such a passage, then the hymen cannot be a sealed marker of virginity. Although belief in it increased from the sixteenth century onwards, so that John Maubray (1724: 39) said that it was 'found in Most, if not All, Virgins', Jane Sharp (1671: 265; Hobby 1999: 201) could still state that 'some do absolutely deny, that there is any such Membrane, or skin'.[25] Marie Loughlin has memorably characterised the doubts of early modern writers as 'This desperate and conflicted search for the hymen as the seal of virginity' (1997: 39).

Most famously, in the early second century AD, Soranos had explicitly denied its existence, on the grounds that no such membrane could be found in dissection; the vaginal probe can be inserted into virgins effectively; and menarche does not produce the same pain as defloration. He accepted that there would be bleeding at first intercourse, but attributed this instead to 'furrows' in the vagina (*Gyn.* 1.5, Temkin 1956: 15; Sissa 1990b: 356). As a sign of virginity, seeing the blood has often been regarded as more important than finding the hymen (Kelly 2000: 28), but it too was open to doubt. Jane Sharp says, within the space of a page, both that 'bleeding is an undoubted token of Virginity' and that 'the sign of bleeding perhaps is not so generally sure' (Sharp 1671: 266–7; Hobby 1999: 201).[26]

Medical writing included not only tests for virginity, often focusing on the content of the patient's urine or her style of urination,[27] but also ways of faking it, by tightening the vagina 'to make a Woman to be as narrow as a Maiden' (Wirsung 1605: 290) or producing blood by other means (Kelly 2000: 32–3).[28] With the hymen being so untrustworthy, the evidence of other parts of the body could be taken into account, as 'secondary signs' of virginity (Loughlin 1997: 39–40); Joubert (Rocher 1989: 220) referred to the neck of the womb as a 'second maidenhead', suggesting that a woman could still be called a virgin if this had not been opened. In ancient Greek thought, because of a homology between the top and the bottom of the body, loss of virginity was thought to deepen a girl's voice (Hanson and Armstrong 1986; Sissa 1990b: 360).[29] The Church Fathers, however, had moved the focus off any aspects of the body, and on to the girl's modest behaviour (Shaw 1998: 166; Salih 1999: 108; Kelly 2000: 18); but, since this was also known partly through bodily demeanour, it was no more reliable than the hymen (Kelly 2000: 30).

While the author of the Hippocratic *On the disease of virgins* was concerned that virginity in those 'ripe for marriage' would lead to serious illness, some medical writers of the Roman empire supported virginity as a healthy option. In his discussion of 'Whether permanent virginity is healthful', Soranos (*Gyn.* 1.9; Temkin 1956: 27–30) noted the debate on this subject. Some medical writers argued that virginity meant no knowledge of desire,[30] and that it is desire which makes 'the bodies of lovers pale, weak, and thin'. Virginity also avoids the debilitating loss of seed, and the exhausting experiences of pregnancy and giving birth. According to other writers, Soranos continued, virgins do not have immunity to desire; merely the lack of opportunity to express it. As for excretion of seed, 'in another respect, namely for the unhindered discharge of the menses, occasional emission at the proper time' may actually be beneficial, relaxing the womb and thus making menstruation easier and less painful. Pregnancy and childbirth may be dangerous, but the reduced efficiency of menstruation in a virgin may be responsible for equally serious health risks.

As for his own views on these matters, Soranos argued that permanent virginity is in fact healthy; women under vows of virginity suffer from less disease than other women, and any menstrual problems they have arise not from their virginity but from lack of exercise. Galen, too, suggested that virginity did not lead to ill health (*Loc. Aff.* 6.5, K 8.425). Christian writers recommending virginity did not cite these medical authorities directly, perhaps – as Jody Rubin Pinault (1992: 132) has argued – because, while medicine suggested that virginity made the present life easier, Christianity argued for the value of preserving one's virginity in terms of the life to come. In medical writing, however, Soranos' message was kept alive through Latin versions associated with the names of Caelius Aurelianus and Muscio; Muscio's version (*Genecia* 1.30, 13.11–13 Rose), probably dating from the sixth century, was read in the Middle Ages and was included in the sixteenth-century compilation, the *Gynaeciorum*.[31] Not all versions of Muscio included the praise of lifelong virginity; in an abbreviated version of Muscio's *Genecia* dating from the late thirteenth century, the recommendation of perpetual virginity as a healthy state was cut from the text (Hanson and Green 1994: 1056). However, even Soranos said that, in the normal course of events, girls should be kept as virgins only until menstruation has begun, which is 'around the fourteenth year' (*Gyn.* 1.10; Temkin 1956: 31). Whatever the benefits of permanent virginity for the individual woman, the 'relentlessly reproductive message' of Soranos still insisted that, for the benefit of the human race, most women must abandon their virginity and produce healthy children (Flemming 2000: 237; cf. Pinault 1992: 131).

Anna is old enough that her virginity has ceased to be 'healthy'; she is 'of marriageable age'. Lange's analysis of what is afflicting her does not use the hymen as the focus of her virginity. Despite echoing his Hippocratic source by acknowledging Anna's ripeness for marriage, in his letter he did not mention the hymen at all; indeed, he actively erased it. Where the Hippocratic *On the disease of virgins* states that blood is unable to escape because 'the mouth of exit' (Greek *to stoma tês exodou*) is not open, Lange shifted to the plural, and 'the mouths of exit being blocked'.[32] The Hippocratic reference to the mouth of the vagina – even if not to the hymen – is thus replaced by a more Galenic reference to the 'mouths' by which the menstrual blood enters the womb from the rest of the body. Looking back to Lange's sources, both translations of *On the disease of virgins* in Calvi used the singular here, as did the translation published in 1546 by Cornarius,[33] so this appears to be an occasion on which Lange saw what a Galenic model of the body led him to expect. Lange's Galenic idea that the blood is unable to move into the womb, rather than being unable to move out through the vagina, was retained in other discussions of green sickness; for example, Jane Sharp (1671: 257; Hobby 1999: 195), who cited Lange (1671: 264; Hobby 1999: 200), focused on the very narrow 'veins about the womb' and described how 'the blood must needs return to the great vessels whence it came and choak them up, and so spoil the making of blood'.[34]

Another difference between the Greek treatise and Lange's letter concerns treatment; in the original Hippocratic treatise, the only therapy given is marriage, yet Lange claims that Hippocrates recommends bloodletting *and* marriage, and then himself adds a third way, 'medicines'. The use of bloodletting, and the reasons for its inclusion in the letter, will be discussed in the next chapter. Nor do all of Anna's symptoms appear in Lange's cited Hippocratic source; in particular, there is no mention of paleness or digestive disturbance in the Hippocratic *On the disease of virgins*. However, in Christian writing, paleness can appear as a further sign of virginity; John Chrysostom lists 'a pale face, wasted limbs, a shabby garment, and gentle glance' (*On virginity* 6.1; Shore 1983: 8) as the outer signs of apparent virginity, which the observer must see beyond if he is to appreciate 'true' virginity, which 'resides not in clothing nor in one's complexion but in the body and soul' (*On virginity* 7.1; Shore 1983: 9). As we saw in chapter 1, the association of paleness both with menstrual suppression and with love sickness further complicates the picture.

According to Lange, Anna's symptoms are due to menstrual blood being unable to enter the womb and instead travelling back to the heart, liver and head. While this internal turmoil is occurring, her external appearance correspondingly alters; she is 'pale, as if bloodless'. This could be suggested to Lange by the reference in his Hippocratic source to menstrual blood moving towards the womb prior to leaving the body; he could be imagining this blood moving inwards from all over the body, away from the surface of the skin. That this interpretation was possible in the mid-sixteenth century is supported by Ambroise Paré (1575: 790), who described the normal skin colour of all menstruating women as being pale, because their natural heat has moved from the exterior to the interior in order to help expel the blood. A similar explanation, but this time specifically directed at the paleness of the disease of virgins, was given by Luis Mercado (1579: 202), who suggested that obstruction of the veins makes heat build up in the affected organs, and leads to a corresponding cooling of the skin. Galen (*On the causes of symptoms* 3.12; K 7.267) believed that the colour of the skin was due to the presence of humours which flooded the skin or sank to the depths of the body, and that such movements were due to emotional upset, heat, cold, excess or insufficiency.

There is, however, a further, textual reason outside the Galenic heritage which may explain why Lange insisted that Anna was 'pale'. The Greek text of the Hippocratic *On the disease of virgins* includes a phrase which should be translated as meaning that the patient wants to hang herself, 'as if this were better or useful' or perhaps 'appropriate behaviour'. The Greek word which I am translating as 'useful' or 'appropriate' is *chreios*, the emendation of the nineteenth-century editor of the corpus, Emile Littré (8.468). In his Latin translation of the Greek text, however, Calvi (1526: 46) followed the majority of manuscripts of this treatise, which read *chroia* here; *chroia* means the skin, and, in particular, the colour of the skin. Calvi's Latin therefore suggests 'and the patient hangs herself, as if this were something better, and her skin colour often changes and alters'.[35] The second, and inferior, Latin translation in Calvi derives from the same manuscript tradition, but makes even less sense: 'indeed she draws to herself various colours'.[36] The Latin translations of the Greek sources which Lange used, and the Galenic tradition within which he read them, combine to make a new disease; here, the manuscripts may have suggested to him that Anna's internal turmoil was reflected by her external pallor.

Other possible Hippocratic sources

Because the Hippocratic *On the disease of virgins* is not a perfect match for Anna's symptoms, some historians of green sickness and chlorosis have tried to find other Hippocratic references to fill in the gaps it leaves. Schwarz (1951: 146) gave up completely with *On the disease of virgins*, arguing that it 'does not contain the faintest hint' of chlorosis; most writers, assuming that the disease they are describing must have been known in the ancient world, have either referred in very general terms to 'Hippocrates', or have identified other treatises which mention whichever symptoms their current clinical picture demands. For example, Stengel (1896: 330–1) claimed that 'The ancient writers, beginning with Hippocrates, looked upon chlorosis as a disease in some way dependent upon disturbance of menstruation. Hippocrates attributed it to the retention of blood in the uterus.' In 1977, Hudson continued to argue for a Hippocratic connection: 'There are descriptions of what could be chlorosis dating back to Hippocrates' (1977: 448). Starobinski (1981: 460) suggested that Lange and subsequent writers simply combined two Hippocratic texts to produce the 'disease of virgins'.

Which other Hippocratic passages may be relevant? Lange did not mention green skin colour; this would support the argument that it was not originally part of the symptom picture of the disease of virgins, but instead moved across from 'green jaundice' and was then reinterpreted in terms of the youth of the sufferer. However, Anna is 'pale, as if bloodless', and elsewhere in the Hippocratic corpus it is said that loss of blood makes the skin 'green' (*Epidemics* 2.2.12; Loeb VII, 34), so it is possible to argue that the concept has a Hippocratic precedent. The other two passages used in this connection are *Coan prognoses* 333 (L 5.656), which mentions a disorder affecting 7-year-olds, involving paleness, difficulty in breathing and the consumption of earth, and *Prorrhetics* 2.31 (L 9.64; Loeb VIII, 280), which gives a brief account of a disorder affecting young people of both sexes, the symptoms of which are a 'bad' colour, headaches, piles, and the consumption of stones and earth (Uzac 1853: 8). *Prorrhetics* 2.31 seems to distinguish this condition from a variant in which the colouring is *chloros* but there is not severe jaundice and, instead of eating stones and earth, the patient has more pain in the region of the hypochondria.

The passage from *Coan prognoses* was understood by a number of seventeenth-century medical writers as a description of green sickness; for example, it was read in this way by Varandal (1619: 9; 1620: 6), who also alluded to the section of *Prorrhetics* (1619: 7; 1620: 4). In his discussion of 'discoloured virgins', de Baillou (1643: 66–7) also referred to *Coan prognoses*: ingeniously, he did not find the mention of 7-year-olds a problem because, according to the principle of 'sevens' found in the Hippocratic text *Weeks*, both 7 and 14, the age of puberty, are highly significant and dangerous ages. It would therefore be logical to apply remarks about 7-year-olds to twice-7-year-olds, since they are in some way equivalent. For Starobinski (1981: 459), the *Prorrhetics* text described chlorosis; indeed, it was identified as 'Chlorose' by its nineteenth-century editor, Littré.

The best discussion of the relationship between chlorosis and classical Greek medicine remains that of Axel Hansen, published in 1931, a time when contemporary writers were observing a dramatic decline in the number of cases of chlorosis. Only once did Hansen mention the Hippocratic *On the disease of virgins*, and then only to say that in none of the Hippocratic gynaecological treatises – specifically including this one – does chlorosis appear (1931: 179). Interestingly, he did not mention Lange's letter and its explicit link with the Hippocratic text, despite the fact that Lange's letter was by then widely accepted as the first clinical description of chlorosis. This is a particularly odd omission in that Hansen, like Lange, set his discussion in the context of the question, 'Do new diseases arise?' Hansen regarded the central feature of chlorosis as its target population of young girls of marriageable age, and it is because of the absence of any mention of this group in the Hippocratic *Coan prognoses* and *Prorrhetics* that he rejected the view that either text provides evidence of chlorosis in Hippocratic times. In addition, he dismissed *Coan prognoses* 333 as chlorosis because it affects too young an age group, and *Prorrhetics* 2.31 because the text explicitly says that 'both men and women' suffer from the disorder which it describes. For Hansen (1931: 177–8), there was no such thing as 'male chlorosis'; chlorosis was an exclusively female disorder.

Unlike many writers on the history of chlorosis, Hansen is a reliable commentator on Hippocratic medicine. He noted, for example, that there are several places in the Hippocratic corpus where diseases are arranged according to the age group or sex of the patients involved. From this he argued that, if chlorosis was indeed prevalent in the ancient world, then it was precisely the sort of disorder which Hippocratic medicine would have appreciated, being linked to a highly specific age/sex category. His argument here is, of course, somewhat circular. He also showed that each of the symptoms associated by the early twentieth century with the 'ideal type' of chlorosis – including green skin colour, swelling, rapid breathing and eating dirt – can be found in the Hippocratic texts, whether individually or in combination with others from the group. Nevertheless, he correctly stated (1931: 179) that the complete disease picture, as known to later medicine, is never found. He did not conclude from this, however, that chlorosis was in some sense an invention of the sixteenth century; instead, he would go no further than to say that it must have been very rare in the ancient world.[37]

'Some unknown monster': the challenge of 'new' diseases

Why was it so important to find classical precedents for the disease of virgins? For both Lange and Hansen, one of the most interesting questions about it was its possible novelty. In the Renaissance, such apparently new diseases as syphilis and the English Sweat challenged the authority of the classical texts on which medical education and practice were based.[38] Faced with the resistance of both Catholic and Protestant world-views to those 'breaking with authority in order to find personal solution' (Hale 1994: 557), one way of preserving the authority of Galen and Hippocrates was to decide that there are no truly new diseases, and to embark on a re-reading of the ancient texts in order to find a description which could be interpreted to fit the apparently novel condition. As Thomas Sydenham, the 'English Hippocrates', put it in the mid-seventeenth century, Hippocrates 'has clearly delivered the symptoms of every disease' and has given 'an exact description of nature' (Sydenham 1753: x, xvii). This was also the position taken by Leoniceno (1497) on syphilis, and by Lange, who believed that all diseases were known to the ancients, and thus that an entirely new disease was impossible, any which seem to be new being best understood as transformations of other diseases (Fossel 1914: 248). In another of his letters, 'On new diseases', he referred to the classical idea that there were over 300 diseases afflicting mankind;[39] surely this is enough, he asked, without any 'new' diseases? If any seem to be new, then traces of them must have appeared in the past. So, if Anna's set of symptoms form a distinct disease, it must be possible to find it somewhere in the classical medical corpus, and Lange believed he had done so in the Hippocratic *On the disease of virgins*. By heading Anna's condition 'the disease of virgins' he underlined this claim of identity.

Lange's position on new diseases is not the only possible one to take up. The question of whether new diseases can arise is not only a medical problem; it affects our understanding of the world, of its stability or otherwise. It is a question which does not go away, as apparently new conditions threaten our faith in medicine, medical texts and medical personnel. To refuse to believe in new diseases is to assume that nature is fixed, or that the world was created once and for all. In this model, change may be admitted, but only in one direction: diseases which once existed may be eradicated by the power of medicine, or simply disappear. This view leaves a steadily declining number of diseases in the world, and gives a satisfying feeling of progress and confidence. To state instead that new diseases are emerging all the time is, on the contrary, to encourage fear; the fear of gradual loss of control over our environment. In the seventeenth century, van Helmont argued that new diseases do indeed arise by the will of God, while old ones change to become more serious. For him and for his followers, this meant that new methods of healing had to be discovered, 'For the Art grows every day' (Pagel 1982: 17; Wear 2000: 376). Those who saw themselves as following in the tradition of Galen and Hippocrates were more likely to deny such novelty; for example, de Baillou, writing in 1574, explained that he was setting down his medical records so that physicians would have 'a knowledge of the progress of preceding and succeeding times and seasons, so that when a disease of this or that character befalls, they will not say that anything new has occurred, and be terrified by the advance and appearance of new diseases, as though by some unknown monster' (Baillou 1640: preface, translated in Lonie 1985: 170).

In their return to the ancient authorities, early modern writers would also encounter classical attitudes to the question of new diseases. In Greek myth, as systematised by the eighth-century BC poet Hesiod, diseases entered the world as part of the 'Promethean incident' in which the culture-hero Prometheus tried to trick the all-knowing god Zeus by stealing fire and giving it to mortal men (Vernant 1974). Before this, men lived on earth free from evils, hard work, heavy sicknesses (Greek *nousoi argaleoi*) and old age. When Pandora, sent by Zeus as revenge for the theft of fire, took the lid off her jar, she released all these evils, and now countless plagues (*myria lugra*) wander among human beings (Hesiod, *Works and Days* 90–2, 100). Diseases strike man by day and by night, acting independently (*automatoi*), without needing gods to inflict them, and in silence, because Zeus took away their voices (Hesiod, *Works and Days* 101–4). This is a terrifying picture, but one which makes diseases an inevitable part of the human condition, part of the group of features separating men from gods and recalling the past Golden Age. It is not, however, the only image in early Greek anthropology. Its corollary is the picture in the Hippocratic treatise *On ancient medicine* (L 1.570–637), in which there is nothing inevitable about disease; on the contrary, all is attributed to an incorrect diet. In the beginning, humans and beasts ate the same types of food: raw fruit, vegetables and grass. People suffered because this diet was wrong for them but, over a long period of time, the present human diet was developed and the savage and unsuitable diet of raw and unmixed foods was abandoned. Disease is thus something which can be defeated, with the aid of the medical profession.

But, regardless of whether diseases are seen as a fixed part of the human experience, or as a challenge to be overcome, could entirely new diseases ever arise? One answer in antiquity was to say that, although the world and its laws did not change, human lifestyles could. Just as improving our diet from raw foods to something better suited to humans could bring disease under control, so a change for the worse could lead to apparently 'new' diseases gaining a foothold. Pliny (*Natural history* 26.6.9–10) wrote that man brings many diseases on himself by his own agency.

According to ancient writers, one source of 'new' diseases was luxury, an aspect particularly blamed in the early Roman Empire. Plutarch, in a dialogue known as the *Quaestiones convivales* ('Table-talk'), features as one of his conversational topics the issue of whether new diseases arise. He puts into the mouth of his speaker Diogenianos the argument that, since there are no really new vices, there should be no new diseases. It is contrary to natural law that anything should arise from nothing, unless one could demonstrate that there was a new kind of air, or water, or food (Plutarch, *QC* 731d). But, we could respond to Diogenianos, there may indeed be 'new' foods, in the sense that the Roman Empire of the first century AD involved contact with new peoples and new luxury commodities from all over the world. In his discussion of Thucydides' account of the Athenian plague which struck the city of Athens in 430 BC, during the war between Athens and Sparta (*Peloponnesian War* 2.47–52), Rhodes (1988: 229) compared this 'deadly import' with the passage immediately preceding it, in which Thucydides presents Athens as powerful enough to import goods from all over the world. The argument that contact with other peoples brings novelty in disease as well as in consumer goods could also be applied to the early modern period, the age of exploration and discovery.

Plutarch's character, Diogenianos, does not agree; he argues that what appear to be new diseases are only a more extreme form of older, known conditions. Entirely new diseases are like the birth of monsters, explained by the mythographers as something which only happened in the past, at the time of the battle between the gods and the giants. It cannot happen any more (*QC* 731f–2a). This is a difficult line to take, because monstrous creatures quite clearly do continue to be born in every age; as 'prodigies', warnings from the gods, they are a concern of the Roman historian Livy, and of the sixteenth-century medical writers, most notably Ambroise Paré (1575; tr. Pallister 1982). Monsters could arise in nature because of imbalances between the four elements of the cosmos (Williams 1996: 178), as a result of 'imagination' – most commonly from the mother gazing on an image of a monster, or being frightened (Sennert 1664: 152–3) – or because of faults in the seed of their parents (Sharp 1671: 117–18; Hobby 1999: 91–2; Pallister 1982: 3–4).

Plutarch and another character in the debate, the doctor Philo, point out that what is really at issue here is the authority of medicine; to argue that there are no new diseases, Plutarch says, is to suggest that the ancient physicians must have been negligent or ignorant, because they failed to mention conditions which are found 'now' (QC 732b). Admitting the possibility of new diseases preserves the authority of medical texts, because their authors can hardly have been expected to know about what had not yet happened, and Plutarch argues for a phased entry of new diseases into the world rather than a once and for all opening of Pandora's jar (QC 732d–e). First, he says, arose the diseases which are caused by deficiency, heat or cold; later – as society developed – came those which arise from luxury and over-indulgence.

As examples of new diseases, Plutarch uses three specific types. First, he discusses the famous plague of Athens (QC 733b). In terms of its influence on later descriptions of plague, it is a highly significant model,[40] but he does not use this stock topic in the same way as other ancient writers do, discussing neither its alleged origins in Ethiopia, nor its progress. Instead, he uses it to counter Diogenianos' argument that there is only a finite number of possible combinations of bodily elements, such as the different substances consumed, and the different movements the body can make. Plutarch argues instead that the number of variables involved in the composition of the body leads to a huge number of combinations, some of which will produce new diseases (QC 733a–b). In particular, he says, idleness can lead to a residue building up in the body and allowing new diseases to breed (QC 732e). Plutarch seems to see the plague not as an import, but as the direct result of imbalance in the bodies of the Athenians.

Second, Plutarch goes on to mention diseases which have attacked only one group; although he says there are many similar examples in addition to the one he gives, his example is a highly localised new condition involving worms in the flesh, which arose near the Red Sea (QC 733b–c). Many diseases in antiquity were believed to be specific to one area, their disease names, such as *morbus campanus*, being formed from topographic adjectives. The first-century BC Roman poet Lucretius (*De rerum natura* 4.1103–8) describes the powerful influence of climate in causing locally specific diseases; the elephant disease (*elephas morbus*, identified with modern leprosy) is found only by the Nile, while in Attica there are foot disorders but in

Achaea it tends to be the eyes which are affected. It is into this category that Lucretius puts the plague of Athens; it was an Egyptian disease, which travelled through the air until it reached those who were not acclimatised to it (*De rerum natura* 4.1141). Other 'new' diseases too were seen as new only in the sense that they had never been found in that particular place before. Pliny says that Egypt is particularly fertile as the 'parent' of new diseases (*Natural history* 26.3.4): he says that leprosy originated there (*Natural history* 26.5.8). Mentagra came from Asia Minor (*Natural history* 26.3.3); carbuncle was specific to Gallia Narbonensis, but hit Italy in 164 BC (*Natural history* 26.4.5).[41]

Plutarch's third category of new diseases is more surprising. It comprises individual oddities like Ephebos of Athens who ejaculated a hairy, many-legged wild creature – reminiscent of the myth of Minos ejaculating snakes, millipedes and scorpions – and Timon's grandmother who used to hibernate for two months each year (*QC* 733c). Such individual oddities are repeated in Ambroise Paré's collection of examples of 'the monstrous'; for example, 'Monsieur Duret assures me that he ejected through his rod, after a long illness, a live animal similar to a woodlouse' (tr. Pallister 1982: 56). Individual conditions, 'one-off' new diseases, also feature elsewhere in ancient medicine; Celsus (Preface to *De medicina*, 49) states that very rarely is a disease truly 'new', but he knows of a case of a woman who died in hours after the descent of flesh from her genitals which remained 'attached' – or, 'unattached', depending on which manuscript is preferred. Grmek (1989) believed this to have been a uterine inversion provoked by a tumour and complicated by gangrene; but, whatever the correct diagnosis, it is noteworthy that Celsus, like Plutarch, classifies this as 'a new disease' on the basis of just a single case.

For Plutarch the main factor causing new diseases is, however, diet (*QC* 733e). Here he agrees with Diogenianos that 'it is the things that sustain life which also cause sickness' (*QC* 731d). Just as diet can eliminate certain diseases, so it can cause others. Honeyed wine and sow's wombs, he says, are new; changes have also been made to the order of courses on the menu, and to drinking habits. So, he concludes, 'the change in our way of life is capable of creating new diseases and making old ones vanish'. A similar view is expressed by Seneca; once mankind started to devise a thousand different sauces (*Epistle to Lucillus* 95, 15) and to mix foods from land and sea (*Epistle to Lucillus* 95, 19), the digestive system gave up in disgust. Seneca says, 'It is not surprising that diseases are beyond counting: just count the cooks!' (*Epistle to Lucillus* 95, 23). Here we have the perfect answer to *On ancient medicine* and its story of the conquest of disease through diet: just as the correct food can bring health, so the wrong food can generate new diseases. Seneca goes even further; because the food being eaten is more complicated, so the resulting diseases are more complex, varied and unaccountable (*Epistle to Lucillus* 95, 29).

Pliny's idea that new diseases could attack very specific groups is also relevant to the original target population of the disease of virgins; *mentagra*, for example, first entered Italy with an affected *eques*, a member of the business class at Rome, and then spread to the nobles (*proceres*; *Natural history* 26.3.3). However, he finds diseases which are specific to a class or age group very odd, noting that usually 'new' diseases attack whole populations indiscriminately (*Natural history* 26.3.4).[42] The disease of virgins, as a disease only affecting young girls at the onset of menstruation, can thus be regarded as acceptable, even if unusual, within the parameters set by the classical authorities. Their sixteenth-century readers who were writing about green sickness or the disease of virgins as 'new' were familiar with the idea that a 'new' disease has strong moral overtones, and can be blamed on idleness, or over-indulgence. In particular, the classical authorities encouraged them to look to diet as the cause, whether deliberately anomalous – as in Bullein's warning that green sickness could arise when women who would 'fayne be fayre' ate particular foods in order to dry up their blood (1558: 115r; 1559: 217) – or simply inappropriate to their age. Dietary aspects of the disease of virgins will be discussed in more detail in chapter 4.

Lange's claim to have found classical antecedents for the disease of virgins, and the use of this name for the disorder in preference to the terms used by 'the women of Brabant', can now clearly be seen as political moves made within wider debates in sixteenth-century medicine. The issue of whether new diseases arise is one concerning the authority of the classical sources on which learned medicine was based. Although there is no Hippocratic source which combines the most commonly named symptoms of the disease of virgins, a concern with the onset of the first menstrual period as a time of great danger is certainly found in the Hippocratic *On the disease of virgins*, and elsewhere in Hippocratic gynaecology. In a sense, then, Lange is correct to call the disease picture he creates 'Hippocratic', even though it cannot be located in any one ancient Greek text. His most significant divergence from his named Hippocratic source is his conversion of a general description into an individualised case history, the story of Anna; a similar manoeuvre was performed by Granville Stanley Hall in his 1904 study of adolescence, where he too used *On the disease of virgins*, but changed the plural subjects into the singular in order to make it into a case history: 'Hippocrates describes a girl who at the dawn of pubescence saw a vision, leaped and tried to throw herself into a well and then to hang herself, deeming death more desirable than life' (Hall 1904: 265). However, Lange also shifts the balance of his source, stressing some features and avoiding others. Further examples of this will emerge in the following chapters, which will investigate in more detail the menstrual and dietary aspects of the disease of virgins.

3

THE MENSTRUATING VIRGIN

When green sickness ceased to be a variant of green jaundice, and became focused on a single age/sex group, in addition to picking up the imagery of the colour green as appropriate to a young girl on the brink of womanhood, it glanced at Trotula's suggestion that menstrual suppression causes a colour like that of grass and, as a result, it moved alongside love sickness. In an article investigating changes in ideas about chlorosis, Chevallier (1955: 5) suggested that its history could be conveniently divided into the era when sexual and menstrual problems were most blamed, and that when digestive factors were seen as the main culprits. Although such a historical division corresponds in general terms to the interests of the sources, and will be broadly followed in the division between this and the following chapter, it neglects two important points.

First, there was no simple shift from one set of causes to the other; in the 1550s, Bullein's 'greene sycknesse' included digestive features while, although regarding blocked menstrual blood as the main cause, Lange included an aversion to food as a prominent symptom of his 'disease of virgins'. In the nineteenth century, when constipation was regarded as a particularly severe symptom and the diet of chlorotics was analysed in minute detail (see chapter 4), discussions of menarche and female puberty make it clear that sexual and menstrual problems remained crucial parts of the disease picture.

Second, at least in the humoral body, it can never be possible entirely to separate one set of factors from the other. Blood is produced from food, and the quality and quantity of food ingested influences the quality and quantity of the blood which is made. Even as models of the body other than the humoral one came into play – with the use of mechanical analogies, and a focus on vital forces or organs rather than fluids – a close connection continued to be made between menstruation and diet. For example, in his lectures for 1748/9 (WMS 6888), John Rutherford, Professor of the Practice of Medicine at Edinburgh, said that 'the menses are never obstructed but a train of bad symptoms follows as there is an immediate connection of the nerves between the Uterus and the Viscera of the lower Belly'. To cure chlorosis, he argued, it was necessary to 'attend to the digestive faculties – get good Chyle sent into the blood'; to bring on a menstrual period by the use of emmenagogues would 'occasion a shewing as it is called by the Common People' but would not benefit the patient. But, even within Rutherford's theoretical ideas, he was combining a mid-eighteenth century interest in the nervous system and the 'excitability' of the nerves, with a Galenic theory of the dietary system, shown in his use of the term 'chyle', meaning food partly digested by the stomach into a milky liquid.

The Galenic physiology of menstruation

As late as the first decade of the twentieth century, in an anti-feminist work on adolescence which was very influential in Britain and America (Dyhouse 1981: 121–3), Granville Stanley Hall (1904: 480) wrote that 'Precisely what menstruation is, is not yet very well known.' The medical texts of the classical world regarded it as an important physiological function, and attributed a range of symptoms to its suppression; from the Roman Empire, through the middle ages, and into the modern era it was the Galenic model of menstruation which was dominant.

In Galenic medicine, disorders of menstruation could arise from faults in the womb, but were often referred to other parts of the body. That 'the liver produced blood from chyle' was 'the fundamental tenet of Galenic physiology' (Wear 1995: 279); the details of the system were challenged by Harvey's discovery of the circulation of the blood, and by anatomical developments later in the seventeenth century, but the connection between the dietary and menstrual systems remained: the liver made blood from food. Lange drew on this connection in the Galenic physiology of his letter to Anna's father, refer-ring, for example, to the menstrual blood flowing down from the liver to the pockets and veins of the womb, and to the 'common bond' linking the heart, stomach and liver.

Although Lange attributed the majority of his material to Hippocrates' *On the disease of virgins*, he also makes direct references to Galen, citing the third book of *On difficult breathing*, Galen's commentary on Hippocrates' *On diet in acute diseases*, and what he calls 'Book 4 of *On the causes of symptoms*'.[1] Lange's description of the cause of menstrual retention, due to the 'narrow mouths of the veins, which are not yet open and which are additionally obstructed by viscous and unconcocted humours and, finally, because of the thickness of the blood itself', is directly Galenic, derived from *On the causes of symptoms* 3.11 (K 7.264 ff.).

In the model of digestion used by Galen in this treatise, food passes from the stomach to the liver, and from the liver to the rest of the body (3.3; K 7.221–2). For Galen, there are three faculties of the body; in ascending order of importance, these are the nutritive, the vital and the logical faculties. Each is associated with an organ; the nutritive faculty with the liver, the vital faculty with the heart, and the logical faculty with the brain. Cooking (Greek *pepsis*) is the dominant metaphor used in the Galenic body (Good 1994: 105–6) and what is eaten is transformed through various levels of cooking into different types of fluid; each of the three central organs also infuses the fluid with a different sort of 'spirit' (Greek *pneuma*). In the nutritive sphere, the stomach 'cooks' food into the semi-refined form of blood called chyle. The portal vein then carries this from the stomach to the liver, where it is further refined into blood by more 'cooking' in which the 'natural spirit' is added (Harris 1973: 326–7). The liver draws in the chyle by 'attraction' (Greek *holkê*), and most of the 'venous blood' which it makes is subsequently attracted from the liver to other parts of the body to nourish them. Some, however, travels on, by way of the vena cava, to the heart where, in a further stage of 'cooking', it takes in 'vital spirit' to become lighter and thinner, becoming what is called 'arterial blood' (Whitteridge 1971: 41–5; Harris 1973: 329). This transmits to other parts of the body the vital faculty, which gives warmth and the power of growth, and which can be measured through the pulse. At the base of the brain, vital blood is further transformed by the addition of 'animal spirit' into the material carried through the nerves, enabling sensation and movement. Before Harvey's unification of the two systems in the theory of circulation, the Galenic body contained veins, with their origin in the liver, carrying food to nourish the body, and arteries, proceeding from the heart and carrying *pneuma*, although they also contain some blood.

In addition to chyle, blood and *pneuma*, there are additional fluid components of the normal Galenic body which may appear in excessive quantities, making it necessary to intervene medically to remove them: normally, the gall bladder purges the blood of yellow bile, the spleen removes black bile, and the kidneys remove water (e.g. *On the causes of symptoms* 3.3; K 7.222; Harris 1973: 330–2). Yellow bile and black bile are by-products of the process by which the liver converts chyle into blood. In his letter on the disease of virgins, Lange imagines Anna's blood moving through the system in the wrong direction: from the womb, back to the heart, and even to the head, so that further venous blood is unable to move on to the heart from the liver. His reference to the motion of the systole reflects the belief, dominant before Harvey, that systolic motion sends 'arterial blood' into the aorta and the rest of the body. In the diastole, when the heart and the arteries dilate, the heart takes in air to cool the innate heat, but also to allow it to continue to burn (Harris 1973: 337).[2]

In general, Galen writes in *On the causes of symptoms*, there are three types of symptoms – those acting through reduction, perversion and lack of completion – and three types of cause: when the parts of the body are too weak to draw in food from the liver; when channels are narrowed by obstruction, or by a tumour caused by the humours settling in one place; and when the blood is thickened and moves slowly, perhaps due to consumption of the wrong foods.

When Galen turns to menstrual suppression in this treatise, he follows this model precisely. One possibility, then, is 'weakness of the part'; here, of the womb itself, which can be unduly compact or hard (*On the causes of symptoms* 3.11; K 7.264–6). This is particularly difficult to cure, because it can be the natural condition of the womb. Another possibility would be narrow channels; again, this can be something present from birth, and thus very difficult to treat, but it may be the result of adjacent parts of the body putting pressure on the channels. Finally, retention may arise from the 'menstrual material' itself being too thick (*crassus*) or sticky (*glutinosus*), or from the presence in it of other humours. He then adds conditions of the whole body which predispose towards menstrual suppression. Too much exercise or a light diet mean that there will be less blood to be lost in this way; too much leisure or an over-abundant diet mean that there will be more to be lost. Finally, if the other parts of the body are too strong, and attract too much blood from the liver, less will be able to reach the womb.

The Galenic model of menstrual suppression is thus a highly inclusive one, making it necessary for the doctor to consider not only the womb, but every other part of the body, in his attempts to explain the cause. It was followed in every particular by Lange's contemporaries; for example Donato Antonio Altomare (1559: 342–4), who supported his argument from his own experience of the case of 'the most illustrious lady, Maria Sanseverina, Countess of Nola'.

Lange, however, although citing Galen and setting his description within a Galenic body, claimed that the best answer to Anna's problem is the one given by 'the divine Hippocrates'. There is certainly a good deal of overlap between the Hippocratic corpus and Galen with regard to the centrality of menstruation in female physiology. The Hippocratic treatise *On generation /Nature of the child* states that menstruation is 'simply a fact of [woman's] original constitution' (*NC* 15; L 7.494; Lonie 1981: 8; Föllinger 1996: 37) and 'if the menses do not flow, the bodies of women become sick' (*Gen.* 4; L 7.476; Lonie 1981: 3); even outside the 'gynaecological' treatises, regular heavy menstrual loss is regarded as a necessity (*AWP* 21; Loeb I, 124).[3] Galen, although seeing retained female seed as a far more serious threat to health, continues to stress this Hippocratic 'correlation between female health and perfect menstruation' (Flemming 2000: 338). In its description of a thwarted menarche, the Hippocratic *On the disease of virgins* suggests that the problems lie with the increased amount of blood in the body – due to 'food and the growth of the body' – and with the blockage of the 'mouth of exit' (see chapter 2). This explanation is consistent with Galen's general picture in *On the causes of symptoms*, which included diet and blocked channels.

Alternative theories of menstruation

In the mid-sixteenth century, Galenic anatomy was simultaneously accepted and challenged by new texts – including the newly available parts of the Hippocratic corpus – and new ways of seeing the human body. Acceptance was supported by the sixteenth-century reprintings of the twelfth-century work discussed in chapter 1, the *Cum auctor* attributed to Trotula, which opens with the Galenic division of causes of menstrual suppression as being due to the womb, the channels, the consistency of the menstrual material, or the woman's individual way of life. The first chapter of *Cum auctor* states that

> Sometimes there is diarrhoea on account of excessive coldness of the womb, or because its veins are too slender, as in emaciated women, because then thick and superfluous humours do not have a free passage by which they might break free. Or [sometimes menstrual retention happens] because the humours are thick and viscous and on account of their being coagulated, their exit is blocked. Or [it is] because the women eat rich things, or because from some sort of labour they sweat too much.
>
> (Green 2001: 73; cf. Spach 1597: 42)[4]

While the Galenic body was continuing to be reinforced in print, it was also being challenged through the same medium, most famously by Andreas Vesalius, who regarded Galenic anatomy as inherently flawed because of Galen's reliance on dissecting animals, rather than human beings. However, Vivian Nutton has pointed out that this challenge to Galen itself relied on a 'deep knowledge of Galenic anatomy'; it arose *from* the Galenic tradition, simply taking it a step further to include the human bodies which it had not been culturally acceptable for Galen to dissect. Furthermore, in his great illustrated work *De humani corporis fabrica*, printed in 1543, 'Vesalius himself had accepted a great deal that was Galenic, particularly in his explanation of the phenomena he claimed to have seen' (Nutton 1988: 116–17). As Andrew Cunningham put it, in terms of his work on animals, too, 'Vesalius as vivisectionist was simply Galen restored to life' (1997: 115). But, despite the presence of an anatomised woman's body as the focus of the title page of Vesalius' *Fabrica*, the new sixteenth-century anatomy altered neither the belief in the centrality of menstruation for female health, nor the idea that most diseases of women stemmed from the retention of menstrual blood (Smith 1976: 101); even dissections of women who died while menstruating could not alter the dominant model of menstruation, since this was a physiological, not an anatomical, issue (Pomata 1992: 72).

In the seventeenth century, a Galenic model of menstruation based on the belief that women's bodies were naturally 'plethoric' – having an excess of blood which needed to be expelled if there were no foetus to use it up – was challenged by an alternative theory which focused on 'fermentation'. This theory, associated above all with the Flemish writer Johannes Baptista van Helmont (1579–1644), regarded all processes in the body as the result of chemical changes. According to van Helmont, the womb dominated the female body as the moon controls the tides of the sea. Women suffer the diseases of men, and also their own diseases; this was seen both as a fitting punishment for the sin of Eve, and as a blessing bringing them closer to the sufferings of Christ (Pagel 1982: 173–4). Thomas Willis's *Of Fermentation of the Inorganical Motion of Natural Bodies*, published in 1659, described 'fermentation in the seminals' leading to the blood becoming volatile and hot: menstruation represented blood which had fermented too much (Brumberg 1988: 53). Where there was sufficient ferment, a woman would have pink skin, but where there was not she would be pale, breathless and lethargic. In his discussion of girls who seemed to be able to survive without eating, John Reynolds (1669: 21) suggested that this phenomenon was most commonly found in girls 'between the ages of fourteen and twenty years when the seed hath so fermented the blood, that various distempers will probably ensue without due evacuations'. If seed lingered for too long in the seminal vessels, it would become acid, and another possibility was that it could somehow supply the fasting body with the nutrition it lacked. In this model, girls' failure to eat could balance out the changes in their blood.

The fermentation theory and the plethora theory coexisted in the eighteenth century but the plethora theory won, at least in British medicine (Lord 1999: 44–5). It was victorious because it implied a whole set of beliefs about women as the weaker sex; these in turn meshed with a growing emphasis both on the idealisation of female puberty, and on its intrinsic dangers, which will be discussed later in this chapter. Many explanations for women's illness hinged on the supposed weaknesses of the female sex and, particularly, of younger women. Simple carelessness could be to blame: Turner (1714: 94) shows a common belief in the insecurity of the menstrual function when he mentions a young girl who developed chlorosis as a result of 'inadvertently putting on a damp Shift, at the Approach of her Menses'. Another eighteenth-century writer, the German physician Storch, treated a maidservant who was suffering from irregular periods, a 'pale and puffed-up' face, and who was 'out of breath, tired, and her feet were swollen' (Duden 1991: 127). Storch did not label this condition – although it has the main symptoms of green sickness – but he accepted her explanation that the symptoms were due to her having accidentally swallowed a pin in the previous year. At least in Britain, however, the main interest of eighteenth-century medical writers on menstruation lay in measurement: the objective quantification of the 'facts' of menstruation.[5]

In the nineteenth century, a further possible role for menstruation was proposed, when it was argued that its purpose was to expel the unfertilised ripe eggs (e.g. Raciborski 1868: 6). An alternative view at the end of the century was that menstruation prepared the surface of the womb so that an egg could implant itself in it (e.g. Hall 1904: 482); this could find a classical precedent in Plutarch's *Dialogue on love* 24, which states that 'Another wounding is the beginning of pregnancy, for there is no impregnation (*mixis*) without hurting each other' (769e).[6] Herophilos had discovered the ovaries in the third century BC (von Staden 1989, fr. 61), but their function was not understood before the twentieth century. In the nineteenth century, analogies with animals 'on heat' reinforced the idea that ovulation occurred during the days immediately prior to menstruation (Raciborski 1868: vii, 43–7; Simmer 1977: 61); this meant that the absence of menstruation could be attributed either to a fault in the ovaries, or to the failure of the womb to respond to their 'call' (Raciborski 1868: xx–xxi). Pomata (1992: 86) has argued that this theory of ovulation led to menstrual blood itself being viewed as pathological, as opposed to the Galenic model in which it was a 'benign excrement' (Varandal 1620: 26), a healthy natural flux of blood serving the useful purpose of regulating the female body and providing the raw material to build and nourish the foetus.[7] For Raciborski (1868: 17), however, menstrual blood remained no different from other blood.

The belief that ovulation needed to occur before menstruation could take place still gave menstruation a central role in the female body, because it continued to suggest that it must occur every month unless an egg had been fertilised. However, it at least meant that a girl who had not yet menstruated, but was of an age when this would be expected, would be spared 'treatment', unless she was displaying the signs of ovulation, which Raciborski (1868: 281) listed as a feeling of heaviness in the lower abdomen, a sensation of heat in the genital area with some white discharge, and a frequent urge to urinate. In the 1870s, the idea that menstruation was dependent on ovulation was challenged (e.g. Jacobi 1877: 64 ff.), but it was not until 1901 that Josef Halban demonstrated experimentally the endocrine cause of menstruation (Simmer 1977: 78), our current understanding of the link between menstruation and ovulation only being reached in the 1930s (Strange 2001: 247).[8]

Letting blood in the Hippocratic and Galenic bodies

Menstruation thus remained at the heart of the economy of the female body, even when the Galenic model started to be challenged by other ideas about why this bleeding should happen. Similarly, treatment for menstrual suppression showed significant continuity. In the case of one treatment, letting blood, its use in chlorosis demonstrates the authority of Galen: because Galen recommended it, the treatment was projected back into earlier texts which had not even mentioned it. The power of the Galenic body for Lange can be illustrated not only by his acceptance of the overall model of digestion and the role of blood, but also by his ability to see, in the Hippocratic text he praises, features which were not originally present. In particular, Lange stated that Hippocrates 'says in his little book *On the disease of virgins*: the patient is cured of this disease by bloodletting, if there are no contraindications. But I myself – he says – order virgins suffering from this disease to live with men as soon as possible, and have intercourse. If they conceive, they recover.' Lange then added his own suggestion: drugs to encourage the menstrual flow.

In fact, only one treatment is mentioned in the Hippocratic text: marriage or, more specifically, in Lange's words, that the sufferers should 'live with men and have intercourse'.[9] Here he was separating out the two meanings of the Greek verb *synoikein*, 'to live together' and 'to have intercourse', which may suggest that he had access to the Greek text;[10] however, in the Latin translation which he used, that of Calvi (1525), the two aspects are also pulled out, so it is more likely that Lange was simply following Calvi.[11]

Lange's claim that Hippocrates recommends bloodletting for this condition is, as I have argued elsewhere (King 1996a), also the result of using Calvi's Latin translations.[12] In the sixteenth and seventeenth centuries, bloodletting, or venesection, was recommended as a cure for many conditions, due to the idea that the artificial release of retained blood would compensate for its failure to come out naturally. Here, however, the original Greek translates as, 'But there is deliverance/release [Greek *apallagê*] from this when nothing prevents the flowing out of the blood.' The text does not suggest that artificial intervention should be taken to remove blood from elsewhere in the body; instead, the Greek would suggest that the removal of the obstruction will result in the natural release of the trapped blood.

The thirteenth- or fourteenth-century Greek manuscript Paris BN 2140 inserts an extra word, *therapeia*, into the sentence, which would make the first part, 'The treatment/cure for deliverance ...', a reading which makes rather less sense, hence its rejection by the great nineteenth-century editor of the Hippocratic corpus, Emile Littré (8.468; Jouanna 1983). The extra word shifts the meaning of the sentence significantly.[13] In the translation of *On the disease of virgins* preferred by Lange, Calvi translated as 'But the deliverance from this, and the cure is – if nothing prevents it – release of the blood [*sanguinis missio*].'[14] The Latin given by Cornarius twenty years later was, 'But the cure in order that they be delivered from this, is removal of the blood [*sanguinis detractio*], if there is nothing which prevents this.'[15] Although these expressions are both ambiguous as to whether the blood loss is natural or induced, they certainly meant 'bloodletting' in the medical Latin of the Roman Empire; the first-century AD writer Celsus used them interchangeably (2.10.17; 4.6.2; 2.10.6). Lange's own phrasing, however, removes any lingering doubt: 'Deliverance from this disease is by cutting a vein [*venae sectio*], if nothing prevents it.'[16]

Once bloodletting entered the tradition, it was there to stay. In Donati's commentary on *On the disease of virgins* (1582: 40–2) it was still present in the Latin translation, and Donati added that, to restore girls with defective menstruation to their original health, he himself would recommend 'quite copious blood-letting'.[17] Stephanus' commentary (1635: 36) gave as the text 'The cure for these, by which they are released, is the drawing off of the blood, if there are no contraindications.' By the publication of de Baillou's study of the condition (1643: 67), the Lange and Hippocratic remedies were simply summarised together as, 'The cure is venesection, the best remedy sexual intercourse'; however, de Baillou also noted the Galenic contraindications to bloodletting (1643: 88–9), which will be discussed in more detail shortly. Other seventeenth-century writers put further restrictions on the use of bloodletting in the disease; the midwife Jane Sharp (1671: 265; Hobby 1999: 200) argued that only if 'the disease is new, and the blood plentiful' should one open a vein, because bleeding when 'the passages are stopt, and the whole body is chilled with raw slimy humours ... will augment the disease'. For Sharp, even marriage – generally the best way to make the menstrual blood come down – may be unwise, if bad humours predominate in the body: 'I have known some that have been so far from being cured, that they died by it' (Sharp 1671: 264; Hobby 1999: 200).[18]

In general, bloodletting plays a very small role in the Hippocratic corpus; as the seventeenth-century surgeon Abraham Bauda (1672: 10) noted, and Brain (1986: 113–14) later demonstrated, although Galen's treatises on bloodletting give the impression that the Hippocratics often recommended this therapy, it is in fact only mentioned about seventy times, most of these references being very brief. Of these, the majority concern bloodletting in male patients: there are very few Hippocratic examples of bloodletting being performed on women. Brain (1986: 114 n. 47) gave only one such example from the three volumes of the *Diseases of women*; Dean-Jones (1994: 142) found a total of three examples, to which Hanson has added one more (personal communication). One case involves letting blood from the ankle, to speed up a protracted labour (*DW* 1.77; L 8.172), while another recommends letting blood from the left arm, as part of a regimen of purging a woman suffering from watery periods in order to encourage eventual conception (*DW* 3.241; L 8.454–6). A further reference in the treatise *On superfetation* 23 (L 8.488) proposes bloodletting twice a year from both the arms and the legs, for a woman who has previously conceived but has not done so for some time. *Epidemics* 2.4.5 (L 5.126; Loeb VII, 72) gives the case of a woman whose lochial flow was suppressed and was released by letting blood from the ankle.

Dean-Jones (1994: 142) argued that bloodletting was only used in the gynaecological texts of the Hippocratic corpus as a last resort, because it was basically seen as 'a remedy for the male body'. Pomata (1992: 81) showed that some early modern texts on bloodletting regarded it as redundant in women who were menstruating normally. The section of the Hippocratic *Diseases of women* which discusses the purging of a woman with watery periods supports the suggestion of a reluctance to let blood from menstruating women; here, bloodletting is indeed a remedy of last resort, only to be performed 'if she is strong enough for it' (*DW* 3.241; L 8.456).

For early modern Europe, Gail Kern Paster (1993: 83) has argued that 'the sign of phlebotomy is menstruation's cultural inversion'. The first is artificial and controlled: the second is natural and uncontrolled (cf. Pomata 1992: 80–1). But this is not the only possible interpretation; it could also be argued that bloodletting imitates or duplicates menstruation, with the means being irrelevant, and the central fact being the identical result. In some Melanesian societies where men practise penis-bleeding, the same word is used for this as for menstruation.[19] The principle that women bleed by natural means only, while men can be given the artificial purgation of bloodletting, was never explicitly voiced by the Hippocratic writers. It is Galen, rather than Hippocrates, who is the major ancient authority for bloodletting; and it is also Galen, in *On bloodletting against Erasistratos* 5 (K 11.164–6; Brain 1986: 26–7), who suggested that this was the principle by which 'Hippocrates' himself operated.

When Galen arrived in Rome in the 160s, he believed in the value of bloodletting. But the followers of the third-century BC Alexandrian anatomist, Erasistratos, who were influential in Roman medical circles, regarded it as contrary to the teachings of Erasistratos. Galen therefore wrote *On bloodletting against Erasistratos*, to argue that in fact Erasistratos had recommended bloodletting. The followers of Erasistratos then took up bloodletting, but more extensively and with rather more enthusiasm than Galen thought appropriate, so he then wrote a second treatise, *On bloodletting against the Erasistrateans at Rome*, to spell out in more detail the situations in which bloodletting was, and was not, good practice. Erasistratos had failed to heal a girl from Chios, whose menstrual blood had gone to her lungs; in *On bloodletting against the Erasistrateans at Rome* (K 11.193–4; Garofalo 1988: fr.285) Galen discussed whether this was due to his failure to let blood in this case. In the same treatise, Galen gave the case of a woman of twenty whose menses were suppressed, causing difficulty in breathing. The doctors refused to bleed her, hoping to cure her by fasting; however, she died 'in a fit of uncontrollable dyspnoea' (K 11.187–90; Brain 1986: 38–9). This may sound like chlorosis, in which menstrual suppression and difficulty in breathing play a central part, but Galen described his patient as having a *red* face, because her diverted menstrual blood had moved up her body. Here we are a long way from Lange's 'pale, as if bloodless'.

In contrast to the other doctors called in to treat this case, Galen recommended letting blood, which he called the remedy of first choice for menstrual suppression (*On bloodletting against the Erasistrateans at Rome* 3; K 11.201; Brain 1986: 45). Like the author of the *Epidemics,* description of letting blood for suppressed lochia, the site he favoured was the ankle, in order to encourage the blood to move down the body, towards the womb.[20] The saphena vein in the ankle was used as part of the cure for menstrual suppression causing cachexia in a case recorded in 1546 by Pieter van Foreest (1595: 132); the patient's body was 'pale, indeed soft, owing to the retention of the menses, and when walking she was only able to breathe with difficulty'. It was also used by Amatus Lusitanus (1556: 39), as the intervention of choice in menstrual suppression in a virgin aged 18.

Even those manuscripts of *On the disease of virgins* which suggest bloodletting as a treatment never state the preferred site for the procedure. Yet, in another striking example of how the influence of the Galenic body prevailed over the Hippocratic texts, the advice to let blood from the ankle also came to be given for cases labelled explicitly as green sickness or chlorosis; for example, the popular health manual known as *Aristotle's Masterpiece* (Anon. 1694: 72–3; Bullough 1972–3; Porter 1985) stated that marriage is the best cure for green sickness but, if this is not an option, then blood should be let from the ankle. The anonymous author added that, in girls over 16, blood could be let from the arm as well. A century earlier, Mercado's discussion of the disease of virgins (1579: 205, and cf. 211), which is heavily and explicitly dependent on Lange, maintained that 'Hippocrates' recommends bloodletting in *On the disease of virgins*, but gave as the preferred site the vein on the inside of the elbow. Galen, however, let blood from the elbow in order to *stop* a heavy menstrual flow, on the basis that it diverted blood to the upper part of the body. Even in classical antiquity, however, there was much disagreement about the best sites for letting blood to control menstruation.[21]

Those passages in which Galen discusses the broad general principles governing bloodletting are helpful here. For example, in *On therapeutics, to Glaucon* 1.15 (K 11.43–6; Daremberg II, 729–31), he listed the different factors which should be taken into account: these include the temperature of the air, the season, individual constitution, complexion and density of the flesh, and the subject's age. He also drew more general distinctions between fair and dark women – seeing dark women as having thicker blood – and between children and adults; he would not let blood in anyone under 14 years of age.[22]

It may have been this last recommendation which led a number of early modern writers to express some caution towards letting blood in cases of chlorosis; Jane Sharp's reluctance has already been mentioned, while Astruc (1743: 60–2) wrote, 'You are never to insist too much on provoking the *Menstrua*, for Nature abhors Violence, nor should unripe Fruit[23] be pulled off too early ... The only *Anchora sacra* is matrimony.' However, despite this preference for marriage, Astruc went on to recommend bloodletting as more generally 'very useful' from either the foot or the arm, the arm being his preferred site. Chlorosis was primarily associated with girls at menarche and, in the classical tradition, menarche was in turn associated with the 'fourteenth year'; that is, the age of 13 (Amundsen and Diers 1969). The target patient for the disease of virgins, although, in the words of the Hippocratic treatise, 'ripe for marriage' rather than 'unripe fruit', would thus be at a difficult age for Galenic bloodletting theory. In addition, Galen adds further contraindications; he explicitly forbids letting blood if 'the complexion of the whole body lacks the colour that indicates an abundance of blood' (*On Treatment by Bloodletting* 9; K 11.279–80; Brain 1986: 81). Since Lange's Anna is supposed to be 'pale, as if bloodless', this too would discourage bloodletting as a remedy. This understanding that, in a strict application of the Galenic model, the age group of chlorosis sufferers and their key symptom of paleness argue strongly against the use of bloodletting, was not, however, always reached by early modern writers. Nevertheless, several early modern medical writers with impeccable Hippocratic or Galenic credentials roundly condemned as bad practice bloodletting in girls with menstrual suppression or green sickness. For example, Guillaume de Baillou (1643: 87), who saw the cause as a dietary defect, an obstruction or the presence of unconcocted humours, argued that the problem always arose from an insufficient amount of 'good' blood, so in most cases one should not bleed the patient, but rather purge the bad humours or remove any obstruction.

In one of his posthumously published case histories, Giambattista da Monte described menstrual suppression in a 15-year-old German girl of noble birth, called Helena.[24] Like Anna, she was pale, but da Monte considered that her constitution was clearly phlegmatic. In addition to menstrual suppression, she had uterine suffocation and a heart tremor. Da Monte died in 1552; if this case had been written after 1554, the date of Lange's letter, it is interesting to speculate as to whether it would have been labelled '*morbus virgineus*'. In Helena's case, da Monte regarded bloodletting as wholly inappropriate. The phlegmatic blood meant that unconcocted humours would be present in her stomach, intestines and venous system; 'both reason and Galen', wrote da Monte, argue against letting blood in such a situation. In his *Medicina Universa*, da Monte listed seventeen 'canons' which should be observed when letting blood. He cited Galen and Avicenna to support his statement that, because nature abhors a vacuum, unconcocted humours would enter the veins to replace any blood taken and would then cause a blockage (da Monte 1587: 938). If the veins were already blocked, then bleeding the patient would be not only ineffective, but positively dangerous. It would cool a body which had no need of further cooling, and would push even more of the unconcocted humours into the veins. Da Monte also condemned the use of mineral baths or drinks of mineral water; these astringents tighten and block the veins even further.

Instead, he recommended commencing treatment with a thorough purge to empty the veins because, in a girl of this age, the most likely Galenic option was simple obstruction of the passages due, in this case, to phlegm. The patient's youth made it unlikely that weakness of the expulsive faculty of the womb was to blame, while her sensible way of life made thick, or insufficient, blood unlikely. Here, bloodletting is presented only as a last resort.

The relationship between the disease of virgins and bloodletting is thus a complex one; the therapy enters the tradition through an extra word in a manuscript, but its entrance is strongly encouraged by the practice of reading Hippocratic texts in a Galenic tradition. One of the passages Lange cites in Greek comes from Galen's commentary on Hippocrates' *Regimen in acute diseases* 4.78 (CMG V.9, 1 p. 336.11–13). The Hippocratic passage which Galen was explaining here, a description of tetanus of the limbs caused by bilious humours blocking the passage of the *pneuma* through the veins, ends with the recommendation of letting blood as the cure.[25] This conclusion, not explicitly noted by Lange in his letter, but one with which he would probably be familiar due to his word-for-word citation of Galen's commentary, would further predispose him to *expect* to find bloodletting in the Hippocratic *On the disease of virgins* as well, as an appropriate remedy for humoral blockage. An alternative scenario was, however, proposed by some writers in the nineteenth century; by weakening the constitution, too much bloodletting could be the *cause* of chlorosis (e.g. Trabuc 1818: 7).

'Marriage is a sovereign cure'[26]

The previous section raised questions about how Lange used the Latin and Greek texts of his classical authorities to create the disease of virgins. Bloodletting entered his letter because it was in a Greek manuscript available to the translators, and because Galenic medicine led Lange to expect its presence. However, the Hippocratic recommendation of marriage as the only treatment for the condition – 'I urge that young girls with this condition should marry as soon as possible' – also needs to be examined in the context of the sources available to Lange.

Lange's letter suggests that Anna's father had two, related, concerns: first, what was wrong with his daughter, and second, should she marry? The solution which Lange proposes covers both of these concerns by arguing that marriage in itself often provides a cure for the symptoms. Within the humoral body, the use of marriage as a treatment is a physiological recommendation rather than some sort of acknowledgement of psychological need. It is anachronistic, for instance, for Guggenheim (1995: 1822) – a nutritionist – to suggest that, by recommending intercourse and conception as cures, 'Lange regarded the condition as psychosomatic or as a neurosis due to suppressed sexuality, which was thus relieved by marriage.' On the contrary, marriage is simply the only socially acceptable situation in which the virgin's body can be put under proper male control, opened, entered and seeded. It is also presented as the *easiest* way to cure the condition (e.g. Dupleix 1626: 103). The rationale for marriage was given different expression as theories of the mechanism of green sickness changed, but it long remained at least a part of the cure. For Sudell (1666: 10), for example, 'Carnal Copulation' was 'much of the Cure', because it enlarged the vessels of the womb. A few years earlier, John Tanner had suggested that it was all a question of degree; only in the more straightforward cases of the virgins' disease was marriage a cure: 'If the Veins of the Womb onely are obstructed, a Husband will cure her' (1659: 315).

These last two examples give some idea of precisely how marriage was supposed to cure the disease: by opening up the veins of the womb. To put it more simply, however, the cure for the disease of virgins was to cease to be a virgin. Loss of virginity was expressed in sixteenth-century male writing through what de Rocher (1989: xviii), writing on Laurent Joubert, has called 'the language of fortification: last ditch, outer wall, gate, assault, combat, battering ram, gaining ground, breaking in, planting one's banner, and so forth'.[27] Such language picks up on numerous classical models linking sex and battle, from both Greek and Latin literature (Fowler 1987). Particularly illuminating here is the early modern use of the imagery of green sickness in a political context, where it complements the common use of the imagery of virginity in geographical exploration and imperial conquest.[28] As Montrose (1993: 184–5) has shown, the naming of England's first American colony, Virginia, was an act which not only recalled its virgin conqueror, but also wiped out the previous inhabitants to make it 'a blank page ... a feminine place unknown to man'. Here, for example, is Sir Walter Ralegh in 1596 encouraging Elizabeth, the Virgin Queen, to undertake the conquest of the New World in his *Discovery of Guiana*:

> Guiana is a Countrey that hath yet her Maydenhead, never sackt, turned, nor wrought, the face of the earth hath not beene torne, nor the vertue and salt of the soyle spent by manurance, the graves have not been opened for gold, the mines not broken with sledges, nor their Images puld down out of their temples. It hath never been entred by any armie of strength and never conquered and possessed by any Christian Prince.
>
> (1848: 115, cited in Montrose 1986: 79; cf. Bicks 2003: 82–3)

The medical interest in green sickness at the end of the sixteenth century may be linked to concerns about the future of the English crown raised by fear of Catholic invasion, a fear made worse by setting 'the virginal, unbreached microcosm of the English body politic' alongside the unbreached but unproductive body of the Virgin Queen (Harris 1998: 45–6). The state needed to be kept virginal, but for that to occur it was also necessary for the succession to be assured; virginity in one quarter depended on its loss in another. At the same time as Ralegh was urging the conquest of Guiana's maidenhood, Shakespeare's Capulet was trying to arrange with all haste the marriage of his 13-year-old daughter Juliet to Paris, because he was concerned that she had green sickness: 'As he sees it, he is taking measures to save Juliet's life' (Potter 2002: 273–4). Here we see again the paradox that, while virginity, as physical integrity, may express autonomy and power, it is highly dangerous to maintain it beyond its proper season; 'the apples being rype, for want of plucking would rotte on the tree' (Greene 1583: Grosart 1881–3: II.36).

The logical result of applying the imagery of conquest is that a country left unconquered too long could develop green sickness, making invasion and settlement almost an act of mercy. An imaginative and complementary picture of Ireland as a green-sick girl is given in Luke Gernon's *A Discourse of Ireland*, a text which, from its allusions to Tyrone's submission in 1603, can be dated to around 1620:

> This Nymph of Ireland, is at all poynts like a yong wenche that hath the greene sicknes for want of occupying. She is very fayre of visage, and hath a smooth skinn of tender grasse. It is nowe since she was drawn out of the wombe of rebellion about sixteen yeares, by'r lady nineteen, and yet she wants a husband, she is not embraced, she is not hedged and ditched, there is noo quicksett putt into her.[29]

The value of marriage to 'hedge and ditch' sufferers from the disease of virgins is a consistent theme of the literature up to the decline of chlorosis at the beginning of the twentieth century; from the certainty of Astruc (1743: 61) – 'The only *Anchora sacra* is matrimony' – to the query of von Noorden (1905: 523–4) – 'The only important point is whether chlorotic girls should be allowed to marry.'

Identical questions about the value of marriage were asked about syphilitics, particularly in the period around the turn of the century.[30] Then, as for Lange when called in by Anna's father to advise on his daughter's marriage prospects, marriage was explicitly a medical issue: for example, Raciborski (1868: xvi) noted that the question, 'At what age should one marry off young girls?' was 'a subject of great importance both for families and for physicians', and used the question of whether girls were fit to marry as a reason why families should allow physicians to carry out examination of the external sexual organs and the womb itself when menarche had not occurred at the normal age (1868: 281, 340–1).[31] The French birth rate had been low from the 1840s onwards, but panic did not set in until after the French defeat by Prussia in 1870 (Nye 1999: 95); I would therefore see Raciborski's concern with marriage as focused more on fears about pubertal girls than on specific anxieties about failure to reproduce the nation. In the early twentieth century, works promoting the eugenics agenda addressed the issue of marriage for chlorotics; Rosin's essay, 'Diseases of the blood in relation to marriage', recommended that the disorder should preferably be cured before the marriage took place but, if this was not possible, then the doctor should still give his consent to the marriage and 'may under certain circumstances actually recommend it' (1907: 189). Here, we can hear an echo of Lange's 'take courage, betroth your daughter: I myself will gladly be present at the wedding'. Raciborski claimed that experience proved that marriage, or indeed childhood prostitution, could bring on menarche, due to the 'direct excitation of the sexual organs' (1868: 281, 327–8, 343).[32] A century earlier, Astruc (1743: 53) had suggested that masturbation had the same effect.[33] This raised delicate questions about what the physician could recommend; the answer was to focus on the patient's ripeness. George Drysdale (1875: 170–3) enthusiastically recommended sexual intercourse, above all in patients whose chlorosis was initially due to masturbation; for them, there was 'a natural habit to be established', and also 'an unnatural one to be eradicated' (1875: 171). In cases of chlorosis, Raciborski considered marriage very useful in patients in the 20–25 age group but, in younger girls, it should be approached with caution, as it could even aggravate the condition (1868: 322–3); excitation of the sexual organs was all very well, but it was possible to have too much excitement.

The recommendation of marriage, even with some caveats attached, largely persisted across all theories of the cause of chlorosis, with the exception of some writers who believed that it was a liver condition; their position will be discussed in chapter 4. For example, Gabriel Andral, whose 'neo-humoralism' gave a central role to the chemical structure of blood (Verso 1971: 56), believed that chlorosis was caused by the nervous system preventing adequate formation of blood, and claimed that

> it frequently happens that by stimulating the nervous system of these chlorotic patients by the physical and moral emotions of matrimony, we produce a more natural complexion and colour of the whole cutaneous surface, thus indicating a corresponding improvement in the process of sanguinification.
>
> (Andral 1829: 106–7)

Although von Noorden considered that chlorosis was a blood disorder, he still regarded regular sexual intercourse as helpful in mild cases: in more severe cases, he thought that marriage should be postponed until the patient was cured, because the strain of keeping house could prove too much (1905: 523–4). Campbell's follow-up study of chlorotics treated at Guy's Hospital suggested that, in any case, 'many chlorotics do not marry, ... if they do the family is not likely to be very large' (1923: 275; *contra* Jones 1897: 28).

But did marriage always work as a cure? As we have already seen, Jane Sharp warned against its use in cases where bad humours dominated the body (1671: 264; Hobby 1999: 200; cf. Sennert 1664: 105–6). François Ranchin, a Catholic physician who was chancellor at Montpellier from 1612, also expressed caution, based on the fact that 'experience teaches' that even marital sex can make some girls very ill (1627: 392). He noted that, although Hippocrates recommended that 'if they conceive, they will be healthy', there was no guarantee that sex would lead to conception, especially as, for conception, it is necessary to have some menstrual blood present to make the foetus, and to have the body in a healthy general condition (1627: 393). Even from within humoral medicine, therefore, the automatically curative power of marriage could come under challenge. A different objection was raised at the end of the nineteenth century by Frederic Coley, physician to the Northern Counties Hospital for Disease of the Chest and to the Hospital for Sick Children in Newcastle-upon-Tyne, who argued that, although 'It is a matter of common observation that chlorosis usually disappears after marriage ... it should be observed that this does not always take place very quickly' (1894: 268). He expressed concern at the possibility that, because the disease was thought to be cured by marriage, chlorosis occurring in young pregnant women would not be recognised, leaving them with a high risk of post-partum haemorrhage because their wombs were not strong enough to cope: they had 'uterine inertia', a phrase which provides the other extreme to the 'wandering womb' of ancient medicine.

This concern with the continued risk of the condition even after marriage is, in fact, echoing Lange's letter, where he wrote that 'of the married, it is certainly the barren who suffer this more'.[34] In its original Greek, this final sentence taken from the Hippocratic *On the disease of virgins* uses the word *êndrômenôn*, which may be translated in two different ways: it can simply mean 'among those who have grown to adulthood', but it can mean 'those who have sexual experience of men'. Calvi's two Latin translations of the Greek text restrict the meaning to that of age, giving 'adult women' and 'grown women'.[35] Lange, however, opts for the second, sexual, sense, giving 'among married women'.[36] Is this evidence that he had access to the Greek original here? This is one possibility, but it is more likely that he was also comparing Calvi with Cornarius' 1546 translation of the Hippocratic corpus into Latin, where the relevant phrase is rendered as 'among women who are joined to a man'.[37]

However, in classical Greek culture, to be a fully grown mature woman, a *gynê*, is also to be a wife; the same word is used for both the physiological status and the social position (see p. 51). To understand the importance of marriage as therapy, it is therefore necessary to go back one stage to investigate how changing ideas of puberty may have fed into the disease of virgins.

The problem of puberty

One of the consistent features of the disease of virgins, through its many transformations, is that it was seen as a crisis of the onset of physical and social maturity. Lange said that Anna's face had 'during the past year blossomed in rosy cheeks and red lips'; her body was showing that she had become marriageable. The full title of Sir Andrew Clark's piece in *The Lancet* of 1887 is significant here: 'Anaemia or chlorosis of girls, occurring more commonly between the advent of menstruation and the consummation of womanhood.' Although 'late' chlorosis is seen here as a possibility, nevertheless the true form ends when 'womanhood' – however defined, but often entered most decisively by marriage (Parsons 2002: 315–16) – is achieved. What did the Galenic tradition, within which Lange wrote, have to say about the specific physiological reasons for an excess of blood in young girls? This question introduces the wider theme of how the Western medical tradition constructed female puberty as a problem, and what solutions it proposed for it.

As we saw in chapter 2, the Hippocratic *On the disease of virgins* clearly regarded puberty as a very dangerous time for the young girls who were the subject of the text. 'Food and the growth of the body' – a phrase used in the Hippocratic text and picked up by Lange – mean there is more blood in the body, but the closure of the 'mouth of exit' makes it impossible for this blood to come out. In terms of the physiology involved, de Baillou (1643: 68) cited the Hippocratic treatise *On generation* to explain that a girl at the time of puberty has naturally narrow channels throughout her body:

> In the case of children, their vessels are narrow and blocked, and therefore prevent the passage of sperm … Girls while they are still young do not menstruate for the same reason. But as both boys and girls grow, the vessels which extend in the boy's case to the penis and in the girl's to the womb, open out and become wider in the process of growth; a way is opened up through the narrow passages, and the humour, finding sufficient space, can become agitated. That is why when they reach puberty, sperm can flow in the boy and the menses in the girl.
>
> (*On generation* 2; L 7.472–4; Lonie 1981: 1–2)

Female puberty could therefore be seen as a medical problem because of the sudden movement of blood through channels too narrow to permit its easy flow. Blockages occur, but sexual activity can open up the channels and encourage the blood to move around. Early marriage is therefore seen as a prophylactic measure; moving girls swiftly from childhood to the status of a married woman was good for their health. The dedication of a girl's childhood toys to the goddesses at her marriage symbolises this rapid shift in status (van Straten 1981: 90 n. 126); there is no intermediate stage of the life-cycle in between.

For modern writers trying to account for the rise and fall of chlorosis, however, one possible explanation has been that its rise could correspond with the idea of 'adolescence' as a distinct life crisis centred on biological puberty. In the history of chlorosis, the period in which the most explicit consideration was given to the dangers of adolescence in girls extended from the late nineteenth to the early twentieth century. For example, Raciborski

(1868: 328) suggested that marriage should ideally take place when a girl was aged between 20 and 24; although he believed that climate had a great influence on the timing, he thought that menarche usually occurred at around 13 or 14. Elizabeth Blackwell (1882: 11) regarded puberty, occurring between 14 and 16, as the necessary preparation for nubility, between the ages of 23 and 25.

Joan Jacobs Brumberg (1993: 102 n. 6) argued that, 'In the nineteenth century, menarche was the critical site for establishing female difference', so that it was the experience of first menstruation which was thought to have the most lasting effects on one's future health as a woman. She suggested that, for middle-class American women, while the age at menarche had fallen from an average of 17 in 1780, to 15 in 1877, and to 13.9 in 1901, the age at marriage had risen to 22 or 23, so that there was increased concern about the proper way to manage the potentially dangerous gap between what was perceived as the onset of sexuality, and its proper fulfilment (Figlio 1978: 177; Brumberg 1993: 104–5, 109). Because of its menstrual focus, Brumberg argued, chlorosis 'represented an entire conception of the female adolescent' (1982: 1468, 1475). It was in the 1880s that the view developed that the use of the brain during puberty would prevent menstruation becoming established and would even damage the future ability to conceive (Dyhouse 1981: 154–5). In addition, formal education – especially if set in boarding schools – created a period of extended dependence on adults (Dyhouse 1981: 119); writers from the late seventeenth century onwards regarded boarding schools as fostering chlorosis (e.g. [Pechey] 1694: 6; Lettsom 1795; Drysdale 1875: 166).

The work of Schultz argues for a strong contrast here with the middle ages, when – as in the ideal of compression put forward in the Hippocratic *On the disease of virgins* – 'the age of marriage for girls will often coincide with the age of menarche', so that 'there simply is no stretch of time between puberty and adulthood' (1991: 528, 530; cf. Lansing 2002: 293). This would suggest an opposition between an adolescence-free classical and medieval world, and a modern world in which, courtesy of both biology and social change, young girls experience an extra stage of the life-cycle, inserted between puberty and adulthood. There is a strong danger here of over-simplification of the classical world for the sake of constructing a binary opposition; as we saw in the last chapter, as early as the second century AD, Soranos (*Gyn.* 1.9; Temkin 1956: 27–30) claimed that some medical writers believed that virgins experience sexual desire, but are not able to express it, making the time at which they are 'ripe for marriage' but not yet married particularly dangerous. Furthermore, even at the modern end this model needs adjustment. In particular, we should not forget about the impact of class; working-class girls of the Victorian and Edwardian periods would have had less experience of 'adolescence', moving straight from childhood to take up adult responsibilities as 'little mothers' within the family (Dyhouse 1981: 119).

But it is also possible to challenge claims that the nineteenth century saw the 'birth of adolescence'. Writers including Ben-Amos (1994), Hanawalt (1992, 1996), Griffiths (1996) and Eisenbichler (2002) have shown that worries about adolescence *did* exist across early modern Europe. Medically, even in medieval sources the humoral model presented puberty in both sexes as a time of excess heat, and therefore of lust, a view which was fed by classical literature and supported by Christian writers (Stoertz 2002: 226–8); by the end of the sixteenth century, there was 'considerable apprehension' about female puberty in particular (Potter 2002: 273), partly because, while young adolescent men were allowed sexual activity, young women were supposed to remain chaste until they married.

In Tudor and Stuart England, various models of the 'ages of man' based on classical and medieval sources[38] were used; while disagreeing on how many age periods there were, writers 'nearly always distinguished a stage of life between childhood and adulthood which they usually called youth' (Griffiths 1996: 20). Some, moreover, also separated out a further category of 'adolescence', but disagreed on whether this should be placed before, or after, 'youth' (Griffiths 1996: 21–2). For women, youth ended with marriage, and the main virtue they were to bring to this marriage was chastity (Griffiths 1996: 29); when women were attacked in the courts, it was their chastity which was invariably the focus of accusations (Gowing 1996).

Hanawalt (1992) suggested an increased concern with adolescence in fifteenth-century English society; during this century of 'disruption and transition, youth became a focus for anxieties about a better future' (Hanawalt 1996: 155), with the middle classes showing a new interest in how children should dress, act and be educated. She argued that this interest was due not to any increase in the number of adolescents in the population, but rather to the low population growth of the time. Until conditions began to improve at the end of the fifteenth century, young rural men had less incentive to migrate to towns as apprentices and, even then, the typical apprentice entered into this role at 18 rather than at 14; he 'needed all the polish that the advice books could give' (Hanawalt 1996: 169; Griffiths 1996: 9).[39] In many guilds, apprenticeship was extended during the fifteenth century, so that young men were often being accorded the subordinate 'adolescent status' associated with apprenticeship until the age of 28; this long 'adolescence' continued in mid-sixteenth-century London (Ben-Amos 1994: 93). 'Youth' continued to be seen as a difficult time in the early seventeenth century; in his investigation of the clientele consulting the astrological priest-physician Richard Napier, MacDonald (1981: 41) suggested that 'Napier's [mentally disturbed] clients, however, found youth much more dangerous emotionally than middle or old age'.

What about women? The stories from popular literature which Hanawalt examined provided positive and negative *exempla* only of the behaviour of boys. In sixteenth-century European cities, guilds – with very few exceptions – were male organisations based on the structure of the male life-cycle and, in most parts of Europe, women's participation from the fifteenth century onwards was very low (Wiesner 1993: 103). The economic decline of the sixteenth century made the situation for women even worse. Merry Wiesner (1986: 191–2) has shown how, in early modern Germany, women's work increasingly came to be seen as 'a temporary or stopgap measure until the women could attain or return to their "natural," married state'. In fifteenth-century London, when the population was not growing, women apprentices were found in a range of skilled crafts and trades: in sixteenth-century London, however, very few women served as apprentices (Ben-Amos 1994: 135–6). If we are to correlate economic conditions with the rise of adolescence, then any concern with female adolescence as a result of changed working practices should have occurred not in the mid-sixteenth century, when the disease of virgins was articulated, but either earlier, or later. In any case, with the numbers involved as apprentices being so small, it seems unlikely that changes here influenced fears about young women's behaviour.

For women, the institution of service, which typically occupied the years between the mid-teens and mid-twenties, would perhaps be a better indicator of a belief that there was a stage of the female life-cycle after puberty and before marriage. Kim Phillips (1999: 5) has argued that this stage could be labelled more appropriately as 'maidenhood', a label carrying the dual meaning of 'young, and virginal'; interestingly, this puts the fifteenth-century maiden under the same tension between sexual maturity and sexual inexperience which characterised Clark's nineteenth-century chlorotic, poised 'between the advent of menstruation and the consummation of womanhood'. Both are seen as highly sexualised and idealised objects – we need only recall the eulogies of the pubertal girl by nineteenth-century writers such as Hollick and Rue (see the Introduction to this volume), while Phillips (1999: 6–10) shows how the heroines of Middle English literature who most encapsulate the ideal of feminine beauty are in their teens – yet the late medieval 'maiden' is not seen as liable to a physical disease, while the nineteenth-century chlorotic is.

Did a 'puberty gap' develop because of later marriage? In mid-sixteenth-century England, around 40 per cent of the population were under 15. The classic work of Wrigley and Schofield suggested peaks in the proportion of young people in 1556, again in 1576, and then 'a sustained rise until 1621' (cited in Griffiths 1996: 5). This was accompanied by a high age at first marriage, as late as 28 for men and 26 for women. This conforms to the north-west European marriage pattern, which has been identified as marriage in the mid- to late twenties, with husbands two or three years older than their wives; in south and east Europe, marriage occurred in the teens, or between a man in his late twenties or early thirties and a considerably younger woman (Wiesner 1993: 57). It was this last model which was the one familiar to the ancient Greeks, and thus to the writer of *On the disease of virgins*. Even if female puberty in the sixteenth century occurred around the age of 14 (e.g. Wiesner 1993: 44), in northern Europe there would still have been a longer gap between puberty and marriage than even in the nineteenth century. However, worries about the prevalence of the disease of virgins were not restricted to the northern countries, and a concern that girls who remain too long unmarried will suffer from green sickness appears constant throughout its history, regardless of changing physiology and social practice.[40] What appears to be specific to certain historical periods, however, is the focus on the onset of menstruation as the key point of danger for women, a time when their bodies and their minds are equally in turmoil.

The philosophy of puberty

However, the driving force making puberty into a medical problem did not only lie in the 'reality' of earlier menarche combined with the 'reality' of later marriage. In the early nineteenth century, before the fall in the age of menarche, French Medical Faculty inaugural dissertations on chlorosis, like the discourse of nymphomania (see chapter 1), were heavily influenced by the philosophical images of female puberty which had been put forward by Jean-Jacques Rousseau (1712–78) and George-Louis Leclerc, comte du Buffon (1707–88) in the previous century. Trabuc's 1818 thesis presented to the Montpellier Medical Faculty included a quotation from Rousseau's *Emile* (first published in 1762) on the title page, while Olive's Paris dissertation of the following year, a discussion of menarche, ended with the traditional Parisian list of Hippocratic aphorisms relevant to the topic, but cited Rousseau in the text (Olive 1819: 7). Trabuc (1818: 5) also quoted from Buffon, who saw puberty as the 'springtime' of a woman's life, but also as a 'general shake-up' in which 'the world changes before her eyes, just as she becomes a new being for the world' (Buffon 1971: 76). This idealisation of puberty continued into the early twentieth century, when G. Stanley Hall wrote of the pubertal girl, 'Each sense is more acute, the imagination more lively, reveries more frequent. In dress she blossoms into colors' (1904: 482).

In the picture he gave of Sophie, who, as the female counterpart to his Emile, 'must be a woman as Emilius is a man' (1768: 4), Rousseau explored the essential difference between the changes of adolescence in the male and the female. In book 5 of *Emile*, he discussed the extent to which the sexes were alike; women have the 'same organs, wants and faculties' except in their specifically sexual parts; there, men are 'active and strong', while women are 'passive and feeble' (Rousseau 1768: 4–5). In childhood, girls and boys are thought to share amusements and tastes, although girls already possess 'a fineness and lightness in their expressions and movements' which hints at what they will become (Trabuc 1818: 5). Echoing these ideas in his inaugural dissertation for the Paris medical faculty, Olive explained that, at puberty, both boys and girls change in ways which enable them to fulfil the roles allocated to them by society, but also to reach the goal for which nature has created them. Girls develop more slowly, and less dramatically, and they stay closer to their childhood form. They are timid, weak and delicate, avoiding amusements which demand much exercise; the main occupation for a girl becomes 'the desire to please, and the search for ways of adding to her charms' (Olive 1819: 6–7). This recalls Rousseau, writing of the 15-year-old Sophie, 'she charms you, and you do not know why' (1768: 74). Olive also cited Rousseau as his source for the statement that girls are more spiritual than boys.

The influence on these texts of Buffon's 'De la puberté', part of the second volume of his *Histoire naturelle, générale et particulière* which appeared in 1749, needs further investigation. The first three volumes of this work were among the best-sellers of the eighteenth century, and were translated for the English, Dutch and German markets (Roger 1997: 184). Buffon generally believed that variation between individuals was more significant than variation from one race to another, but he was interested in the effect of climate on the human race (Roger 1997: 178–80), and saw puberty as occurring at a younger age in those who were well fed, lived in towns or were from the wealthier classes; however, his limits were not set very far apart, 12 being seen as 'early' for girls and 14 as 'late', although in particularly hot climates puberty could occur as early as the age of 9 or 10 (Buffon 1971: 83–4). In boys, puberty occurs two years later, because men need longer in order to grow their extra muscles, stronger bones and more compact flesh.

Buffon's views on virginity were unusual; he regarded it as a moral, not a physical, state, and attributed its reification as a 'favoured idol' to a male interest in possessing everything 'exclusively and for the first time' (Buffon 1971: 85). He summarised sixteenth- and seventeenth-century debates on whether or not the hymen existed as a sign of virginity, and proposed that in fact both sides were correct; some girls have a membrane, others have a few 'caroncules', and others have nothing (Buffon 1971: 86–7). In any case, virginity is more properly seen as a moral state than as a physical object (Roger 1997: 168).[41] As for bleeding at defloration, Buffon argued that intercourse with a girl below the age of puberty rarely causes bleeding unless there is a serious disproportion between the male and female parts, or undue force is used; with a strong and healthy girl at puberty, there is often some bleeding because her genitalia are swollen with the blood needed for their growth and development. If there is a gap of some months between first and second intercourse, the parts can reunite and then bleed again, so that 'virginity' can be renewed four or five times over the years between the ages of 14 and 18 (Buffon 1971: 87–9). Buffon believed that it was possible to become pregnant without having menstruated, because menstrual blood was only 'accessory matter' in the process of reproduction, the 'essential matter', seminal liquid, being contributed by both partners (1971: 96).

At puberty, Olive believed, the womb awoke as though from a long sleep; under its influence, a girl's body developed 'soft and malleable contours, a voluptuous plumpness' which was only found in pubertal girls (Olive 1819: 8). This almost voyeuristic approach to female puberty is characteristic of the early nineteenth century;[42] as we have already seen (p. 6), writing in the same year, Rue (1819: 13–14) believed that menstruation 'gives to this young beauty, no matter how sad or languid, the freshness and sparkle which mark the dawn of her life'.

Chlorosis has a complex connection to physical appearance. Blushing was seen as a feature of puberty (e.g. Hall 1904: 482), and also of chlorosis (e.g. Ashwell 1836: 533; Bramwell 1899: 32, cited on p. 7). In the early stages of the disease, von Noorden wrote (1905: 357), girls may be 'admired for their rosy complexions', but pale mucous membranes would indicate the true nature of the illness. The external appearance may be misleading: along with the extreme pallor of a chlorotic girl, 'A *deceptive* red flush is not infrequent' (Ward 1914: 307; my italics). Here, then, the outside is deceptive, but the inside tells the truth; this recalls the classical Greek image of the first woman, Pandora, whose beautiful appearance concealed 'the mind of a bitch' and a ravenous appetite which compelled her unlucky husband to work day and night in order to satisfy her (King 1998: 26–7).

In his report to the British Medical Association Scientific Grants Committee in 1897, the pathologist Ernest Lloyd Jones wrote that the girls most likely to be affected with chlorosis are 'generally fair, with pretty pink and white complexions, blue or light eyes, fine hair, with a goodly amount of subcutaneous fat' (1897: 16–17).

He argued that chlorotics tend to come from large families and, when they have recovered, to exhibit high fertility themselves; the chlorotic is perceived as 'pretty' because of this underlying fertility (Jones 1897: 28). In this analysis, the erotic chlorotic becomes even more desirable; her future fertility is shown in her appearance, which here becomes a true guide to the underlying reality.[43] However, the fertility of chlorotics was challenged by the work of J.M.H. Campbell (1923: 275).

Town and country

During puberty, a girl was seen as highly vulnerable; nineteenth-century male authors who seem barely able to resist her charms speak explicitly of threats to her health other than those which they themselves pose. The girl must be carefully prepared for menarche by taking plenty of fresh air and country walks, while avoiding the many activities associated with urban life and believed to cause 'nervous excitement'; these dangerous stimuli included perfume, sexually explicit paintings, novels, 'libidinous conversations', masturbation, tea, coffee and spirits (Trabuc 1818: 8; Olive 1819: 14–15, 25; Rue 1819: 14–17).

The idea that chlorosis is 'almost wholly confined to town life' (Tait 1889: 282), and therefore that 'the country' is good for chlorotics was repeated many times in the urbanised nineteenth century; for example, James Hamilton (1805: 5) wrote of the need to 'foresake the haunts and habits of fashionable life; to leave the crowded city' and 'to court the country, pure air, moderate exercise, and simple diet' while Samuel Ashwell (1836: 538) recommended to sufferers 'Change of air, a residence in the country, and more natural and out-of-door avocations' which would encourage the onset of puberty and thus the menstrual function which was so necessary.[44] This belief in the countryside as encouraging menarche was not, however, universal. Clark (1887: 61) said that the incidence of chlorosis was independent 'of country or of town' (cf. Ward 1914: 320), while Raciborski (1868: 210) demonstrated statistically that, in general, girls in towns menstruate at an earlier age than country girls. But, here too, there was a moral message behind the opposition between town and country. In a work first published in 1869, but which continued to be reprinted for several decades after his death in 1875, the influential home-opath Edward Harris Ruddock (1892: 26) claimed that the menstrual function itself was 'due to enervation incident to civic life and a highly artificial state of society'.[45] The language used here, of civilisation as an 'artificial state', suggests the legacy of Rousseau, and the image of the 'noble savage' (Whorton 2000: 31–2). Raciborski believed that puberty came earlier in towns because of the daily meetings between children of both sexes in public spaces, which could stimulate ovulation; abandoning one's doll in favour of playing with a young brother or male cousin led to jealousy and rivalry between girls for male attention, and provoked desires with which their bodies were unable to cope (Raciborski 1868: 211–12, cf. 288).

By the end of the nineteenth century, surveys of sufferers from chlorosis were increasingly common, as medicine more generally moved from the individual case to the general 'type'. Bramwell (1899: 23) considered, from the 314 cases he himself had seen, that the condition was most often found in young servants, particularly country girls in service in the towns.[46] Stockman's views were much the same (1895b: 1475) and in his study of sixty-three cases (1895a: 416), he found thirty-eight domestic servants, thirteen factory girls, two shop girls, two dairymaids, three fieldworkers and three girls who lived at home. However, Stockman did not regard his findings as statistically significant, pointing out that the figures would depend on the local economy; both his and Bramwell's figures were from the Edinburgh region, where Stockman was assistant physician at the Royal Infirmary. The pattern of a country girl moving to the town, and soon becoming ill, was also found towards the end of the history of the disorder, in cases cited in Patek and Heath's work of the 1930s (1936: 1466; cf. Cabot 1908: 641).

Figlio (1978) argued that nineteenth-century chlorosis was a middle-class condition, linked to men delaying marriage in order to establish themselves in a career. He suggested that doctors, themselves from the middle class, projected the condition on to upper-class girls, linking it to their indolent and vain behaviour (1978: 179–80) while, for working-class girls, the diagnosis of chlorosis served as an attempt to deflect attention away from their poor working conditions (1978: 181–7). Turning to writers contemporary with chlorosis, John Tanner (1659: 315) linked it both to those who 'go to Feasts, and upon a full Stomach, dancing and sporting all Night, disturb the naturall Frame of the Body, and want Rest' and to those who 'sleep too much, and sit long at their work, as Seamsters, Bonelace-makers, and the like'. At the very end of the history of the condition, similar groups were singled out. Von Noorden (1905: 350) suggested that chlorosis could be caused by too much, or too little, exercise, so that servants would develop it from too much work, while seamstresses were in a sedentary job providing insufficient exercise. As for poor nutrition as a causative factor, this could occur as often in well-off families, where diet may be poor due to 'childish whims', as in poor households (1905: 349).

Despite their eulogies of the pubertal girl, a note of concern also enters into some of the early nineteenth-century dissertations. Olive (1819: 10–12) says that, at menarche, a girl becomes melancholic, seeks solitude, and bursts into tears without knowing why she is crying. This mental disorder may lead her to feel that only men can fill the gap in her life. This again recalls Rousseau's Sophie, whose bouts of tearful melancholy are signs of her need for a lover (Rousseau 1768: 93–4). For Olive, the girl's symptoms of lassitude, hot flushes, skin eruptions, a powerful pulse, vomiting and palpitations will cease when her menses start to flow, and she will feel renewed. But, if the menses are suppressed, she will suffer from chlorosis.

Independently of social changes leading to earlier puberty and later marriage for girls, medical writing from the middle and end of the nineteenth century shows very similar concerns about female puberty. Medical professionals saw it as a 'violent storm', a period of mental instability and 'extreme nervous sensibility' (Mezière 1846: 15), 'this most important change' (Ashwell 1836: 535), when enormous strains are placed on the body, particularly on the organs which form blood (Bramwell 1899: 25). Analogies were drawn between animals on heat and women about to menstruate; the nervous system was considered to be under great stress, making a woman irritable, and prone to the passions of jealousy, anger and vengeance (Raciborski 1868: 83). Some writers regarded the entire body of the young woman as susceptible to changes at menarche; for example, development of the vocal organs made her more likely to suffer from laryngeal catarrh, while all her bodily secretions and excretions were liable to be disturbed (Bretheau 1865: 14; Mezière 1846: 14). Yet they also saw the

start of menstruation as offering a complete – but never permanent[47] –
cure for some conditions; Mezière presented it in these terms for girls with
hysterical symptoms.

Regardless of the real extent of the 'puberty gap' in any historical period,
the classical medical texts contained the materials to support the suggestion
that the onset of menstruation was a medical problem. The concern about
girls 'ripe for marriage, but remaining unmarried' is found in the
Hippocratic *On the disease of virgins* as much as in Lange's letter about Anna;
by the nineteenth century, such constant concerns were particularly vividly
expressed by constructing female puberty as both attractive and threatening,
femininity as inherently capricious, and virginity as a disease. Medical explanations accounted for observed changes in the body by proposing theories
about what is taking place unseen, inside the young girl, and applying these
more widely in order to prescribe the social roles appropriate to women. In
particular, the early nineteenth-century texts built on connections between
blood and growth which can be traced back to the Hippocratic corpus.

4

DIETARY FACTORS

In the Hippocratic *On the disease of virgins*, it was on account of 'food and the growth of the body' that an excess of blood was present in young girls at puberty. This phrase was open to a range of interpretations in medical writers which were explored from Lange onwards, and which allowed the disease of virgins to retain the digestive symptoms that had been part of green sickness before it became a condition specific to young girls around the time of the first menstrual period.

The previous chapters have already given some sense of the complex nature of Lange's contribution to the disease of virgins, and to chlorosis. In order to understand the development of the disease picture of these conditions, we need to read the Hippocratic *On the disease of virgins* in a context which takes into account not only the Galenic theory of the body dominant in 1554, but also Lange's significant reinterpretations of the Greek text. Some aspects of Lange's disease of virgins derive from the particular manuscripts available to those who produced the Latin translations he used; the interest in a changed skin colour, found in the folk categories of the 'women of Brabant', is reinforced by the manuscript choice of *chroia* over *chreia*, while the manuscript insertion of *therapeia* encourages Lange's very un-Hippocratic recommendation of the release of blood through bloodletting. Both of these examples are also fully consistent with reading a Hippocratic text within a Galenic model of the body; and, of course, the manuscript readings themselves derive from copyists working in cultures in which that model ruled. The full extent of the power of the Galenic model is best illustrated by Lange's shift from the 'mouth of exit' of the Hippocratic text – suggesting the vagina – to the 'mouths' of the channels emptying into the womb, a move which is made in direct opposition to the Latin translations he was using.

The later picture of chlorosis included three further symptoms which are found in Lange but not – or, at least, not on first reading – in the Hippocratic *On the disease of virgins*.[1] These are difficulty in breathing, dietary disturbance and swelling. In Lange's letter, he says that the girl Anna 'has an attack of dyspnoea when dancing or climbing stairs; her stomach turns away from food (Lat. *cibum fastidire*), above all from meat; her legs – especially near the ankles – swell with oedema at night'.

Difficulty in breathing is not directly mentioned in the Hippocratic original, where sufferers from the condition are, however, described as 'feeling strangled' and also as hanging themselves or jumping down wells. I have argued elsewhere (King 1983; 1998: ch. 4) that, in their original fifth- or fourth-century BC context, these references may best be understood in terms of the imagery of closure and opening, reflecting ancient Greek beliefs about the role of the virgin goddess Artemis – known in one myth as the 'Strangled Goddess' – in initiating the maturation of the female body. Attempting suicide does not feature as a symptom in Lange's list of Anna's problems; however, in scholarly commentaries on the text of the Hippocratic *On the disease of virgins*, there was considerable discussion of this feature of young girls' behaviour, and attempts were made to find other classical texts to help make sense of it. In particular, the sixteenth- and seventeenth-century commentators linked the Hippocratic text to Plutarch's *On the virtues of women* (249b–d), where a mass suicide by girls in Miletos took the form of hanging.[2] However, they proposed that the cause of this event could properly be understood only in the light of Hippocratic medicine; as Donati (1582: 38–9) put it, commenting on the Hippocratic comment that virgins 'desire death as a lover',

> But our most ancient and prudent author [i.e. Hippocrates] expresses the opinion that all the blame for those diseases should be traced to the holding back and suppression of menstrual blood.[3]

In trying to make sense of the Hippocratic references to suicide in virgins with suppressed menstrual blood, Donati also mentioned a more recent mass suicide, a mass drowning by women in Lyons in 1508 (1582: 36–8). As his source, he cited Pietro Crinito, *De honesta disciplina*. Crinito (1504, Book 3: ch. 9; Angeleri 1955: 112–13) explained this event by looking to the descriptions of the plague of Athens given by Thucydides (2.49.5) and Lucretius (*De rerum natura* 6.1172–8); sufferers were so hot that they jumped into water to cool themselves. This is not incompatible with menstrual suppression, since blood is humorally 'hot' and 'wet', so that its retention makes women – normally the colder sex – become hotter and, as we shall see, cooling diets were recommended to young virgins. Crinito also mentioned the virgin Neera, who jumped into a well; her story, he said, was told by Giovanni Pontano (1490). Thomas Heywood's collection of stories about women, printed in 1624, gave a different version of Neera's story; he explained her suicide as the result of disappointment in love, and claimed that she killed herself by opening her veins (1624: 212).

Medical writers such as Mercuriale (1587: 284d) and Varandal (1619: 98–9; 1620: 96–7), whose work was published after the appearance of the first of these commentaries in 1574, picked up additional classical examples such as the story of the virgins of Miletos, and incorporated them back into their discussions of the medical implications of the Hippocratic *On the disease of virgins*. Varandal saw female weakness, leading to the retention of menstrual blood, as lying behind both the Milesian girls hanging themselves, and the women of Lyons drowning themselves; he added that this was also the condition Hippocrates described in *On the disease of virgins*. However, if commentators were bringing in suicidal thoughts and attempted suicide as symptoms, then they more commonly placed their analysis of the Hippocratic text not in a section on menstrual suppression or chlorosis, but under the categories of 'uterine fury' – where the reference to jumping down wells could be seen as an action to quench the heat of lust – or 'melancholy' (e.g. Mercado 1579: 180, 182). Jane Sharp (1671: 326; Hobby 1999: 241–2), following Sennert (1664: 119), described virgins and widows suffering from a 'melancholy distemper' who 'grow mad … see fearful spirits, and dead men … wish to die; and when they find an opportunity, they will kill, or drown, or hang themselves'. The theme of seeing ghosts is also taken directly from *On the disease of virgins* (see p. 50 of this volume), and Lange mentions 'fancied terrors of spectres'. It featured in the later medical tradition of chlorosis; for example, de Baillou (1643: 67) repeated the relevant section of the Hippocratic text, while Clifford Allbutt claimed to know of a chlorotic girl who suffered a relapse after thinking she had seen a ghost (Loudon 1984: 33). A further example of this multiple use of *On the disease of virgins* occurs in the work of Mercuriale (in Bauhin 1586–88, vol. 2: 155; Mercuriale 1591: 186–7), who included passages from it in his section on uterine fury; Varandal (1619; 1620) also devoted his first chapter to chlorosis but his fifth to melancholy and uterine fury, there quoting extensively from *On the disease of virgins*, and only there discussing the girls of Miletos. Similarly, Sennert's *Practical Physick* (1664: 115) used *On the disease of virgins* in the chapter on 'the Frenzie of the womb', claiming that Hippocratic girls 'follow men, and sollicite them shamelessly'. One ancient text could therefore provide the raw material for more than one sixteenth-century disease category.

Lange, however, did not mention attempting suicide in his picture of Anna and of the disease of virgins. Instead, later in his letter, he described how veins blocked with blood put pressure on the diaphragm, causing rapid, shallow breathing: here, the Hippocratic references to strangulation have become a medical symptom with an organic cause, rather than a mode of suicide.

Swelling of the lower limbs, with lassitude in the feet and legs, mentioned by Lange, is also characteristic of seventeenth-century descriptions of chlorosis such as that of Sydenham: it too could derive from a misinterpretation of another section of the Hippocratic text, in which an analogy is drawn between the oppression of the heart due to the misplaced menstrual blood, and the numbness (Greek *narkê*) caused in the feet by sitting still for a long time. The writer of *On the disease of virgins* goes on to say that, when blood has collected in the feet, the way to make it return to its proper place is to immerse the numb feet in cold water to just above the ankles. He never claims that the feet and ankles themselves swell in a case of retained menstrual blood; his point is merely to compare the relative ease of dispersing excess blood pooling in the feet, with the difficulty of reversing a surplus of menstrual blood located in the more critical and complex area of the heart, where the channels through which the blood passes are 'at an angle'. But, in the chlorosis tradition, an analogy used to explain something internal and invisible by reference to something external and visible is transformed, and the feet came to be seen as directly affected.

Difficulty in breathing and swollen feet can thus be seen to derive – indirectly, at least – from reading the Hippocratic *On the disease of virgins*. Turning 'away from food, especially meat' is far more complex, but an interest in digestive disturbances persists throughout the history of the condition. For example, Maubray (1724: 44) considered that the symptoms all 'proceed[ed] from a deprav'd Nutrition', while a century and a half later Habershon (1863: 518) suggested that the pallor and amenorrhoea of chlorosis 'are preceded by defective nutrition and by impaired or capricious appetite, and the changes in the blood itself appear to be secondary to the imperfect absorption and assimilation of food … chlorosis and amenorrhoea are slowly induced by defective nutrition'.

A whole class of symptoms of chlorosis could be grouped together under the headings of 'defective nutrition' and 'impaired or capricious appetite'. These disturbances include not eating at all; a poor diet; the avoidance of foods believed to encourage the production of blood; and pica, consumption of non-food substances such as chalk and clay, which were thought to block the internal channels of the body. 'Obstruction of the passages' seems to be implicated in green sickness from an early date, suggested by Lange's recommendation of 'medicines for provoking the menses and for opening up obstructions' to treat the disease of virgins, and by Langham's list of effects of 'Blessed Thistle', good 'for green sickness, griping and pain of belly, to open obstructions, cause passage of urine' (Langham 1597: 82 no. 48); diet was one possible cause of such blockages. Constipation, seen as the result either of a poor diet, or of inadequate power to expel food waste, also needs to be considered here. The liver, the seat of blood production in the Galenic body and therefore implicated in menstrual theories of the disease of virgins, was also blamed in the dietary explanations for the disease.

Aversion towards food, *fastidium*, could be understood as a symptom of love sickness which, as we have already seen, overlapped with green sickness and chlorosis; Martinez (1995: 353–4) cites Galen (*In Hippocratis Prognostica* 1.4.18; CMG 5.9.2, 207), who described 'those who grow gaunt or pale or lose sleep or even get fevers for reasons of love', while the love-sick character

Philetas, in Longus' novel *Daphnis and Chloe* (2.7.4), says 'I could not think of food or take drink or get sleep'. But it could also be classified as a symptom of menstrual suppression in general, for example in the sixth-century AD writer Aetius of Amida (16.52). In medieval medicine, the Trotula treatise, *Cum auctor*, included craving for 'earth, coals, chalk, and similar things' as a possible symptom of menstrual disturbance, whether excessive or insufficient (Green 2001: 72), while a commentator on ps-Albertus Magnus' *On the secrets of women* 12 also stated that, in pregnant women, it was the retained menses that led to bad humours, which in turn produced food cravings (Lemay 1978: 397; 1992: 141). This connection was not only found in traditional Galenic medicine; for example, Astruc (1743: 50) went one step further, regarding pica as a normal sign before any menstrual period starts, 'through the Vice of the digestive Ferments from the universal Plethora'; in other words, the excessive amount of blood present in the body before a period sends the digestive system into confusion, so there would be no surprise in finding that retained menses in a girl at puberty caused unusual dietary behaviour. The idea that normal sexual maturation in a girl could lead to an erratic or capricious appetite continued into the late nineteenth century (Brumberg 1988: 174–5).

The womb could also be seen as having some role in this dietary upheaval. In his list of symptoms of menarche, Olive (1819: 13) suggested that it is the concentration of vital forces on the womb which leads to digestive disturbances, including a taste for salt, plaster, vinegar, or bitter, green fruits. As we shall see shortly, lists of this kind are common in medical literature on women; Olive's list is little different from that of Joubert in the sixteenth century, listing 'paper, plaster, ashes, coals, wheat, flour, pure vinegar, pepper and other spices, green and sour fruit, etc.' (Rocher 1989: 154–5), while 'green fruit' is included in Jane Sharp's list of 'crude raw things' to be avoided in the regimen for sufferers from green sickness (1671: 263; Hobby 1999: 199). Vinegar, in particular, had other associations, as it was thought to be used by women if a menstrual period was due on the occasion of a social event; Mary Gove (1846: 253) gave the example of a girl who took vinegar because she wanted to attend a ball, and who then failed to menstruate for seven months. For some nineteenth-century writers, however, a focus on digestion accompanying a shift from the womb to the liver as the central organ involved allowed chlorosis to be seen as a condition affecting not only girls at puberty, but also older women – including pregnant women – boys, and even adult men.

Food and the growth of the body

As we have seen in chapter 2, diet played an important role in ancient discussions of the origin of 'new' diseases; this was often phrased in terms of the dangers of luxury, as part of an attack on the new imports available to

Romans living under the Empire, which were thought to have overturned the simplicity of life in republican Rome idealised by writers of the early Empire. As we saw in the previous chapter, in the Galenic humoral body, the type of food eaten affects directly the quality of blood produced: as a sixteenth-century writer put it, 'such as the food is, such is the bloud: and such as the bloud is, such is the flesh' (Cogan 1584: A3^v– A4^r, cited by Wear 2000: 172 n. 51). The 'qualities' of the food eaten – its heat, coldness, wetness and dryness – needed to be matched to the humoral temperament of the eater, so that diet 'symbolised the individualised treatment of learned physic' (Wear 2000: 225), but early modern handbooks on regimen also gave detailed lists of foods and their qualities to enable lay people to follow Galenic guidelines.

Like so many other aspects of the disease of virgins and chlorosis, digestive disturbances originate in the Hippocratic *On the disease of virgins*. The key phrase here is a simple one, the suggestion that 'more' blood is flowing to the womb 'on account of food and the growth of the body',[4] but it is its very simplicity which allows it to carry such a range of different meanings. What did an ancient Greek writer mean by this, and how in turn would a sixteenth- or seventeenth-century medical writer understand it?

In Hippocratic terms, as for Galen, food is the direct origin of blood. From Homeric times onwards,[5] it was believed that food produces blood, so that more food would mean more blood. In Aristotle, semen, menstrual fluid and milk are all forms of surplus nutriment, but the scientific expression of the idea that blood is the agent of nutrition goes back much further, to the pre-Socratic philosophers of the fifth century BC (Longrigg 1985). As for 'growth', in *On the disease of virgins* this could be connected to the idea, found elsewhere in the gynaecological texts, that a girl's body has to be 'opened up' inside, so that extra spaces are created in her flesh to hold the accumulating menstrual blood before it moves to the womb each month (*Diseases of women* 1.1; L 8.10–14). This is compatible with the Hippocratic text *On generation* 2 (see p. 84 of this volume), which argues that the internal channels through which blood moves to the womb are 'narrow and blocked' in girls, and need to 'open out and become wider in the process of growth'.

But why does 'more' blood flow to the womb on account of food and the growth of the body? The simplest option in terms of Hippocratic gynaecology is that the girl is eating normally, but her internal channels have now grown to the point where, for the first time, the blood she is producing can reach her womb. For the Hippocratic writer, the problem resides not in the 'food and growth of the body', but in what happens when the blood reaches the womb; as the rest of the sentence makes clear, the 'mouth of exit' is not open, and the blood cannot flow out, instead moving upwards to the heart and diaphragm. The girl has reached a stage of maturity sufficient that her blood can reach her womb but, from there, it has no way out of her body.

The greater detail of the Galenic body and its recommended food intake meant, however, that other interpretations of the Hippocratic text became possible. A variant interpretation of 'food and the growth of the body' was offered by de Baillou (1643), in his chapter '*De foedis virginum coloribus*', concerning the ugly colours of virgins. This disorder seems to be yet another variation on chlorosis; like Lange's 'disease of virgins', to which it does not refer, it is largely dependent on the Hippocratic *On the disease of virgins*. De Baillou saw the disorder as affecting 'virgins who are already mature, especially when the time of the menstrual purgation is close'. When blood is being used both for nourishment and for growth – that is, for 'food and the growth of the body' – there is no excess to lose; but, when growth to maturity is completed, there is suddenly a surplus of blood which is no longer needed. The symptoms occur, he claimed, because the soft and tender body of the virgin is ill prepared for the movement of this blood through it. This is very close indeed to the Hippocratic view of the process of opening up channels and spaces in the female body as it matures; and, indeed, de Baillou cited *On generation* 2 to support his argument.

This interpretation may also be found in the anonymous but influential popular work, *Aristotle's Masterpiece* (Anon. 1694: 2–3), which said that, in girls at puberty, the blood 'which is no longer taken to augment their Bodies, abounding, incites their Minds and Imaginations to Venery'. If a girl affected in this way does not marry, she will suffer from a 'Green and Weasel Colour, short Breathings, Tremblings of the Heart, &c'.[6] Here again, the problem is not menstrual blood which is unable to get out, but blood which is no longer needed for growth. This would suggest that the solution is for girls who have completed their growth process to reduce their food intake so that only the minimum amount of surplus blood will be produced. This can be achieved by cutting down on all food, or by avoidance of selected foods only. Clark (1887: 61) suggested that a girl 'In the period between the advent of menstruation and the consummation of womanhood' would, in any case, start to worry about putting on weight, so that 'Afraid of getting fat, she stints herself in food, and eats only of dainty things.' For him, the onset of the problem lay here; the girl was reducing her food intake too radically.

But fear of fat was not the only motivation possible, particularly when the humoral system still ruled. Lange, while translating 'on account of food and the growth of the body' in the section of his letter in which he quotes directly from the Hippocratic text, adds in his earlier list of Anna's symptoms the point that she turns away from food, 'especially meat'.[7] The second-century AD writer Rufus of Ephesus recommended that girls approaching menarche – a time which he thought could be detected from a reduction in their speed of growth and a lack of interest in children's games – should avoid meat and strong foods, and should drink wine only after the addition of plenty of water. These measures would reduce the risk of the body becoming overfilled with blood and, as a result, developing disease; the diet would ensure that virgin girls remained virgins until their marriage (Rufus, in Oribasius, *Collectiones medicae, libri incerti* 2; Daremberg 1862: 82; Aly 1992: 138, 188; Shaw 1998: 163). In the fourth century AD, Basil of Ancyra recommended in considerable detail a 'cooling' diet for a virgin to follow. The aim of this diet, based on Galenic principles, was to control the production of humours but also to guard the sense of taste, as one of the sensory portals through which pleasure could enter the body (Shaw 1998). In Galenic theory, meat is the food which is most completely converted into blood, leaving the least residue (*To Glaucon* 1.15; K 11.46; Brain 1986: 5). The logic of food containing blood also being food which produced blood was unassailable. Jane Sharp (1671: 326, Hobby 1999: 241) advised unmarried women and nuns to avoid meat and eggs, so that only the minimum amount of seed may be produced, and sexual desire be reduced. Until the late nineteenth century, medical texts continued to recommend restricting the consumption of animal flesh in order to delay menstruation and reduce sexual desires, so that Brumberg (1982: 1473–4) has suggested that 'good' girls would make the rejection of meat 'a positive social virtue'; the avoidance of meat was indeed found in many chlorotic patients in the second half of the nineteenth century (Brumberg 1988: 176–8). The other side of this idea is found in the recommendation of meat in the *treatment* of chlorosis; according to Jane Sharp (1671: 293; Hobby 1999: 219), menstrual suppression was best treated by fattening up the sufferer 'with nourishing meats and drinks', while two centuries later Raciborski (1868: 285) prescribed a diet which was 'tonic, substantial, composed of roast meats, wine, etc., etc.'

One possibility is therefore deliberate avoidance of food: taken within a Galenic model of dietary behaviour, Anna's rejection of meat could be her own choice. She needs less blood now that she has completed her growth to puberty, and so she follows Galenic dietary advice and avoids blood-producing foods. There may even be a religious dimension to her behaviour. 'Excessive fasting was a spectacle' (Vandereycken and Van Deth 1994: 218), but one which was open to different cultural interpretations. As the work of Caroline Walker Bynum (1987) has shown, due to the particular roles of food in medieval Christianity, where fasting and feasting were part of the calendar, women in the high Middle Ages could define themselves as 'good' by fasting; Bynum further argues that food was one area of life over which women had control – 'women cooked and men ate' (Bynum 1987: 277) – and was thus an appropriate area in which they could show autonomy. But Christian food practice also involved the community sharing the consecrated elements in the Eucharist; such extreme behaviour as refusing to take any food but the consecrated Host could be seen as commendable devotion, but it often met with opposition from family and spiritual advisers (Vandereycken and Van Deth 1994: 219). By the late Middle Ages, food behaviour within the context of piety became less about the unity of the community in the shared Eucharist, and more individualistic (Bynum 1987: 65). More generally, in pre-Christian cultures fasting was also often seen in very negative terms, as a way of setting oneself apart from normal human behaviour, and thus from the wider community (Martinez 1995: 342–3). Brumberg (1988) and Vandereycken and Van Deth (1994) have shown how, in sixteenth- and seventeenth-century Europe, medical writers started to challenge miraculous eaters. Some proposed physiological explanations for how a body – particularly a female body – could survive with no food intake;[8] others suggested that miraculous eaters were taking food surreptitiously so that, as with chlorosis, the issue of deceit came to the fore.[9] One could further argue that, by restricting the production of body fluids at puberty, Anna is trying to resist a natural process: the description of her as 'now of marriageable age' could imply that she has shown her maturity by menstruating but, if she has not yet menstruated, or her menstruation is not fully established, then she is too young to be limiting her diet in this manner.

There have, however, been several other ways of interpreting these two concepts of 'food' and 'growth' and linking them to chlorosis. In complete contradiction to de Baillou and the *Masterpiece*, Ralph Stockman (1895b: 1473) – one of the most influential of those late-nineteenth-century physicians who regarded constipation as the cause of chlorosis – argued that puberty put the whole body under great strain. During this period of rapid growth, girls suffered from dyspepsia and constipation, which reduced their appetite, 'so that an inadequate amount of food, and consequently of iron, is consumed'. He analysed the diet of fifteen girls, and found that one girl ate only bread and milk for three months (1895b: 1473–4). For Stockman, although chlorosis sometimes began with particularly heavy menstrual blood loss, the subsequent amenorrhoea served a protective function, sparing sufferers from further haemorrhage (1895b: 1474). Hudson (1977: 456–7) regards menarcheal blood loss as the final event precipitating chlorosis in a girl already at risk because of limited iron reserves, the pubertal growth spurt and poor diet (*contra* Loudon 1984: 28). Cabot (1908: 642; cf. Figlio 1978: 173) also saw the onset of chlorosis as being 'in the period immediately *after* the establishment of menstruation' (my italics). Putting these suggestions together, it would then be possible to argue that 'food and the growth of the body' should be glossed not as a normal diet suddenly being more than the newly full-grown body requires, but as 'poor diet and the pubertal growth spurt', combined with loss of blood in menstruation.

Some writers on chlorosis, however, wanted to locate the condition not at the onset of menstruation, when blood loss began, but at an even earlier stage. Clifford Allbutt (1909, cited in Siddall 1982: 255; cf. Brumberg 1982: 1471) argued that the condition was more likely to develop 'prior to the onset of the menses'. Writing in the late nineteenth century, Raciborski (1868: 379) suggested that 'Chlorosis usually begins on drawing near to puberty' and regarded it as a factor delaying menarche by about eighteen months:

> It is not unusual to find young chlorotic girls of 15 or 16 years of age, who have not yet begun to menstruate, even among girls coming from wealthy families, and living in large cities.[10]

However, he did not regard the absence of menstruation as the direct cause of chlorosis (1868: 380–1). We can thus see a shift from the belief that the blood loss of first menstruation causes chlorosis, to the idea that chlorosis delays first menstruation; the link between menstruation and the disease takes many different forms, which in turn require different readings of the respective roles of 'food and the growth of the body'.

Pica

In *Aristotle's Masterpiece* (Anon. 1694: 2–3) we read that young girls at the age of puberty further increase their chances of developing chlorosis by eating 'salt sharp things' such as spices, which heat up the body and additionally stimulate the sexual appetites. So, another way of interpreting the Hippocratic reference to 'food and the growth of the body' would be to understand by 'food' a reference to particular foodstuffs deemed unsuitable. For the *Masterpiece*, such substances make the body too hot, but other writers suggest that the main problem with unsuitable foods is their effect on the channels which carry blood around the body. For example, in de Baillou's account of the 'foul colours', the veins of the otherwise mature young girl are often made narrow by 'perverse foods or a leisured and idle life' so that the route the blood needs to take is blocked. The reference to life style picks up another common theme in ancient Greek gynaecology: women menstruate not only because they have naturally more spongy flesh which retains excess blood, but also because they have a more sedentary life style than men.[11] A certain level of idleness is normal to women – indeed, part of their socially defined role, as guardians of the home[12] – but if they are downright idle then a plethora of menstrual blood or seed will inevitably build up (Paré 1575: 787–8). As in the Hippocratic *On the disease of virgins*, medicine here defines women's roles and threatens them with the consequences of rebellion against their assigned tasks.

Where Lange shows us a girl whose refusal of meat could be interpreted as an attempt to delay menstruation and thus avoid womanhood, de Baillou implies that the deliberate ingestion of specific substances is partly to blame for the disorder. What could he mean by 'perverse foods'? The *Masterpiece*'s statement that hot foods increase sexual desire was repeated widely in medical writing of this period, and continued to be expressed up to the nineteenth century (Hudson 1977: 457). Rebello, who wrote in the thirteenth century and whose handbook was printed in 1550, claimed that 'hote meates [i.e. foods] and such as do encrease much seed' are responsible for lust in both sexes. Hot foods can therefore be to blame for chlorosis, if it is seen as the result of an excess of passion without a suitable outlet.

But an alternative dietary aetiology also exists elsewhere in the *Masterpiece*, in a list of non-food substances such as 'Ashes, Coals, old Shoes, Chalk, Wax, Nut-shells, Mortar, Lime, Oat meal, Tobbacco-Pipes' (Anon. 1694: 72; cf. Tanner 1659: 314; Sennert 1664: 101; Sharp 1671: 263, Hobby 1999: 196). Other works of this period describe how these substances block up the blood vessels and obstruct the menstrual flow (*Aristotle's Compleat Midwife* 1659: 237–8). Some descriptions of chlorosis use more than one type of eating disorder; for example, Mercado (1579: 201, 211) follows *On the disease of virgins* and Lange by saying that the disorder strikes 'when virgins are already ripe for a man' but adds that it may affect younger girls if they eat perverse foods. He thus extends the vulnerable age group, if the other contributing factors of excessively blood-producing foods or blockage caused by non-foods are present. In the nineteenth century, Fogo (1803: 44–5) included lime, chalk, ashes and salt in his list of substances consumed by the green-sick girl, but made them into a form of self-help rather than an aggravating cause, suggesting that they were eaten to absorb the 'acrimonious ... liquor secreted by the stomach'. Anorexia and pica were linked by Stengel (1896: 348), who said that the patient 'often loses the desire for meat and substantial foods', but added that she may eat earth or 'chalk, plaster from the walls, slate pencils'. Walter Johnson (1849: 4) imagined a personified Chlorosis 'tempting the maiden with a savoury morsel of slate-pencil'; Trabuc (1818: 8) included dirty linen in his list of foods consumed by chlorotic girls, and Johnson (1849: 34) also imagined a patient 'eternally nibbling the contents of her work-basket'.

Current theories about pica in medical anthropology encompass the views that it is a cultural phenomenon – even considered normal in certain groups – that it is psychological, done in order to gain attention; that it is a response to hunger, or to a shortage of a particular nutrient; that it restores the normal intestinal pH; or that it dries the mouth when there is excessive production of saliva (Lackey 1978: 121–8; *contra* Loudon 1984: 30). It has also been suggested, on the one hand, that it is the result of iron deficiency, and, on the other hand, that – if clays are consumed – it exacerbates the problem of iron deficiency by preventing the proper absorption of iron (Hudson 1977: 454).

However, Starobinski (1981: 460) has cited seventeenth-century sources which clearly show that girls were thought to be eating these substances for another reason; to give themselves the pale complexion which was considered socially attractive. In the early eighteenth century John Maubray (1724: 43) commented on the disease label 'Foedus seu pallidus Virginum color', 'the ugly pale colour of languishing Virgins', that 'I have seen many women, in France, and in Germany, who have been so far from thinking it an ugly Colour, that they have esteem'd it most Beautiful; and have used very pernicious things to gain and appropriate this Colour to Themselves: Esteeming Fresh-Looking-Women, of a fine sanguine Complexion, mere Rusticks'. Maubray gave a town/country slant to his description, but the suggestion that vanity lay behind the condition was not a new one. As we saw in chapter 1, William Bullein (1558: 115r; 1559: 217), whose work was not known to Starobinski, gave the earliest explicit statement of this kind, when he described girls who 'would fayne be fayre' eating foods which dried up their blood, and then contracting green sickness. Walter Cary (1583: 40–1) claimed that green sickness affected 'maidens, who either of follie desire to abate their colour, and to be over fine; or otherwise of childish appetite feed upon such things, as change the state of their bodies, which are these: apples, pears, plums, cheries, and generallie all rawe fruites and hearbs; also oatmeale, wheat, barlie, rawe milke, and manie other things of like nature'. Varandal (1619: 5; 1620: 2) similarly claimed that the epidemic of chlorosis in his own time was due to 'virgins and weak unmarried women'[13] trying to gain a more beautiful appearance by changing their diet to become more pale. A further intrinsic contradiction in chlorosis becomes apparent here: on the one hand, a pale complexion was regarded as attractive, and girls would abuse their bodies in order to achieve it, while on the other hand girls with greensickness were described as having a 'bad' or even 'ugly' colour.

In Victorian thought, Brumberg (1988: 175) has suggested that 'nonnutritive eating constituted proof of the fact that the adolescent girl was essentially out of control and that the process of sexual maturation could generate voracious and dangerous appetites'. Strange food cravings were seen as normal for girls at this age, and were regarded as evidence of their emerging sexuality; indeed, the dietary signs of the young female masturbator overlapped with those of chlorosis, Mary Wood-Allen citing 'desiring mustard, pepper, vinegar and spices, cloves, clay, salt, chalk, charcoal, etc.' (cited in Brumberg 1988: 175). Brumberg therefore argues that a woman's appetite acted as a moral barometer (1988: 182). Following dietary fashions was also regarded as a cause of chlorosis; in the eighteenth century, drinking too much sweet coffee was thought to be involved (James 1743: s.v. chlorosis). By the late eighteenth century, attention turned from coffee to tea; for example, Lettsom's discussion of outbreaks of chlorosis in boarding schools[14] recommended that tea should be taken only as a special treat (1795: 17), and feather beds avoided at all costs (1795: 29). But coffee too remained a target for medical writers (e.g. Johnson 1849: 17). By the end of the nineteenth century, it was argued that sufferers used tea as a substitute for a nourishing meal, or took tea with food to reduce the appetite (Stockman 1895b: 1476).

Although Lange made no reference to pica in his letter, and merely mentioned an aversion to food and, in particular, to meat, there is another aspect of his description which could suggest that dietary behaviour blocks the veins. As we have seen, in ancient Greek theory, the channels inside a young unmarried girl's body are seen as very narrow. To this, Lange adds the extra factor of abnormally thick blood.[15] In Galenic theory, fasting causes the blood to become thicker, so that it flows less quickly; in *On bloodletting against Erasistratus* 3, he states that 'in fasting the blood is dried up and becomes thicker, and hence is rendered less free-flowing' (K 11.205; Brain 1986: 47). Anna is described as having an aversion to food; according to this theory, then, fasting in itself could be enough to block the veins. Paré (1575: 789), writing only a few years after Lange, in 1561, discussed how blood which is too 'thick and sticky' can cause menstrual suppression, but he goes on to give an extra reason why blockage would more readily affect girls of this age. He suggests that the blood of a girl who has only recently started to menstruate is 'still undigested, and not cooked' (Paré 1575: 792) and goes on to describe how, if such a girl waits too long for marriage, suffocation of the womb will ensue, together with a weakness of the heart and the rotting of unused seed. He lists as further symptoms palpitation and depraved appetite, inability to sleep, a pale and yellowish colour, and swelling. He ends, 'So then, to avoid such occurrences, I advise the family and friends of the girl, that if she is of the right age and maturity, they should marry her to a man who has enough to pay, so that he won't defraud the merchants.' This is heavily dependent on *On the disease of virgins*, but the debt is not acknowledged. I would suggest that the position of pica in lists of symptoms from the later history of chlorosis is largely due to Lange's idea, of sluggish blood blocking the veins, being reinterpreted in terms of a deliberate practice on the part of the patient being responsible for the blockage.

In medical writers, pica in chlorosis is acknowledged to be a particular problem because it is more commonly associated with pregnancy. When the sixth-century AD Aetius of Amida (16.10) explained the cravings of pregnancy, he envisaged a bloody humour, normally expelled every month, rising up and attacking the stomach. To satisfy this humour, women would crave salty or acidic foods, sand, oyster shells and ashes, up to the fourth month of pregnancy. 'Sharp' humours (*vitiosi humores*) were also held responsible for pica in young girls; for example, Amatus Lusitanus (1556: 296–7) described a girl of 12, 'pale in face, thin in posture, who suffered from a morbid appetite'. She consumed indiscriminately pebbles, earth, chalk, cotton, wool and similar substances. In pregnant women, the humoral material could be removed by vomiting – this accounted for morning sickness in the early months of pregnancy – and by the growth of the foetus, the condition coming to an end when the foetus is drawing more blood to itself for nourishment.

But was the pica of a pregnant woman the same as that of a green-sick girl? Jane Sharp describes green-sick girls as 'longing after hurtful things' (1671: 257; Hobby 1999: 195), while pregnant women 'desire unnatural things' (1671: 292; Hobby 1999: 218).[16] In the eighteenth century, Turner (1714: 91) proposed a similar way to distinguish between two types of pica: the pica of pregnant women, who 'crave Things rather difficult sometimes to be obtain'd' and that of virgins, who long for 'Things absur'd or unnatural'. Whereas it was common knowledge that to refuse a pregnant woman what she craved would cause her to miscarry,[17] girls with green sickness were to be kept away from the foods they desired (Sharp 1671: 263–4; Hobby 1999: 199). Such distinctions did not meet with universal acceptance. A century later, Rue (1819: 7) and Trabuc (1818: 10) noted that the dietary symptoms of chlorosis resemble those of the first months of pregnancy; doctors must therefore be on their guard, Trabuc warned, as there are some girls who try to conceal an unwanted pregnancy behind a diagnosis of chlorosis. If these girls are treated with emmenagogues or other ways of 'exciting' the womb, the doctor will be causing an abortion – which could endanger his reputation. The use of emmenagogues on girls at menarche was condemned by Raciborski (1868: 280) because they would irritate the stomach and the digestive function. Von Noorden (1905: 360) claimed that 'chlorosis resembles the early stages of pregnancy', and added a further source of confusion, the suggestion that the symptoms of chlorosis are worse in the morning (1905: 357); it was, he said, the 'family and friends of the patient' who were most likely to assume that an unmarried pregnant girl is in fact suffering from chlorosis (von Noorden 1905: 475–6). Here, the doctor moves from being the kindly father-figure of Lange treating Anna, and becomes the bearer of the unpalatable truth which those around the girl deny.

'Food' can then be understood as a poor diet, or anorexia thickening the blood, or unsuitable foods blocking the veins, overheating the body or producing excess fluids: 'growth' can imply the additional needs posed by the onset of pubertal growth, or its completion leading to an unused surplus of blood. The vagueness of the Hippocratic phrase allows for its reinterpretation as ideas about disease causation and cure change over time.

Green sickness as a liver disorder

A further possibility is that Anna's aversion to meat is caused by another part of her body; this would suggest that the disease should be classified as a dietary disorder, thus returning it to its origins in 'green jaundice' (see chapter 1). When Lange discussed the opinion of the other physicians who had been called in to treat Anna, he said that some believed a 'defect of the liver has caused an aversion [towards food] in the stomach'. The idea that the liver was the organ responsible could be given Hippocratic authority; in his discussion on 'De foedis virginum coloribus', de Baillou (1643: 146) drew attention to a passage of Epidemics (2.1.10; L 5.82) stating that 'colours, yellowish, greenish, dead white are to be observed, since everything of this kind comes from the liver'.

The Galenic idea of the liver as the central organ in the process by which food becomes blood – discussed in chapter 3 – tended to shift into the background when chlorosis was established as a medical diagnosis inextricably linked to menstruation and to virgins, and best cured by marriage. It was not, however, forgotten; Walter Cary regarded the liver's inability to make good blood as the real cause (1583: 40), while Jane Sharp suggested that there was a risk that green sickness could develop into a more severe form in which 'the liver grows hard like a stone that it can make no blood' (1671: 258; Hobby 1999: 196). In medical disputes over the construction of the disease in the late eighteenth and early nineteenth century the liver again played an important part. If chlorosis was regarded as a liver disease, then this would automatically raise as a possibility the existence of male chlorosis.

A significant figure in medical classification in this period was William Cullen, the Professor of Physic at Edinburgh. His classification of diseases, used in the *Edinburgh Practice of Physic*, placed chlorosis in class II, the neuroses. Within this class it was further distinguished as lying within order II, the *Adynamiae*, characterised by 'A diminution of the involuntary motions, whether vital or natural'. Chlorosis itself appeared as genus *xlvii*, being listed after Hypochondriasis, and embracing only one idiopathic species, called either *chlorosis virginea* or *chlorosis amatoria*. It was said to occur a little after puberty; its most distinctive symptom was given here as the consumption of non-food substances such as lime, chalk, ashes or salt, but it also led to symptoms of sluggishness, lassitude, debility, dyspepsia, a pale or yellowish face, swollen feet, breathlessness at any exertion, palpitations and – sometimes – headache (Cullen 1786: 34–5). According to the second volume of the *Edinburgh Practice of Physic* (1803: 361–2), it could be caused by 'love and other passions of the mind', and cured by the stimulus to the womb provided by 'indulgence in venery'; the appearance of the menses was regarded as evidence of a cure.

In Cullen's work, menstruation remained central not only to the cure of chlorosis, but also to its origins (Risse 1986: 130). Elsewhere, Cullen (1786: 33; Hamilton 1787: 126–8) distinguished between menstrual retention – the absence of menarche in a girl of the right age – and menstrual suppression, in which the menses ceased to appear in a woman who had previously had them for some time, and who was not pregnant. He believed that chlorosis was a condition 'hardly ever appearing separate from the retention of the menses' (1786: 36), which meant that his definition acted to reinforce its place as a disorder of female puberty. Indeed, Cullen's theory of the causes of normal menarche itself, which described a process of 'topical congestion', made chlorosis fit most naturally into this time of the female life-cycle. He rejected the theory of 'plethora', by which it was thought that more blood was present than the body could cope with, either because of a surplus of blood being produced, or because the vessels through which it passed were constricted (Hamilton 1787: 55).

In order to explain why menarche occurred, Cullen replaced the theory of plethora with 'topical congestion'. He argued that the system of blood vessels begins to develop into its mature form from the top of the body downwards. Once vessels have reached their mature size, they resist further growth and push blood on into parts as yet undeveloped. In time, this downward pressure reaches the vessels of the womb, causing them to pour out blood (Hamilton 1787: 56). As in the Hippocratic text *On generation/Nature of the child*, menarche thus marks maturity. In the eighteenth-century model of chlorosis, blood should pour out to mark the completion of the internal vessels, but is retained because of the weak actions of the vessels of the womb (Cullen 1786: 34–5); this contrasts strikingly with sixteenth-century Galenism, in which da Monte insisted that a girl of 15 could not possibly have a womb too weak to perform its expulsive faculty effectively (see p. 78). However, Tardy's commentary on the Hippocratic *On the disease of virgins*, written in 1648, suggested that 'Certain virgins are in fact the most exposed to disorders of the womb, because their wombs grow feeble or remain very weak on account of being exempt from, and deprived of, their own characteristic functions.' He adds that even the strongest girls will suffer in this way at puberty or a little later if they do not marry. For him, the function of a woman is to give birth and, if she fails to fulfil this function, her unemployed womb will naturally weaken. For Cullen, the cure for a weak womb was either to restore tone to the whole system, by tonics, cold baths or electric shocks, or to stimulate the vessels of the womb itself by compression of the iliacs (Cullen 1786: 38–40; Hamilton 1787: 126–8).

According to Cullen's theory, menstrual blood is simply ordinary blood: the challenge is to decide first why women have so much blood that they need to lose some every month, and second why menarche occurs at a particular time in the development of a woman. Neither the nature nor the quality of menstrual blood were, however, something on which medical writers of the time were agreed. For example, the surgeon Andrew Fogo, who in 1803 published an attack on Cullen's theories of amenorrhoea and chlorosis, refers to an alternative theory by which the menses are thought to be a specific secretion of the uterus, and not to be composed of blood at all (Fogo 1803: 10).

Fogo represents part of a wider challenge to Cullen's proposal that the womb was the central organ in the causation of chlorosis, a challenge which not only opened up the possibility of male chlorosis but even led to the suggestion that there was no such thing as a discrete condition of 'chlorosis'. In his *Observations on the opinions of ancient and modern physicians, including those of the late Dr Cullen on Amenorrhoea, or green-sickness* (1803), Fogo described how he moved to Newcastle and found there

several unfortunate instances of the injudicious treatment of young
women, who were thought to be labouring under the supposed
diseases called chlorosis, green-sickness, obstructions, &c.

(1803: introduction, p. 2)

In the main body of his text, he refers to green sickness as just one of the many
names for an 'imaginary disease' also known as 'suppression of the menses, the
want of *them*, *those*, the courses, the flowers, &c.' (1803: 1).

This amenorrhoea, he says, is not the cause, but merely one effect of the
true cause, which lies with the liver. How can retained blood possibly be the
cause, he objects, when one of the symptoms is a pale complexion (1803:
82)? Fogo uses many plant analogies based on the common idea that the
menses are popularly called the 'flowers' because they appear at the proper
season and wither when the 'fruit' sets, in that they cease when a woman is
pregnant; 'flowers promise fruit' (1803: 25).[18] Based on a tabular comparison of their symptoms, he equates dyspepsia, chlorosis, chronic
inflammation of the liver, 'cachexia Africana' and scrofula in children;
'cachexia Africana' is the consumption of earth and other forms of 'dirt'.
Fogo (1803: 45) argues that the consumption of chalk serves the purpose of
absorbing 'the acrimonious ... liquor secreted by the stomach' in the
absence of bile. It is the inflammation and obstruction of the vessels of the
liver which are really responsible for the symptoms of young girls diagnosed
as being chlorotic; enlargement of the liver puts pressure on other organs to
cause back pain and difficulty in breathing, while obstruction of the liver
leads to a yellow complexion (1803: 46, 83).

As for cures, Fogo vigorously attacks Cullen's recommendation of sexual
intercourse to stimulate the system, which he says echoes popular ideas of
chlorosis:

> Her female as well as male visitors are often telling her of a remedy,
> I am ashamed to mention, which would cure her; but which Dr
> Cullen mentions in tolerable plain English.

(1803: 64–5)

James Hamilton, too, found Cullen's label of *chlorosis amatoria* 'offensive
to the modesty of the fair sufferers' (1805: 99–100). The specific idea that
'the common people' continue to recommend marriage as a cure, while
medical opinion has separated itself from this, is also found in Trabuc (1818:
12). But sexual activity, Fogo argues, is the last thing possible for a young
girl who has been diagnosed as suffering from chlorosis; the suggestion
would only be a practical and sensible recommendation if made to married
women, but they are never given the diagnosis of chlorosis because it is so
clearly defined by Cullen himself as exclusive to girls at the onset of
menarche, 'for let a married woman labour under any disease whatever, she is

never suspected to labour under chlorosis' (1803: 80–1). Besides, Fogo adds, when a girl is pale and breathless, 'There is never a man will look at her, except to laugh and make a jest of her' (1803: 81).

Fogo is particularly firm in his condemnation of Cullen's suggested cure of compression of the iliac artery, which he claims was 'invented by some wicked practitioner, to try what a young woman would submit to, for the sake of recovering her health' (1803: 78–9). Fogo's explicit acknowledgement of the circular nature of the condition, in that the label 'chlorosis' is by very definition only applied if the appropriate symptoms appear in *young* girls, is noteworthy. As we saw in chapter 3, at the end of the nineteenth century Frederic Coley (1894: 268) also raised the concern that a 'chlorotic young woman' could marry and then become pregnant, but if this happened then 'her chlorosis is very apt to be overlooked' due to the common assumption that married women could not possibly have it.

In the nineteenth century, then, we can see attempts to extend the category of chlorosis from its original constituency of pubertal virgins, drawing in married women and even pregnant women. Another surgeon who attacked Cullen was Samuel Fox who, like Fogo, argued that chlorosis is not exclusively female, nor 'limited to any particular period of life', but should be understood as deriving from the liver and digestive system. Fox qualified as a member of the Royal College of Surgeons of England on 6 August 1802, and then worked as a naval surgeon before entering general practice at 219 High Street, Shoreditch some time after 1822.[19] In 1839 he wrote *Observations on the disorder of the general health of females called Chlorosis: shewing the true cause to be entirely independent of peculiarities of sex,* the only title credited to him in successive editions of the London and British Medical Directories. He seems to have died in 1854, but his son Oscar Harger Fox (MRCS 1842) continued to practise from the Shoreditch address.

Unlike Fogo, Fox did not give any explanation for his interest in chlorosis. In order to attack Cullen, both men cited their target's work at some length. Fogo tended to read Cullen through Hamilton's *Outlines, Theory and Practice of Midwifery*; Fox made it much clearer when he was using Cullen, and when he was citing Hamilton's commentary on Cullen's ideas.[20] Fox (1839: 52) regarded ill health in young women as most likely two or three years prior to menarche; he rejected any claim that menstruation is essential to health, arguing that women are often in better health after the menopause than they were before it (1839: 27). As for cures for chlorosis, since it is caused by 'a peculiar functional arrangement of the liver and digestive economy' which can occur in women of any age as well as in 'young and delicate' men, he rejected drugs intended to bring on menstruation as 'disgusting and often dangerous' (1839: preface) and regarded the traditional idea that marriage can cure a patient as 'an absurdity, and I must say, obscenity' (1839: 117).

Fogo and Fox were thus saying much the same thing. What is the relationship between their treatises? An answer may lie in the manuscript notes on the text of Fogo held in the Wellcome Institute for the History of Medicine. Unfortunately the text has been cropped, so sentences are incomplete. The annotator comments on Fogo's identification of the liver as the true cause:

> Fogo is perfectly correct in this statement. I flattered myself I alone had discovered the true cause of these symptoms and intended to publish ... Fogo has treated the subject in a more entertaining and equally full manner. He treats the learned ... Physiologists with merited ridicule ... whose stories ought to be consigned ... [21]

Who was the owner of the text who made these notes? Could it have been Fox himself, whose very similar arguments, written in a style far less entertaining than that of the choleric Fogo, were in fact eventually published?[22] Some support for this tentative suggestion may come from the notes on page 90: 'Admiral Darby died of this disease ... Fox Charles Fox ... the same.' Here Fox could be supporting the argument that symptoms of chlorosis can be found in men, as well as women, by referring to a male member of his own family, and to a colleague from his days as a naval surgeon.

Constipation

In the eighteenth century, the lectures of John Rutherford (WMS 6888) delivered in 1748/9 suggested that one aspect of chlorosis was the retention of food for too long in the stomach, and that weakness of the intestines led to constipation because 'the intestines are weak and so can't propell the faeces at their proper times'. The patient under consideration here, Margaret Muckleroy, also had 'a lowe diet', mainly oatmeal and water. The association of constipation with chlorosis was not new; for example, Barker's case notes for 1596 mention Mrs Basnett's daughter, suffering from *morbus virgineus* or green sickness, and describe her as 'Cold and costive',[23] while in 1666 Sudell had stated that the cure began with the correction of the 'distemper of the bowels', using a purge which included mugwort, before going on to bloodletting and other drugs (Sudell 1666: 8).[24] However, what was different in discussions of chlorosis from the eighteenth century onwards was the proposal that constipation was the underlying cause of the problem. It could be linked with menstrual retention, with both being attributed to weak muscles or to a general 'sluggishness' (Reece 1826: 52); Fox (1839: 53–4) stated that the stools were 'of a dark greenish cast' and that exercise was needed to keep the bowels moving. In terms of 'food and the growth of the body', constipation was thought to be exacerbated by a poor diet (e.g. Hurst 1919: 79–80).

Both defecation and menstruation could be placed under the heading of 'excretion', one of the six 'non-naturals' in the Galenic body. Excretion had long featured as one of the aspects of the body requiring careful control to safeguard health, but James Whorton (2000: 15, 38) has suggested that an increased medical concern with waste disposal within the body corresponded with public health improvements, and with the rise of the factory, starting in the 1840s. The body's own sewage system, and its efficient use of materials, soon became an obsession; even before the development of germ theory from the 1860s onwards, constipation came to be feared as the source of foul miasmatic gases rising up the body and causing illness (Whorton 2000: 17). Germ theory simply provided what Whorton (2000: 56–7) has called 'the scientific glamor' which allowed constipation to become the source of the terrifyingly named 'auto-intoxication', a medical fad which peaked in 1900–20.

In the final decades of the nineteenth century, a number of British physicians looked to the end process of digestion to explain chlorosis. Foremost among them was Sir Andrew Clark, who suggested that the cause of chlorosis was 'faecal poisoning', or 'auto-intoxication by faecal products' (Clark 1887: 55).[25] Following James Hamilton (1805: 89), he claimed that sufferers had bad breath, with even a faecal odour; the appetite was irregular; they experienced flatulence, sinking feelings, and pain, often on the left side of the colon; they suffered from constipation or inadequate emptying of the bowels, and 'the faeces, usually scanty, hard, dark, and lumpy, occasionally consist of showers of scybalous masses, embedded in an offensive mucus swarming with bacteria' (1887: 56). Clark regarded the menstruation of these girls as 'usually normal' (1887: 57). As we have already seen, he blamed a new awareness of the body in girls between menarche and womanhood, whose concerns about becoming fat led them to restrict their food intake (p. 100); in addition, their fashionable sense of modesty encouraged them to ignore the urge to open their bowels (Clark 1887: 61; cf. Burne 1840: 162). Clark's advice to sufferers therefore included the suggestion 'do not notice or distrust yourself' (1887: 62–3). The physiology of his theory suggested that the mucous membranes of the bowel, irritated by accumulated faeces, produce 'new substances, ptomaines[26] and leucomaines' which are absorbed into the blood and cause the symptoms (Clark 1887: 62).

What was new about Clark was his concentration on constipation to the complete exclusion of menstrual disorder. Other writers of the second half of the nineteenth century, including the homeopath Ruddock (1892: 75), regarded constipation as a central feature of chlorosis, accompanied by bad breath. However, Ruddock (1892: 78) pointed to the dietary cause of these symptoms: 'Bread-and-butter forming the staple diet, the relish for animal food of every kind almost completely ceases.'

Following Clark, Ralph Stockman (1895a: 415; 1895b: 1473) found moderate or severe constipation in around 50 per cent of chlorosis patients.

Of these, most had 'weak digestions', while some of those who reported no dyspepsia 'ate very little … or were extremely careful in their diet' (1895a: 416). However, Stockman (1895b: 1473) argued against Clark's constipation theory, in which constipation caused ptomaines to break down the red blood cells, and by 1919 this theory was thoroughly discredited (e.g. Hurst 1919: 242). Instead, Stockman believed that the problem was that constipation led girls to eat less food; indeed, 'a totally inadequate amount of food' (Stockman 1895b: 1473). Brumberg (1988: 178) has suggested another sense in which constipation was the reverse side of the Victorian girl's failure to eat; both symptoms were part of the ideal of femininity as something divorced from bodily demands.

Some physicians who saw constipation as the root of all evil believed that women were more likely than men to suffer because their more sedentary life style left them with weaker muscles (e.g. Hamilton 1805: 102; Burne 1840: 167). Others focused on the use of corsets (Whorton 2000: 65–7). For late-nineteenth-century constipation fetishists, the pressure exerted on the colon made it sluggish, reducing natural muscle tone – which was, in any case, weaker in the weaker sex. Twentieth-century scholars trying to explain the apparent rise of chlorosis in the eighteenth and nineteenth centuries, and its subsequent disappearance, have often blamed pressure on the internal organs from corsets (Vertue 1955; Hudson 1977: 457–8), while Hansen railed against 'the deplorable habit of tight-lacing' (1931: 184). This victimisation of female dress also occurred in the remarks of contemporary observers (e.g. Johnson 1849: 13–15), but it becomes clear that fashion shifted many times in the period identified, as well as being different for women of different social classes; Lettsom, writing in 1795, believed that stays cramped the growth of the womb, and praised the looser clothing of his own time (1795: 17).[27] Raciborski (1868: 310–11) saw nothing wrong with corsets, only with their abuse, if the compression they produced became too heavy and prevented proper digestion. But he believed that 'coquetry, which sacrifices everything to fashion, including reason and even health' led girls to adopt an inadequate diet, which was the most common cause of 'chlorosis or the pale colours, a very common disorder among young girls … at the time of puberty' (Raciborski 1868: 285). Even the constipation expert Sir William Arbuthnot Lane, who pioneered the total removal of the colon as a cure for constipation, suggested that some corsets could be beneficial; he and his followers believed that pregnancy was helpful in women sufferers, because a gravid uterus acted as a 'natural' corset, lifting up a sagging bowel and holding it in a better position (Chapple 1918: 323; Whorton 2000: 67). The advice-writer Mary Wood-Allen, who regarded constipation as a problem in young girls because of the pressure it placed on the pelvic organs, recommended wearing a cotton flannel bandage during the day to support the bowel (1898: 123–6).

For other medical writers, chlorosis remained the main problem: constipation was only a symptom, but the toxins it produced exacerbated the symptoms of chlorosis (e.g. Hurst 1919: 242). Constipation 'aggravated and protracted' chlorosis (Burne 1840: 5). The overlap of symptoms included difficulty in breathing, languor (Burne 1840: 96–7) and the skin colour, described by Lane as 'staining', leading to a 'dirty-looking' appearance (Lane 1909: 30, 51–2).

Constipation theory thus represented the final variant on the idea that diet – inadequate, or perverse – lay behind the manifestations of chlorosis. However, this interest in constipation reiterated older themes such as the weakness of the female sex, their vanity, and their coquetry. Even in the writings of Arbuthnot Lane, in the midst of his recommendation of colectomy as the cure for constipation and all its attendant ills, female sexuality remained central. Lane suggested that a woman with good intestinal drainage could be healthy without sexual intercourse but, in a discussion of breast cysts, he claimed that a woman with 'imperfect drainage will of necessity undergo changes of varying severity in her sexual organs if she remains a virgin. Regular sexual intercourse would appear to oppose this cystic degeneration of the breast' (1909: 33). A shift in focus from chlorosis to constipation did not necessarily change the medical insistence on the dangers of virginity.

5

'THE LABORATORY CAME TO THE RESCUE'

Technology and chlorosis

The revived theory of the liver as the origin of the symptoms of chlorosis, and the consequent extension of the category to women of all ages and even to men, was not the end of the story. As the anatomical structures of the body continued to be studied, even chlorosis in girls was sub-divided into new categories. For example, Ashwell argued that, rather than thinking of any incident as 'a common case of green-sickness', one should concentrate on the organ most seriously affected, as chlorosis would head for the weakest organ in the patient (1836: 539). The most difficult variety to cure was when the cerebellum was affected, even though the structures of the brain would remain unaltered (1836: 542). Should chlorosis affect the lung, it would cause previously latent lung diseases to surface (1836: 545). By the end of the nineteenth century, chlorosis had been reinvented yet again, this time as a blood disorder: hypochromic anaemia. In its earlier incarnation as the disease of virgins, blood was responsible for the symptoms because it was too thick and sticky to pass through a virgin's narrow channels into the womb; its thickness could be due to a faulty diet. Because, in the Galenic body, the liver made blood, the idea that the blood was inadequate could be traced back to the liver. In the nineteenth-century version of chlorosis, however, the new science of blood testing involved looking into the blood itself, and measuring its constituent parts to explain the symptoms.

As Joan Jacobs Brumberg (1982: 1469) noted, however, the nineteenth-century refiguring of the condition as hypochromic anaemia does not mean that we can now dismiss the disease of virgins or chlorosis as simply 'a curious, archaic name for iron deficiency anaemia', something which can affect people of either sex and any age. It is clear that, throughout its history, 'chlorosis' could cover far more and, even in the nineteenth century, there remained a strong pull drawing it back to its position of a disease found only in young girls. In the Introduction, I have suggested that, in early modern medicine, academic debates over translations of Greek and Latin texts acted as substitutes for laboratory results, making control of the classical sources into the dominant medical technology. In this chapter I want to concentrate on the diagnosis and treatment of the disease of virgins, and to examine the role played by technological change, in particular in the latter part of its history. The development of new medical technology, above all for blood testing, over the course of the nineteenth century, gave a new life, and increased sophistication, to the idea that chlorosis was in some way related to the blood.

Histories of chlorosis have tended to regard the laboratory as the place where all, finally, became clear. For example, Hudson (1977: 449) claimed that 'it was advance in laboratory medicine which would finally bring physicians close to consensus on the nature of chlorosis', and stated that 'the laboratory came to the rescue' (1977: 451 n. 38), while Campbell (1923: 293) used the phrase 'cases "proved" by blood examination'. The 'rise of the laboratory' is conventionally dated to the period from around 1850 onwards. Clinical writers on chlorosis have shown many areas in which the laboratory was eventually able to distinguish between chlorosis and its imitators. Cabot (1908: 647), for example, looked to blood testing to exclude from the diagnosis of chlorosis those cases which were better described as neurasthenia. Looking back at the prevalence of chlorosis in the nineteenth century, Patek and Heath (1936: 1465) credited tests for detection of occult blood in the stool – developed between 1900 and 1904 – with making it possible to distinguish between chlorosis and peptic ulcers, and X-rays as allowing physicians to separate chlorosis from tuberculosis (cf. Guggenheim 1995: 1823). Ward (1914: 308) suggested that X-rays showed a displacement of the heart in chlorosis. This increasing differentiation could suggest that the mystery of the disappearance of chlorosis was simply due to there being nothing left which had not taken on another name. But, Patek and Heath insisted, 'even with the elimination of such faulty diagnoses there probably did exist a large number of cases of chlorosis' (1936: 1465).

More recent work on medical, and other, technologies suggests that their role is not so benign. For example, Donna Haraway argued that 'Technologies and scientific discourses can be partially understood as formalizations, i.e., as frozen moments, of the fluid social interactions constituting them, but they should also be viewed as instruments for enforcing meanings' (1991: 164, cited in Kelly 2000: 12). Writing on chlorosis and other blood disorders, Keith Wailoo suggested that technologies – glossed here as 'knowledge-producing tools', a reading which allows us to include under this umbrella the classical medical texts which were the instruments of medicine in the early modern period – are still 'constituting, creating and complicating diseases in our time' (1997: 13 and 2). His account links the disappearance of chlorosis not only to the changing politics of American womanhood but also to a decline in the family doctor, in favour of the hospital as the place where medical knowledge is produced. Certainly, in nineteenth-century medical writing, we can detect increasingly insistent claims that the physician should be invited to participate in ever more intimate areas of the patient's life; such claims could be read as a rear-guard action against the increasing prestige of the laboratory and of the hospital. For example, Raciborski (1868: 278–9) was adamant that the interests of the family would best be served by involving the physician in 'all the business of health within the family' from the choice of a wet-nurse onwards. Taken with Haraway's work, this would suggest that chlorosis was increasingly defined out of existence by the laboratory, but that this occurred within a context in which the meaning of chlorosis, as a pressing reason for early marriage and as grounds for medicalising a stage of normal physical development, was no longer needed. The disappearance of chlorosis in the early twentieth century coincided with changed roles for women, including their entry into all levels of the medical profession and medical science; however, as I will show in the final section of this chapter, being a medically trained woman did not necessarily mean regarding chlorosis, and its causes and treatments, any differently.

The pulse

What technology was available to the physician trying to diagnose the disease of virgins before the nineteenth century? Most diagnosis relied on the senses (Bynum and Porter 1993), but above all trust was placed in the testimony of the patient. John Johnston's description of menstrual suppression (1657: 75) stated that 'The SIGNS are afforded from the relation of the woman herself'; it was only 'if they wil not confess' that the physician needed to go further. Hearing the symptoms of the sufferer and, in incidents of this condition, simply noting her status as a young unmarried girl, the physician could confidently assume that this was a case of the disease of virgins. But the disease picture given by Sydenham (see p.14) also included some symptoms which may seem amenable to quantification: in particular, 'feverish pulse'. A fast and frequent pulse was thought to be characteristic of the disease of virgins (e.g. Mercado 1579: 202), but also featured in the history of the cousin of the virgins' disease, love sickness; most famously, Galen diagnosed the passion felt by the wife of Justus for a man beneath her social class, after detecting a change when the name of the beloved was spoken in the presence of the sufferer (Nutton 1979: 103; Wack 1990: 7–9).[1] But Galen denied that 'love sickness' was a somatic disease due to humoral disturbance, and in this case the pulse was only described as erratic. A general statement of a 'quick' pulse is found in early descriptions of the signs of the virgins' disease; for example, John Tanner (1659: 315) wrote that 'the Pulse is swift and quick as in a Feaver', and François Ranchin (1627: 382) included a rapid pulse, arguing that this implied the disease was a 'hot' one.

Although an interest in the pulse as an indicator of health and disease was part of Galenic medicine (Bylebyl 1971), particularly important in showing whether bloodletting was needed (Fissell 1991: 101), quantification in taking the pulse was not an ancient concept, but developed only in the eighteenth century, when it was stressed that the frequency of the pulse was the one aspect which could be agreed between two commentators (Gibbs 1971: 189). This point about technology facilitating comparison was also made in the period in which the sphygmomanometer was introduced, after 1890. But the new technology met with resistance; in the early days of quantification it was difficult to know where the boundary between normal and abnormal lay (Evans 1993: 784–5), and medical instruments were additionally seen as reducing medicine from the status of a profession, to that of a trade, bringing in negative nuances attached to factories and machines (Evans 1993: 802).

Even when the pulse was being described in quantitative terms, other, more qualitative, aspects of what was felt with the physician's finger continued to be described. In *The Physician's Pulse-Watch* Sir John Floyer used Chinese techniques of feeling the pulse, combined with a special watch made for the purpose; he believed that 'Our Life consists in the Circulation of blood, and that running too fast or too slow, produces most of our Diseases' (1707: preface). However, despite his interest in his 'New Mechanical Method', he believed that the tool was a way of improving the senses of the physician, rather than a substitute for them. He continued to use concepts such as the 'vermicular pulse' – slow and small, like a worm crawling – and the 'formicant pulse' – weak, small and frequent, like an ant (1707: 50–1). He believed that the pulse in a woman is weaker, because of her cooler nature and more sedentary life (1707: 70), and would be higher in a woman carrying a male child than in one pregnant with a girl (1707: 310). In white fever or green sickness, however, the pulse rises to 90 beats per minute (1707: 225) because 'the Menses are suppress'd, which makes the Pulse quick and frequent; and the Pulse appears beating violently in the neck. Most suppressions of Humours naturally evacuated, ferment the Blood; and the Stop of the Menses produce the *febris alba*' (1707: 122).

A generation later John Rutherford (WMS 6888) said of his chlorosis patient Margaret Muckleroy, 'her pulse is weak and frequent but this I don't take to be a very bad symptom in her case; for such a pulse generally attends a chlorosis'. A quick, but feeble, pulse was also expected by the medical men who discussed chlorosis in nineteenth-century medical journals (e.g. Ashwell 1836: 534) and features in self-help manuals for women (e.g. McMurtrie 1871: 219). But it had never been the subject of universal agreement; while her source, Sennert's *Practical Physick* (1664: 101) described the pulse in green sickness as 'little and often', Jane Sharp characterised it as 'little and faint' (1671: 258; Hobby 1999: 196), while Walter Johnson (1849: 40) noted that the pulse could be very slow in chlorosis, down to 40–50 beats per minute, and Gordon Ward (1914: 308) suggested it was only in some patients that the pulse rate went up. Measuring and counting were regarded with mixed emotions by the medical profession. As a way of avoiding being deceived by the patient, they were to be welcomed, but there was often a sense that the figures could be trusted even less than the words of the patient. The insistence on qualitative aspects could be interpreted as a way of maintaining a role for the trained physician; if numbers alone could be used to diagnose, then lay people with access to the technology would be able to manage their own health.

The stethoscope

The stethoscope was introduced by René-Théophile-Hyacinthe Laennec in 1816, and his work was translated into English in 1822. Uneasy about the propriety of putting his ear to the chest of a young woman patient, Laennec used a rolled-up piece of paper to distance himself from direct physical contact, and then went on to develop a wooden cylinder (Reiser 1993: 828–32).

The stethoscope could be seen as a further move towards objective measures of quantity – how many beats, and the pattern of the beats – rather than subjective quality. However, as with the pulse, a subjective sense of what was heard continued to dominate, with users resorting to creating analogies with other sounds in order to communicate the subtleties of what they heard with the new instrument. There was nothing obvious about the sounds of the body; Malcolm Nicolson (1993: 135) has shown how 'we must distinguish between two groups of nineteenth-century commentators on stethoscopy – those whose senses were educated in the use of the instrument and those whose senses were not … the ears of the participating doctors had to be retrained' (cf. Youngson 1979: 20).

Patients were awed, terrified and baffled by this new technical tool to aid the sense of hearing (Reiser 1993: 832), but during the nineteenth century doctors too often questioned its reliability. Samuel Ashwell explained his own rejection of the stethoscope as a diagnostic tool in chlorosis because, 'I am fearful of [the practitioner] attaching too much importance to the absence of physiological evidence of this disease' (1836: 579). If the physician were to wait until 'auscultation[2] affords proof that organic change is actually commencing' then it would be too late for effective treatment. Here, reliance on the technology could damage the patient by preventing an early diagnosis. Trousseau, who regarded chlorosis as a nervous disease (1872: 106), raised many, more general, doubts about the value of the sounds heard by auscultation; they do not, he warned, have 'the semeiotic value hitherto attributed to them' (1872: 102).

A particular sound labelled *'le bruit de diable'*, a 'soft, continuous humming heard by the stethoscope over the veins of the neck' (Cabot 1908: 645) was first associated with chlorosis by Bouillard in 1841 (Trousseau 1872: 100). Clark (1887: 1004) identified several different sounds: 'a systolic bruit is heard within the pulmonary area; … rarely a bruit may be heard over any of the orifices, and even at the diastolic time; ... the larger vessels are liable to attacks of local throbbings, and ... slight compression of their walls elicits a systolic and sometimes also a diastolic murmur; ... the pulse, varying in frequency, quickness, and force, is deficient in tension, and moderately full'. Most characteristic, however, was the sound at the neck, which could be glossed as 'a venous hum' (Bramwell 1899: 41), or described as resembling the sound of the sea heard in a shell (Johnson 1849: 40). At Guy's Hospital, this sound was known as the 'tearing-cotton murmur' (Johnson 1849: 41). Although Trousseau (1872: 95, 102) presented a 'blowing murmur in the vessels of the neck', attributed to a spasm in the veins, as characteristic of chlorosis, he nevertheless argued that there was a danger that this sound could also occur in patients with tuberculosis or syphilis, or could still be heard in cured chlorotics. He therefore urged that only a very intense sound, resembling 'the purring of a cat when it is being caressed, or the noise of a spinning-wheel' (1872: 100), could be regarded as truly significant.

In 1894 Frederic Coley, who worked at the Northern Counties Hospital for Diseases of the Chest, and also at the Hospital for Sick Children in Newcastle, published an article in *The Practitioner* on the physical signs of chlorosis. His particular concern was that it was difficult to distinguish between heart disease and chlorosis, due to shortness of breath being a symptom of both. He rejected the *'bruit de diable'* as 'having little clinical value' (1894: 264), but argued that the sounds heard in the pulmonary region provided a useful guide as to how far the disease had damaged the heart. In particular, he suggested that damage to the mitral valve was very common in chlorosis. In favour of his theory that this damage was often caused entirely by the chlorosis, he argued that treatment always led to the abnormal sounds disappearing. However, severe chlorosis did not invariably mean intense sounds. By 1914, Ward dismissed systolic murmurs as 'here one day and gone the next', and said that the *'bruit de diable'* was found in only half the cases seen (1914: 308). The search for diagnostic certainty by means of the sense of hearing was abandoned.

Blood testing

Ever since the introduction of the microscope, in the seventeenth century, the idea that what is visible to the researcher is the final level which exists has been questioned. Roe (1981a: 84) argued that the use of microscopes actually encouraged the idea of 'invisible structures' at an even lower level, which only a better microscope would make visible. The quest for access to a world beneath the senses led to the development of better lenses, and more complex technology for viewing the body. Blood, seen as the life-force within the body, was studied with particular care; early experiments with blood transfusion between animals by Richard Lower in the seventeenth century, and James Blundell's first use of transfusion between humans in 1825, eventually led to a classification of blood types. Such work was not, of course, exempt from a social agenda. By the 1920s, aspects of women's blood were used to support their different role in society. In England, the 1923 Report of the Board of Education used the lower haemoglobin level in the blood of girls as an argument against equality of access to education (Dyhouse 1981: 133); in fact this is an entirely normal biological difference between the sexes, women normally having 14 per cent less haemoglobin than men (Bartels 1982: 262). Blood chemistry was also used to provide a rationale for treating adolescent girls with great care; for example, a deficiency in calcium – which, again, is normal for women, who have a 10–15 per cent lower level in their blood than men – was thought to make girls more excitable than boys (Dyhouse 1981: 132–3). Medical writers who acknowledged that healthy women had blood different from that of healthy men nevertheless argued for a form of inferiority: 'Their blood is therefore less able to withstand any drain on it' (Stockman 1895b: 1473).

The first blood counts were performed in the mid-nineteenth century by Karl Vierordt of Tübingen, but his techniques for measuring the number of red cells were quickly developed by other researchers trying to make the process both faster and more accurate (Verso 1964). The French physician Georges Hayem published a method for measuring haemoglobin in 1875–6 (Verso 1981: 7), and in 1877 Sir William Richard Gowers developed what he claimed was a more reliable method of counting which became popular; he invented a haemocytometer, a device enabling the user to count the number of red corpuscles in a diluted sample of blood, and a haemoglobinometer, in which 'blood was diluted until it matched a picrocarmine standard' (Verso 1971: 62–4). Writing in the *Lancet*, Gowers (1878: 675) described his gadgets as being more accurate than 'the observation of the colour of the skin and mucous membranes' in judging the efficacy of remedies administered to improve the blood. But he readily admitted that there were several possible sources of error in the equipment he used; for example, the diluting solution altered the appearance of the red cells, making them more difficult to distinguish from the larger white cells (Gowers 1877: 798). Other difficulties lay in transferring the right amount of diluted blood from the pipette, and distributing it evenly across the flat surface on which it would be counted using a squared plate. With a haemocytometer, the blood needs to be distributed evenly in the counting chamber (Verso 1964: 156); with other methods, such as the haemoglobinometer, it is necessary to rely on subjective elements such as the colour of the blood and its closeness to the colour of the tube, or on judging the degree of abnormality of the shape of the cells, another factor which was considered significant in chlorosis (Stockman 1895a: 415). As with the stethoscope, it was necessary to retrain the senses, and testing could still be combined with traditional sensory evidence. Bramwell (1899: 38–41, 53) discussed the use of the sphygmograph and the haemoglobinometer but used old-fashioned observation and touch alongside; he claimed that the '*bruit de diable*' could not only be heard, but also felt with the finger in some cases, while 'A flickering pulsation ... in the dilated external vein' (1899: 41) could often be seen. Alongside the use of increasingly sophisticated technologies, the insistence on the direct first-hand evidence of the medical gaze – 'I actually saw a woman turn green' – remained intact.

Raciborski (1868: 285) considered that 'the nature of chlorosis consists in the impoverishment of the blood, and more particularly in the reduction – more or less considerable – of the ... blood corpuscles'. He cited the work of Andral and of Gavarret as demonstrating that the reduction of corpuscles in chlorosis was unique to this disease. Medical writers were quick to latch on to the significance of the level of the red cells in chlorosis so that, by the 1890s, 'a striking deficiency of red corpuscles' was considered to be characteristic of the condition (Stockman 1895a: 414). Taylor (1896: 720) also blamed the condition on 'a defect in the formation of the corpuscles'; Ward (1914: 315; cf. Heath and Patek 1937: 326) regarded the red cells of a chlorotic as smaller than normal red cells. Bramwell (1899: 32–3) stated that, in sufferers, the red cells would be as low as 2,500,000–3,500,000 per cubic millimetre, or even 1,500,000 in rare cases, with haemoglobin down to 20 per cent or below. These figures were disputed: Ward (1914: 315) thought that chlorosis was implicated with red cells below 4,000,000 per cubic millimetre and haemoglobin at 20 to 30 per cent: 'this is very characteristic of the disease as a similar disproportion is seldom seen in any other condition'. In a healthy young woman, the average figure for red cells was considered to be 4,500,000, with haemoglobin at 80–90 per cent. Campbell's discussion of chlorosis used a number of different criteria based on the blood; he argued that it was necessary to have a haemoglobin level of 60 per cent or less to count as 'chlorosis' (1923: 256), while blood volume would be high, being double the normal amount of 3.2 litres (Campbell 1923: 262), and specific gravity low as a result of the deficiency of red corpuscles (1923: 265). The haemoglobinometer was also used to monitor the effects of treatment (e.g. Bramwell 1899: 53).

Although Keith Wailoo (1997: 29) is correct to note that the label of hypochromic anaemia shifts the focus from the sufferer's moral behaviour – her dietary foibles, her flirtations with new fashions, her excessive interest in her own appearance – and on to the objective qualities of the blood, this transformation should not be overstated. The idea that the blood of sufferers was in some way 'weak' or 'pale', 'watery' and 'impoverished' (Drysdale 1875: 166), containing an insufficient number of red cells, replicated the observation of weakness and paleness in the patient herself. Menarche, dressed up in the language of blood testing, returned as the root of the problem; at the end of the nineteenth century, for example, in a report to the British Medical Association Scientific Grants Committee, the pathologist

Ernest Lloyd Jones (1897: 9, 57–8) argued that chlorosis was indeed properly associated with pubertal girls, because the onset of menstruation led to a fall in the specific gravity of the blood. While rejecting 'menstrual defects' as the ultimate cause of chlorosis, Frederick Taylor, a lecturer at Guy's Medical School, nevertheless argued that the disease was restricted to 'the female sex, and the age of puberty and early womanhood' (1896: 719–20). Beneath the new language of blood testing, the traditional image of the disease of virgins showed little change; instead, the laboratory reinforced Lange's picture of the girl who is 'pale, as if bloodless'.

Treatments

To what extent did the laboratory lead to change in the treatments offered to sufferers? In chapter 3, I discussed the two main therapies applied to the disease of virgins within the Galenic model of the body, and beyond: marriage, and bloodletting. As a substitute for bloodletting, cupping glasses – those 'deputies of bleeding' (Johnston 1657: 75) – could be used. From Lange onwards, a combination of remedies was usually applied: Lange himself brought together the Hippocratic recommendation of marriage, the Galenic use of bloodletting, and 'medicines for provoking the menses and for opening up obstructions, to refine the coarse blood'. Bloodletting continued to be used for chlorosis throughout the nineteenth century; one remedy suggested by Edward Tilt (1853: 116) consisted of applying six to eight leeches to 'the cutaneous parts of the labia'. Although no longer using leeches, letting blood was still being recommended for chlorosis in 1914 (Ward 1914: 322). Dietary adjustments were used from the sixteenth century onwards, with behavioural therapy: the rest cure, and exercise. Surgery, in the form of operations to perforate the hymen and let out the retained menstrual blood, was used for chlorosis in the eighteenth century (Lord 1999: 51–2), but the operation was rarely performed because parents did not want their daughters to have it done, regarding it as a loss of virginity.

In the nineteenth century, electricity was also used to treat chlorosis. Static electricity was employed in medicine from the mid-eighteenth century onwards, but electricity became more popular still in the mid-nineteenth century, when direct current (galvanic) and alternating current (faradic) electricity were developed (Whorton 2000: 153–4; Rowbottom and Susskind 1984). Cadwallader Evans (1757: 83–5) gave the case of a girl of 13, with obstructed menstrual flow thought to be due to 'exposing herself to cold'. The patient herself decided to try electricity, and visited Benjamin Franklin in Philadelphia. After two weeks there, she went home with 'a glass and bottle, to electrify myself every day for three months' (cited in Evans 1757: 85): she was then cured. The use of electricity in treatments for chlorosis peaked in the 1880s–90s. Reece (1826: 56) considered that gentle electric shocks would stimulate the womb, while Habershon (1863: 552) also claimed that, in some cases of chlorosis, electricity 'has been followed by a speedy cure'. Trabuc (1818: 16) doubted the value of magnetism, but still recommended the use of electricity to increase the 'animal heat' and to provoke the menses and other secretions.

In retrospect, we can argue that all forms of treatment could also have caused illness. Siddall, for example, linked the apparently high incidence of the condition in the nineteenth century to the popularity of bloodletting for gynaecological disorders, and suggests that, in this period at least, chlorosis was 'an iatrogenic syndrome' (1982: 254). However, as bloodletting was used for the condition over a much longer period of time, this argument cannot be supported (Loudon 1984: 28). Hudson (1977: 454) pointed out that, even where iron deficiency may have contributed to the picture of symptoms, the sufferers' reported practice of eating chalk or clay would sometimes have prevented this treatment from working, and chalk was also prescribed for chlorosis; the hydropathist Sebastian Kneipp recommended as 'an excellent remedy against green sickness ... a pinch of powdered chalk in four to six spoonfuls of water twice daily' (1893: 135). The laxatives given to ease constipation contained substances, such as magnesium salts, which would bind ingested iron so that it could not be absorbed (Hudson 1977: 454). James Oliver (1893: 35), for example, insisted on the need to clear up the constipation first, because otherwise iron would not work. Chlorotics were also thought by Coley (1894: 268) to be in particular danger of developing phthisis, and Trousseau considered that the administration of iron for 'false chlorosis' in tubercular girls may even have encouraged their tuberculosis to move from latency to an active condition (1872: 97).[3]

Many of the drug treatments used in pre-modern medicine would have had an obvious effect; they would have made patients sweat, vomit, and void blood, urine or faeces; as George Drysdale wrote, 'there is a popular prejudice in favour of "a good active purgation"' (1875: 170). What could not be known by physicians was whether these physical effects were also curing the disease (Risse 1986: 365). But producing a visible result was obviously impressive; in this, emmenagogues and bloodletting were equally 'effective' in a humoral body because, if the condition was thought to be due to retained blood, then letting the blood out would be thought to produce relief. As we have seen in chapter 3, however, John Rutherford's lectures for 1748/9 warned against using drugs to 'occasion a shewing as it is called by the Common People', because these did not reach the real cause of the problem (see p. 68). He hints here at a conscious distancing of academic medicine from the ideas of the 'Common People', the latter continuing to feel that a good humoral evacuation is what is needed. This idea seems to have persisted among lay people into at least the mid-nineteenth century, when writers continued to feel it incumbent upon them to warn of the dangers of emmenagogues, arguing that it was not in fact the sexual organs, but 'the entire system' which was at fault (Ashwell 1836: 533). Dr Samuel Ashwell said that it was 'the family', but even more commonly 'the female friends', of the patient who pushed for this treatment, as they insisted that 'If the catamenial function were but established, all would be well' (1836: 536).

As these passages suggest, the drugs used for chlorosis would be those also employed in cases of simple menstrual suppression. John Tanner's *The Hidden Treasures of the Art of Physick* explicitly states that the cures recommended for green sickness are equally applicable to menstrual suppression (Tanner 1659: 319). Jane Sharp similarly noted in her discussion of green sickness that, 'to save you the labour of much reading and me of writing too often of the same thing, under several heads, you may find what is to be done almost in all respects, where I write of the stopping of the Terms' (1671: 259; Hobby 1999: 197).

Deciding which drugs to use was, however, difficult, even in straightforward menstrual suppression. The treatise on menstruation by the Galenist Jacques Dubois was first published in Latin in 1555, then translated into French in 1559 by Guillaume Chrestien, physician in ordinary to the Duke of Bouillon, then to King Francis I and to Henry II, and subsequently corrected by Alexander Arnaud and included in Latin in the 1566 *Gynaeciorum* collection (Dubois 1555; 1559; Wolf 1566a). Dubois insisted on the importance of deciding which of the Galenic causes of suppressed menses applied in an individual case; for example, if the suppression were due to insufficient blood, because it was being lost by another route, then strong emmenagogues would be very dangerous. Dubois stressed the importance of starting with gentle emmenagogues, before trying something stronger, and he listed the drugs available to him in ascending order of strength (1559: 169–78). All categories include items with a strongly 'red' message – red seeds, and also *ruscus* (butcher's broom), which has spikes and bright red berries. The weaker remedies include *phaseolus* beans, 'mainly the red'. As we saw in chapter 1, the English writer William Langham also used a number of red plants in his remedies for green sickness. The stronger remedies in Dubois include betony, *aristolochia* (birthwort), mint, oregano, rue and valerian, but also butcher's broom. The very strong remedies include bryonia, both types of hellebore, pyrethrum, cyclamen root, squirting cucumber and its fruit, faeces, mithridatum and theriac.

Combinations of therapy were normal in humoral medicine. Tanner said the condition was

> cured by opening the Obstructions, evacuating the filthy Humours, and strengthening of the parts. The Obstructions are opened, by such medicines as are mentioned in the cure of the Obstructions of the Liver and Spleen: you may add to them such things which respect the Womb ... open the Saphaena or Ancle-Vein, but first, if the Maid be full of blood, open a Vein in the Arm.
>
> (1659: 315–16)

Pieter van Foreest (1595: obs. xxv) described the case of his uncle's daughter, Cordelia Johannis, whom he treated for cachexia due to menstrual retention in 1546; that is, before the establishment of the disease of virgins, green sickness or chlorosis as disease categories, although he could perhaps have called it 'white fever'. 'Her whole body was pale, indeed soft, owing to the retention of her menses.'[4] He began treatment with a syrup containing oxymel, squill and honey water, followed by a purgative, and then let blood from her ankle. She was then given to drink wine containing artemisia, camomile flowers, juniper, sugar and cinnamon; this brought on her period. However, the most significant part of this case history may be the ending, where we are told that she married soon after, and subsequently gave birth to many children.

Sixteenth-century writers recommending treatment drew on all the classical authorities they cited. For example, in his list of cures for menstrual suppression, Mercuriale (1587: 284d) mentioned the Hippocratic cure (sexual intercourse), the Athenian plague cure (cold baths) and, from more recent medical theory, the avoidance of wine, hot foods, meat, and anything else which can lead to an excess of blood. He also included shaming the sufferers; this derived from the classical story of the virgins of Miletos who committed suicide *en masse* (see chapter 4), an epidemic which ended when the bodies of the girls were displayed naked in the market-place. In similar vein, Turner (1714: 94) gave the case of a young girl who was treated by vomiting, tincture of steel and being frightened with 'Thoughts of Death'.

Jane Sharp also believed in starting with mild remedies for young girls: 'Tender natures (as maids) must have but gentle remedies' (1671: 295: Hobby 1999: 220).[5] She gave a regime of therapy which followed a similar pattern to that of Dubois, starting with a gentle purge using a drink based on rhubarb, then another using succory, madder, liquorice roots, aniseed, fennel, Harts tongue, borage and sassafras;[6] then the liver could be anointed with 'opening' ointments using lavender oil and bitter almonds, rue and mugwort. This was followed by bloodletting, and steel powder could also be used for 'stoppings' at this stage.

Steel is made up of at least 98 per cent iron, meaning that iron therapy was used well before the discovery of iron in blood gave a chemical basis for its use, or the need for iron in the formation of haemoglobin was understood (Heath and Patek 1937: 268, 287); however, the taste of blood would empirically suggest iron as a remedy to strengthen it. Sydenham's 'steel pills' date to the 1660s (Sydenham 1753: 658; Loudon 1984: 31; McFarland 1975: 251), while Sennert's *Practical Physick* (1664: 102–4) and Nicholas Sudell (1666: 9) also recommended steel filings to open obstructions. These were often taken in sugared wine, as in 'The Old Countesse of Arundels prime powder for ye greene sicknes', which uses steel filings, ginger and sugar, from a manuscript recipe collection of a similar date (WMS 1323, *A Book of Receipts Phisicall and Chirurgicall*: 149).[7] An earlier recommendation of steel in cordial water or in wine appeared in Varandal (1619: 28). Writers on chlorosis tried to find Hippocratic precedents for the use of iron (e.g. Uzac 1853: 9), while purveyors of alternative remedies had to set their wares against it. For example, the anonymous pamphlet extolling the virtues of 'the Bermudas Berries Imported from the Indies', published in 1694 and attributed to John Pechey, gives a case of a patient who was not helped by steel, but was cured by the berries ([Pechey] 1694: 5–6). At the beginning of the twentieth century, Ward (1914: 318) stated that the role of iron in treating chlorosis was so important that 'to withhold it is malpraxis'.

In nineteenth-century commercial medicine, advertisements for Dr William's Pink Pills for Pale People – 'a medicine aimed at the chlorotic market' (Brumberg 1988: 173) – claimed that its target market consisted of 'Young Girls Fading Away'. The most common commercially available remedy for amenorrhoea was Blaud's pills, developed in France in 1832 (Heath and Patek 1937: 268), which contained sulphate of iron with potassium carbonate. Julie-Marie Strange (2000: 619) has noted the apparently successful use of these pills in a case in 1866. Byrom Bramwell (1899: 52), physician to the Edinburgh Royal Infirmary, commented, 'Personally, I have been most successful with Robertson's Blaud's pill capsules'; these, he wrote, were particularly well absorbed. He started with the highest dose, the no. 3 capsule, and increased the dose until, in the fourth week of treatment, four no. 3 capsules – the equivalent of thirty-six Blaud's pills a day – were being taken daily (1899: 53). In an exceptional case which he treated in hospital, he gave the equivalent of ninety pills a day. Because Blaud's pills were available over the counter for self-dosage, some medical writers were unhappy about their use: Ward (1914: 319) wrote about those who used them to counteract constipation 'in quantities dictated by their financial circumstances and passing fancies'.

In early modern medicine, the timing of drug treatment was a further important consideration. Liébault (1597: 10) believed that all remedies for retained menses – letting blood, herbs, exercise, and rubbing the thighs and legs[8] – should only be used at the end of the month or at the new moon, otherwise they would not work. A Latin proverb ran: '*Luna vetus vetulas, iuvenes nova luna repurgat*' (Dubois 1559: 129; cf. Varandal 1619: 32; 1666: 32).

In Chrestien's French translation this appears as 'Femmes agées purge la vieille Lune, Comme elle faict jeunes quand elle est jeune'; Dubois therefore claimed that young women menstruate at the first quarter of the moon, and older women at the end of the lunar month, and recommended that bloodletting should be carried out on lunar principles, with younger women only being bled in the first or second lunar quarter (Dubois 1559: 165). Sharp insisted that remedies for menstrual suppression be given to all women 'a little before the Full Moon, or between the New and the full, for then blood increaseth; but never in the Wane of the Moon, for it doth no good' (1671: 296; Hobby 1999: 221).

Shall we dance?

Sharp included in her regimen for menstrual suppression the six Galenic 'non-naturals', discussing alongside the drugs, sweating and bathing, 'meats of good digestion, and good nourishment' (1671: 263; Hobby 1999: 199), temperately hot air, and moderate sleep. One of the non-naturals was exercise: menstrual suppression called for an increase in physical activity, because 'motion makes heat, and helps to distribute the Nutriment through the body' (1671: 264; Hobby 1999: 199–200; cf. Sennert 1664: 105). Even those recommending new treatments could add that exercise was essential in conjunction with their favoured remedy (e.g. [Pechey] 1694: 6). Housework, conveniently, was a particularly good therapy; this made sense in terms of increasing the level of exercise in order to use up the excess blood which could not escape by the normal route. The sixth-century AD writer Aetius of Amida (16.61) suggested that women who have ceased to menstruate, a condition attributed to too much leisure, 'must be put to work'. Fontanus (1652: 1), echoing the classical Greek text, ps-Xenophon's *Oikonomikos*,[9] opened his work *The Womans Doctour* with the words, 'Women were made to stay at home, and to looke after Household employments.' Housework activities remained appropriate exercise for women into the late eighteenth century; in the clinical notes of James Gregory (1779–80), for example, Janet Anderson was put to polishing the floor to bring on her menses, but in her case this was not successful (Risse 1986: 220).

For nineteenth-century writers, the ideal exercise, bearing in mind the chlorotic girl's natural aversion towards anything unduly strenuous (Rue 1819: 12), was commonly thought to be dancing; Olive's explanation of the benefit of dancing was that it combines 'movement and pleasure' (1819: 25). Trabuc (1818: 13) suggested that it encourages humours to flow to the womb, and thus provokes menstruation; on similar grounds, he also recommended horse-riding, or rides in a carriage, provided that the carriage had poor suspension and travelled over rocky terrain. Raciborski (1868: 313) also favoured horse-riding, provided that there was no prior inflammation of the sexual organs; he considered it useful at puberty, because it gave a light stimulation to these organs, and could encourage the onset of menstruation.

We may note here that Lange's Anna suffered difficulty in breathing specifically when dancing or climbing stairs: how should this be interpreted? We could understand it as a deliberate refusal to take part in the social or community activity of dancing (Ben-Amos 1994: 195); however, while sixteenth-century writers did recommend dancing as a suitable exercise for young girls, helping to keep their blood flowing (e.g. Liébault 1597: 10–11), it could have very different associations in the conduct books of early modern Europe (Bell 1999: 188–90; Potter 2002: 282). In the imagery of the late sixteenth century, a brothel could be called 'a dancing-school' and dancing itself was condemned as 'an introite to al kind of lewdenes'.[10]

Even in the terms of nineteenth-century medicine, however, Anna's failure to dance would have appeared as a contributory factor in her failure to menstruate. Raciborski (1868: 205) notes, in a discussion of the social influences on the age of puberty, that statistical tables cannot answer the question of whether young girls who have learned to dance start to menstruate at a younger age than those who have not; he implies that this was a genuine debate of his time, although one which he rejects as irrelevant. Like many writers in Europe and America at this period, he regarded dancing as the best possible exercise for young girls, giving grace to their movements;[11] however, the early modern association between dancing and inappropriate sexual expression remained a concern. Raciborski therefore stressed that, for younger girls, dancing should only take place within a group of close friends or family members. 'A young woman should not be taken to great social gatherings, to balls, until around 18 or 19 years of age' (Raciborski 1868: 314): such events would over-stimulate her emotions in a dangerous way. While recommending dancing, Trabuc (1818: 8) too had condemned balls. Similar unease about the correct social location for dancing appeared in the popular 1898 advice manual *What a Young Woman Ought to Know*, written by the social purity lecturer Mary Wood-Allen, who agreed that dancing was 'a pleasant and graceful exercise' (Wood-Allen 1898: 187) and suggested that, 'If dancing could be conducted in the day-time, out of doors, among well-known home friends and companions, in proper dress, and with *no round dances*, there would be much to commend, and little to condemn' (1898: 188; cf. 74).[12] In an earlier nineteenth-century advice manual, Catharine Sedgwick (1845: 61) encouraged dancing as 'a cheerful and useful exercise; but in heated rooms, and at late hours, [it] does more harm than good'. A male self-help writer, Henry McMurtrie, recommended dancing to women as a cure specifically for chlorosis, but cautioned that it should only be carried out in the day-time (1871: 220).

Von Noorden's 1905 study of chlorosis marvelled at the way in which 'young women who scarcely feel able to perform the lightest housework in the morning dance without difficulty for hours in the evening, and are admired for their sparkling vivacity' (1905: 359). This claim raises once again the issue of the sincerity of the chlorotic girl. One way of coping with this was to place 'variability of spirits' on the list of symptoms; for example, Clark (1887: 60) suggested that, 'At one time languid and indifferent, the patient at another time is interested and active. Sometimes capable of great temporary exertion, she is at other times exhausted by the slightest effort.'

Rest

Trends in chlorosis treatment were, of course, influenced by wider shifts in medicine. The 'rest cure' developed in America by Silas Weir Mitchell was influential in the last decades of the nineteenth century, while exercise once more eclipsed rest after the rise of the physical culture movement from the 1890s onwards (Whorton 2000: 145–9).

But the nineteenth-century focus on the inadequate red cells in the blood had its own impact on treatment for chlorosis. Whereas a sixteenth-century sufferer from the 'disease of virgins' would be advised to marry, be subjected to blood letting to remove the excess of blood in her body, and given purges to encourage her menses, a nineteenth-century girl who was thought to have 'chlorosis' would be given iron, and – although some writers would still urge her to take appropriate exercise, such as country walks and supervised dancing – others would now insist that she should rest. The aim was not to use up, but to strengthen, the blood. Gowers (1878: 675) gave the case of a chambermaid aged 18, who had been pale since she started to menstruate at 15, and was now breathless, with 'a slight greenish-yellow tint' to her skin; blood examination showed red corpuscles 'reduced to 26 per cent of the normal'. In this case, he measured and examined the corpuscles regularly, commenting not only on their number, but also on their shape and size. The treatment, he considered, was rest, 'an albuminous diet' – strong beef-tea and four eggs daily – and chloroxide of iron three times a day.

Instead of exercise and fresh air, which he feared would exhaust the corpuscles, Frederick Taylor similarly recommended iron and prolonged rest of up to three months; he noted that both 'patients and friends' would not like this treatment, and would object that 'they want to dance, or play lawn tennis, or ride horses, not to say bicycles', but the results would justify the treatment (1896: 724). The imposition of total bed rest, despite the anticipated objections of patients, is also found in von Noorden's 1905 essay; he also insisted on a detailed timetable of meals, walks and rests in less severe cases. Although the shift to hypochromic anaemia diluted some of the moral content of chlorosis (Wailoo 1997: 29), moral management remained an essential part of orthodox medical treatment. Control of the patient remained the key (von Noorden 1905: 517, 510–12).

Alternatives to orthodoxy

In the late seventeenth and early eighteenth centuries, quack doctors were also advertising their wares in the medical market-place. Often their advertisements singled out the 'embarrassing' conditions, where a patient was expected to feel less shame in buying a patent remedy than in visiting his or her local doctor. Even though the disease of virgins was usually seen as something for which the patient should not be blamed, as a menstrual condition it was something which patients and their families may have felt embarrassed to mention, so that green sickness was often included in the lists of illnesses advertised. In a collection of medical advertisements dating from the period 1675–1715, a German doctor claimed that he could 'cureth Women and Maids of many Infirmities, as, the Green Sickness, Stoppage or Overflowing of the Courses of

Nature', while Salvator Winter's 'elixir of life' cured 'all obstructions of the Stomach, Liver, and Spleen, The Jaundice, Scurvy, Green sickness' and 'All distempers incident to women', and Rose's balsamic elixir helped young women 'that are troubled with the Green Sickness to a Miracle'.[13] Other advertisers specifically linked green sickness to 'Virgins (though never so weak)' and to 'Maids'.[14] In an advertisement extolling the virtues of 'The Grand Balsamick', it was described as 'an Excellent Remedy against Barrenness, the Green-Sickness, and those other Obstructions incident to women'.[15] Here, green sickness seems to float between the menstrual condition of chapter 3, and the digestive obstructions of chapter 4.

Although some advertisements imply that everyone knew what green sickness was, some focus on the symptoms rather than the name. For example, Stephen Draper 'M.D. and Man-midwife' said that he could cure those who had 'lost and spoiled their Stomachs, from whence proceeds a paleness in their Faces, and the Maids get a desire for strange and unnatural things'.[16] The advertisement for 'Mr Elmy's pilula homogenea' explained,

> The Green Sickness is a Disease arising from the Obstructions of the Veins about the Womb, Liver, Spleen and Mesentery, causing various Symptoms in young women, the course of Nature being stopt, producing a Cachexia or evil habit of the Body, and alters the Complexion, sending ill Vapours to the Brain, causeth a Loathing of Meats that are good, occasion swellings in the Belly and Legs, with unwillingness to exercise, attended sometimes with difficulty of Breathing, and universally indispose the Body, so that most Distempers incident to Women may arise from it.[17]

Such advertisements therefore played an important role in keeping the green sickness in lay consciousness and, indeed, in teaching more people to identify it.

In descriptions such as this, it is clear that the purveyors of quack remedies operated within an entirely Galenic model of the body, in many ways identical to that of orthodox practitioners (Wear 1989: 319). Some of the healers selling their services in this way were women, who often announced themselves as widows of doctors; for example, Elizabeth Russell, widow of Dr George Jones, selling his 'Friendly Pills', electuary and balsam, Sarah Gardiner, the late wife of William Kellitt, and Sarah Cornelius de Heusde, daughter and widow of doctors.[18] As well as using this connection with the male world of medicine as a selling-point, such women also played on the modesty of their sex. Sarah stated that her father and husband had referred on to her their female patients who were ashamed of their illnesses;[19] she claimed to be able to cure 'the pale Colour' in maids. A 'Gentlewoman' who was 'Wife to an Eminent Physician almost Twenty Years, now Deceased', could cure diseases which women – out of 'Modesty' – were unable to reveal to a male doctor, including green sickness.[20] A German healer, Ann Laverenst of Arundel Street in London, used as a banner outside her home 'a Red-Cloth hang out at the Balconey, with Coagulated Stones taken out of the Bodies of the Female Sex'. She specialised in the diseases of women and, although she did not name green sickness, she listed among the symptoms she could treat 'absence of Courses', 'loss of appetite', 'a Paleness or unusual Yellow' and the desire on the part of maids to eat chalk, coal and so on. She diagnosed from urine alone, thus obviating the need for modest patients to pay her a personal visit.[21]

Another woman quack healer stressed the value of travel in her claims to cure — amongst other things — green sickness; she attributed her success to the discoveries made by her father in his travels around the world.[22] Travel represented another motif used by woman healers as well as by men; it is also found in the handbill for a woman practising in late seventeenth-century London who called herself 'Agnodice: The Woman Practitioner, dwelling at the Hand and Urinal, next Door to the Blue Ball in Hayden-Yard in the Minories, near Aldgate.'[23] She claimed to have 'Travelled for many Years in Forreign Parts' and to be able to cure diseases of infants, children, and of her 'own Sex', adding that 'the Diseases in particular I shall forbear to mention, they being not proper to be exposed to the public'. However, she stated that she could cure venereal disease, test for pregnancy and aid conception, and that she could treat green sickness.

Two important alternative movements in nineteenth-century medicine also drew heavily on orthodox theories of the cause and treatment of chlorosis: homeopathy, and hydropathy. Homeopathic views of chlorosis repeated much of the current orthodoxy on menstruation in general; for example, that early menstruation was due to spicy foods, and too much novel-reading and dancing (Ruddock 1892: 27). As for late menarche, in both homeopathic works and self-help manuals this was regarded as something requiring no treatment, provided that the general health of the girl remained good (Ruddock 1892: 30; cf. McMurtrie 1871: 218). Chlorosis was attributed to 'nervous causes' (Ruddock 1892: 74), and was distinguished from anaemia (1892: 76); poor ventilation and light, and lack of exercise, were thought to predispose one to the condition. In addition to homeopathic remedies chosen according to whether cachexia, nervous symptoms, menstrual symptoms or digestive symptoms were dominant (1892: 78–80), patients were managed with a nourishing diet and plenty of exercise, which would encourage the proper oxygenation of their blood. Cold baths were thought to diminish the 'extreme sensitiveness of chlorotic patients' (Ruddock 1892: 80).

A more complicated approach to baths was found in another branch of alternative medicine. 'Taking the waters' had been used for chlorosis since the seventeenth century; the *Bath Memoirs* of Robert Pierce recommended it (1697: 188–9), and George Cheyne too argued for their purgative value in this condition (Guerrini 2000: 101). The hydropathy movement, a variant of 'natural' healing, was most strongly associated with Vincenz Priessnitz, who practised his form of treatment at a spa he set up at Gräfenburg in 1829. The water cure involved drinking water to flush out bad fluids, and also opening the pores to sweat out noxious substances. Sebastian Kneipp (1893: 134–5) discussed the 'distressing picture' presented by sufferers from green sickness, and recommended in addition to the water cure plenty of fresh air and moderate outdoor exercise. 'Three to four times weekly let the patient rise from bed, and having washed the whole body, return there quickly; standing in water up to the calves for one minute, succeeded by holding the arms in water two to three times weekly.' If the patient was very weak, salt or vinegar should be added to the water, which should also be warmed.

In England, Malvern became a centre for 'establishments' offering the water cure (Bradley and Dupree 2001: 430); Walter Johnson set up a hydropathic establishment in Edgbaston (Johnson 1852: advertisement at end of book), and published on hydropathy with his father and brother (Johnson 1856); like many writers on hydropathy, he was interested in other forms of natural healing, and also wrote on homeopathy. In the 1860s, the Johnsons set up another establishment at Malvern, where Florence Nightingale was one of Walter's famous patients (Smith 1982: 89).

Some of the treatments could also be carried out at home. Edward Johnson described in his *The Domestic Practice of Hydropathy* (1856: 153–6) the home treatment of chlorosis; a patient would be given a 'tepid washdown' twice daily for the first two days; then, if she was suffering from menstrual suppression, she should have 'the sweating blanket, and the half wet sheet for thirty minutes, on alternate mornings' (1856: 155). The wet sheet 'became the early trademark of the cold water cure' (Bradley and Dupree 2001: 418). If the patient's menstruation was normal, then the sweating blanket would not be needed. In either case, shallow baths and sitz baths should also be used. In the sweating blanket, a patient was wrapped up like 'an Egyptian mummy' so that her body was hermetically sealed; she would then sweat for several hours (1856: 18). In the 'half wet sheet' she would be wrapped from her armpits to her mid-thighs, but with an inner layer of a well-squeezed-out wet sheet (1856: 20, 27). These measures were seen as serving to purify the blood, removing 'poisons' through the pores. Hydropathy, like orthodox medicine of its time, looked to the blood as the key to chlorosis (Bradley and Dupree 2001: 420).

Women physicians and chlorosis

In the second half of the nineteenth century, when women first entered the medical profession, they used the same rhetoric of modesty and shared womanhood as the women who advertised their cures for green sickness in the early modern medical marketplace. How did such women regard menstruation and chlorosis?

I have argued in chapter 3 that a concern with avoiding very early menarche, and with preventing too much 'excitation' of young girls, seems to be particularly characteristic of the late nineteenth and early twentieth century; in particular, it is found in many writers who were opposed to the equality of women. Granville Stanley Hall (1904), for example, who saw adolescence as the time when an individual 'recapitulates' the savage stage of the race's past (Prescott 1998: 17–21), wanted to prolong 'the green stage', not letting girls 'blossom' too early (Dyhouse 1981: 122–3). This is the same language as that of the early nineteenth-century French medical dissertations influenced by Rousseau (see pp. 88–92). The adolescent girl is seen as sexually desirable, and attempts are made to control the period of her 'bloom', with the avowed intention of preserving her health and, in eugenic discourse, safeguarding the future of the race. However, the message is different; from the second half of the nineteenth century until the 1930s, this language was structured around the debate concerning the education of women. Some writers considered that girls should be educated, but preferably segregated from boys, while others argued that the education of girls should cease entirely during the years when menstruation was becoming established, otherwise the use of the brain could permanently damage the developing reproductive system (Dyhouse 1981: 154–5). Hall, for whom chlorosis was a 'neurosis of menstruation' (1904: 499), idealised the sensation of menstruation, so that he presented women as completely absorbed in the experience, having no time nor need for education: 'The flow itself has been a pleasure and the end of it is a slight shock ... When her cycle is complete, her whole life must be regulated to prepare for the next' (1904: 493). Such a woman learns so much by 'intuition and experience that her way of wisdom is larger and must always seem more esoteric and mystic to man ... Every day of the twenty-eight she is a different being' (1904: 493–4).

As Regina Morantz-Sanchez (1985: 217–18) has shown, especially after 1880, the first generations of women doctors in America had a very similar social background and training to those of men. However, the same language, and the same medical activity, could hold different significance for a woman in the medical profession. Women and men doctors 'acted alike in most therapeutic situations, but for very different reasons and with meanings both different to themselves and to their patients' (Morantz-Sanchez 1985: 231).

In the late 1840s, Elizabeth Blackwell was the first American woman to qualify as a doctor; she moved to England in 1869. Coming from a strongly Christian, progressive family, she argued for the improvement of society by the realisation of 'Nature's true intention, viz.: the equality of the sexes in birth and in duration of life' (Blackwell 1882: 25). Although she used the same language as male physicians, for whom women were more 'delicate' than men, she interpreted this as a factor in favour of women physicians, because this 'delicacy' meant that patients would be more likely to accept treatment from one of their own sex, while women's greater compassion would make them particularly good doctors (Morantz-Sanchez 1985: 52). Like male writers, however, she warned of the dangers of stimulating too soon the sexual 'faculty'; this could endanger the future fertility of a woman (Blackwell 1882: 10–11). The faculty of 'secretion' was seen as one particularly strongly influenced by the mind, so that secretions of 'the genital system' would increase if the mind were focused on an object of passion (Blackwell 1882: 16–17). She regarded menstruation and male nocturnal emissions as equivalent, representing 'the natural healthy actions of self-balance'; both occur spontaneously in healthy people, and can frighten young people if they are not given proper preparation by their parents (Blackwell 1902: 25, 28). Hall (1904: 480) argued that, by equating these two phenomena, she viewed menstruation as a way of relieving sexual desire.

Blackwell cited with approval *The People of Turkey*, a two-volume work published in 1878 and based on the experiences of 'A Consul's Daughter and Wife' (Lane-Poole 1878a; 1878b). This book, 'worthy of careful consideration' (Blackwell 1882: 20), showed the degrading conditions of life in a harem, where women were treated 'as a valuable horse or dog', and sensuality went hand in hand with the 'moral degeneration of female character' (Blackwell 1882: 21, 55–6). 'A Consul's Daughter and Wife' did not discuss green sickness, although it told the story of 'a young beauty of sixteen' suffering from love sickness, in which the sufferer's young brother plays the role of Galen, naming the object of desire (Lane-Poole 1878b: 88–9; see also p. 118 of this volume). She also wrote of 'the ladies of the harem, when permitted to escape from their cages', roaming through the pleasure gardens of the seraglio 'like a troop of school-girls during recreation hours' (Lane-Poole 1878a: 246); she added that 'The treatment these girls received seemed to be very kind, but sadly wanting in decency, morality, and good principle' (Lane-Poole 1878a: 253). She concluded that 'until the harem system, and with it polygamy, are finally abolished, the condition of Mohammedan women can never be anything but degraded' (Lane-Poole 1878b: 100).

The later nineteenth century was intrigued by tales from the harem (Said 1978), and writers on chlorosis argued that it was particularly widespread here. In his discussion of the geographical spread of the condition, August Hirsch (1885: 495 n. 2) referred readers to the work of Rigler (1852), who found a 'very considerable amount of the sickness in Turkey and adjoining countries of the Levant'. The idea that women in hot climates did not menstruate as heavily as those in Europe was an old one, found for example in Varandal (1619: 31; 1666: 32).[24] Hirsch's survey of medical journals also suggested that chlorosis was widespread in Mexico, the West Indies, Brazil, Algiers, India, China and Japan (1885: 497–8). He concluded that the condition was more common in tropical regions, and was more likely to strike women having insufficient exercise in the open air, 'leading an indoor life' (1885: 499); again citing Rigler, he noted that the disease was 'especially common among those Oriental women who led an inactive and purely sensual life in the harems' (1885: 501; Rigler 1852: 412). Here the motif of the 'disease of virgins' has been forgotten; from a condition affecting those who have no experience of sex, chlorosis has become something affecting the sex-sated women of the East.

In his book *Sex in Education: A Fair Chance for Girls*, published in 1873, the American physician Edward Clarke argued from his own experience in medical practice that women should not enter higher education; he listed a range of negative consequences for health. Opponents of women doctors rallied round this book (Morantz-Sanchez 1985: 54–5), but the prize-winning essay of Dr Mary Putnam Jacobi, 'The Question of Rest for Women during Menstruation' (1877) rebutted his assumptions.[25] Although she urged employers to allow women who experienced difficult menstruation to rest (1877: 232), Jacobi demonstrated that normal healthy women did not automatically need rest during menstruation; however, this did not end the debate. Granville Stanley Hall, who offered some support for women as doctors to other members of their sex (1904: 505), thought that the real problem for female health was the rapid evolution of 'modern woman': in particular, 'puberty for a girl is like floating down a broadening river into an open sea'. The only solution was for women to 'assert their true physiological rights' by 'regularly stepping aside at stated times for a few years till it is well established and normal' (1904: 511); in other words, to rest.

In her essay on the treatment of women suffering from anaemia, Jacobi was not impressed by iron, bed rest or electricity; although an electrical current applied to the womb could induce 'a slight oozing of blood' (Jacobi and White 1880: 6), this was not enough. Instead, she recommended the 'cold pack', in which the patient was wrapped in a wet sheet, surrounded by a dry sheet and six blankets, for an hour every other day. This, she believed, would 'accelerate tissue metamorphosis – to increase waste and the products of oxidation – thus indirectly promoting assimilation' (Jacobi and White 1880: 1). It is noteworthy that, while occasionally using the label 'chloro-anaemia' (1880: 27, 34–5), she carefully avoided the label of 'chlorosis', even in cases such as that of a girl of 16 with anaemia, 'loud venous humming', 'pallor of skin and mucous membranes', amenorrhoea and anorexia (1880: 7).[26]

Even in the early twentieth century, when more women were becoming more involved in the medical profession, many educated women continued to present female adolescence as a time of dramatic change and instability. In this period, they would cite Hall's work as authoritative, although they focused more on the experience of the girl.[27] In a lecture delivered to the Childhood Society in November 1904, 'Miss M.E. Findlay B.A.' suggested that the girl of around 12 or 13 feels 'lank, clumsy, hoydenish, and, like moulting birds, they are inclined to shun society' (Findlay 1905–7: 84). Her sensitivity 'should not be rudely scarred, for it has the value of the sheathing leaves round a bud'. Once a girl crossed the line between girl and woman, defined here as the 'radical change' of menarche, 'a period of storm and stress', she should take great care to avoid 'exposure to damp, excitement, and over-strain', and should pay careful attention to her diet (1905–7: 86). Anaemia and chlorosis, described as 'maladies peculiar to this period in girls', show that one should not divert the energy required for physical development into intellectual activities; girls using their brains during this period ran the risk of sterility, and so they should not take public examinations between the ages of 12 and 18, but should instead take time to learn household tasks from their mothers (1905–7: 87, 90–1). As Regina Morantz-Sanchez (1985: 61) has pointed out, the first generations of educated women were already acting as pioneers in their own fields, without taking on every possible feminist cause; as those in the medical profession had enough to do to prove that they were capable of being doctors while remaining 'feminine', and would not take time off every month for menstruation, we should not be surprised that they continued to emphasise the importance of marriage and motherhood, and the nurturing skills of women.[28] Jacobi, for example, regarded celibacy as an 'evil' (1877: 211); insisted on the importance of 'marriage at a suitable time' in preventing menstrual pain (1877: 62); and mentioned what she called 'chloro anemic girls' who could often be cured by pregnancy (1877: 211).

The technology of the laboratory and of diagnostic development made little difference to chlorosis. The attempt to objectify what was felt when touching the pulse, and the enhancement of the sense of hearing with a stethoscope, produced no definitive sign: even the *bruit de diable* came to be widely challenged. Agreement on the signs of chlorosis came closer with the development of blood testing, but even here it was acknowledged that there must be a subjective element in reading the results. Furthermore, the claim that this was a disease of the blood only reinforced the association with menstruation, and in particular with menarche. From being one of the proffered treatments, rest became also a prophylactic measure for girls in their first years of menstruation, and took on political dimensions, since such extensive rest made it even more difficult for girls to receive anything above a basic education. Even 'alternative' forms of medicine emphasised the dangers of puberty in girls, and an early marriage continued to be seen as the best resolution of the problem. Medical women supported these views. It was only with the entry of women into new roles during the First World War, and the abandonment of ideas of menstruation as an 'illness', that attitudes began to shift, particularly as studies began to focus not on women whose experience of menstruation was centred on pain and incapacity, but on surveys of a wider sample of girls and women (Strange 2000: 623; 2001: 254–6).

CONCLUSION

The disease of virgins was a condition with a 'father' – Lange, who also acted as a father-figure to the nubile Anna – and a 'godfather' – Varandal, who gave it its most long-lived of names, chlorosis. Yet its origins lay with women, with the 'matrons of Brabant' who had called it 'white fever, on account of the pale face, as well as love fever, since every lover is pale' (Lange 1554), and in the mid-nineteenth century, as 'green sickness', it still remained a 'homespun term, familiar to mothers and nurses' (Johnson 1849: 30). The varied symptoms of the condition, however, rarely included a fever. It was classified as a 'new' disease, at least in 1558, when William Bullein described green sickness in such terms; this meant that it was perceived as a challenge to the stable order of creation. For classically trained commentators, this novelty suggested that it should be understood as a moral issue, and be attributed to the faults of the sufferers, above all to diet, idleness and luxury. But, from Lange onwards, attempts were also being made to show that it was 'old', with writers striving to provide it with a long classical pedigree.

What was the disease of virgins? In modern terms, it was a label embracing a wide range of conditions, encompassing dietary, hormonal and behavioural disturbances. As Sennert's *Practical Physick* (1664: 101) commented on the long list of symptoms, 'These are not all in all people, but most are in most, and in some all.' The broad symptom picture meant that it could include what we would currently want to label as anorexia nervosa, irritable bowel syndrome, or M.E.(myalgic encephalitis), but the idea of such a disease could also account for vague feelings of tiredness or malaise, provided that they occurred in a young girl.

So, what was the disease of virgins for? Why was this collection of symptoms linked to young girls at, or soon after, the onset of menstruation? I have suggested here that the condition began when the English vernacular condition of green sickness became narrowed down on to young, 'green', women and shifted at the end of the sixteenth century from a predominantly digestive, to a menstrual, disease, a step made easier by the moving fluids of the Galenic humoral body. This process was accelerated by Lange's bid to

139

colonise for academic medicine the Dutch folk disease known to women as white fever. This label already suggested Ovid's 'pale' lover, but Lange found his much-needed classical precedent elsewhere, in the Hippocratic *On the disease of virgins*; the concentration of this text on trapped menstrual blood as the underlying cause helped to focus green sickness on to young girls. Meanwhile, in the same year that Lange's letter describing Anna's diagnosis was published, the possibility of wider access to Sappho's 'greener than grass' and its Catullan version brought the connection with love sickness, already made by the matrons of Brabant, more emphatically into play. In addition, green, pale and discoloured virgins were made more plausible, and the menstrual origin of the symptoms was underlined, because they recalled Trotula's imagery of menstrual suppression. In sixteenth-century green sickness, menstruation became so important that the diagnosis had to be abandoned if the patient were subsequently to menstruate.

The peak period of chlorosis has often been seen as the second half of the nineteenth century, either because of a longer 'puberty gap' between maturity and marriage, or because of a more general 'age of anxiety'. But many of the worries about young girls expressed in this period drew on eighteenth-century ideas about the process of puberty in the female sex, and can equally be found in the early modern period. Why, in particular, was there so much creative cultural activity around menstruation and virginity in the mid- to late sixteenth century? It is possible to link this to the rise of Protestantism making marriage even more firmly the proper destiny of a Christian woman, while, certainly in England, concerns about the future of the state under a virgin queen also played their part. Virginity was 'good to think with': and, while conquest of virgin lands was in progress, such conquest could be seen as doing a favour to the health of the girl, or the territory, being invaded. Insistence on marriage as the ideal cure for sick girls could thus underpin the State rhetoric of the benefits of invasion.

Lange's use of the Hippocratic text on virgins, with its picture of the physical and mental effects of remaining unmarried despite being 'ripe', was complex but inspired. He read it within a Galenic model of the body, adding in elements which were not in the Greek text, but merging the whole into a story which did not close down any subsequent reinterpretations. The condition continued to oscillate between digestion and menstruation right into the nineteenth century. The fragile boundaries between green sickness, the disease of virgins and other disease concepts of the early modern period – in particular, the lines separating green sickness and white fever from love sickness – were a source not of weakness, but of strength: flexibility led to longevity.

But, despite debates over its novelty or its antiquity, and different theories as to the underlying cause, not all aspects of the condition were so fluid. Throughout the period studied here, the condition resisted reassignment away from its original target group of virgins observed to be at, or near, menarche, and considered of marriageable age. Menstruation normally led to a revision of the diagnosis, while marriage would remove the disease of virgins or chlorosis from the list of suspects: Cullen wrote, 'for let a married woman labour under any disease whatever, she is never suspected to labour under chlorosis' (1803: 80–1). The Western medical tradition constructed female puberty and virginity as problems, and proposed solutions for them; von Noorden recommended that girls should 'be treated as children as long as possible'. But when the grass is ready for the scythe, it needs to be cut immediately. While virginity was difficult to define and to monitor, the symptoms of the disease of virgins provided further empirical evidence that girls were indeed ripe, and that they should be harvested in the interest of their own health. The disease was averted by keeping girls innocent, but cured by ending their maidenhood. Exacerbated by being near other girls or women, as feared in the boarding school as in the harem, it reveals a deep unease about the proper management of puberty in girls.

The disease of virgins, green sickness, chlorosis and the white fever were 'the same thing' inasmuch as they were expressions of these same anxieties about female puberty, which functioned by making it 'a disease'. As 'a disease', it should not have been seen as the girl's fault, although some aetiologies proposed that some feature of her behaviour was to blame. Nor was it her family's fault: Lange's letter exonerated Anna's father, supporting his feeling that it was time that she was married. As 'a disease', it was also amenable to treatment. The implications for treatment could vary: the disease of virgins and green sickness both suggest within their names themselves that marriage will cure the condition, but chlorosis too – by evoking Sappho's lovesick shade of *chloros* – can contain the same idea. But even with the development of diagnostic technologies in the nineteenth century, and new treatment methods, marriage and childbirth remained the ideal final chapters to the chlorotic story.

Emerging from popular notions of the body, and reinforcing these, the version of the disease of virgins developed in academic medicine also came up against popular ideas about treatment. Where lay people made jokes about 'ease in a green gown' as the best cure, or demanded a good bleeding, academic medicine tried to discover other ways to ease the symptoms, or at least to find some rationale for the popular remedies. Whether authority was believed to lie in the texts of classical antiquity to which Lange had first linked the condition, or in the laboratory, the disease of virgins was adjusted to fit into changing ideas about the female body, and constant concerns about puberty. A condition with roots deep in the classical tradition, its rise corresponds to the Renaissance rediscovery of the ancient Greek medical texts, while its fall occurred as those texts finally lost their power over medicine.

APPENDIX

Johannes Lange (1554) *Medicinalium epistolarum miscellanea*, Basel: J. Oporinus, pp. 74–7.

De morbo virgineo

Conquereris mihi, ut tuo fido Achati, filiam tuam Annam primogenitam, et iam nubilem, a multis procis, virtutum integritate ac stemmatis claritate, opumque facultatibus, auito tuorum maiorum generi non imparibus, in coniugem desiderari: quos tu, ob filiae imbecillitatem, abdicare cogaris. Nec id adeo tibi esse molestum, quam quod hactenus nullus Medicorum internam morbi causam et essentiam explicare, simulque curam praescribere potuerit. Nam unus esse cardialgiam ait, alius cordis palmum, hic vero dispnoeam, ille matricis suffocationem: nec defuisse, qui ex vitio epatis esse ventriculi fastidium suspicarentur. Quorum discors de filiae tuae morbo iudicium, ac de nuptiis consilium fidele, pro veteri amicitia efflagitas: simulque quibus morbi symptomatis affligitur, recte primum declaras: cuius nempe faciei indoles, quum anno praeterito roseo genarum labiorumque rubore floruisset, ea modo velut exanguia, pallescere triste, cor ad quemvis corporis motum contremiscere, arteriasque temporum sensibiliter pulsare, et in choreis ascensú ue scalarum dispnoea corripi, stomachum cibum, ac praecipue carnem fastidire: et crura, praecipue iuxta thalos,[1] ad noctem oedemate intumescere. Ex his sane accidentibus, et signis morbi pathognomicis,[2] quae morbi causam et substantiam produnt, eiusque curam designant, miror vestrates Medicos morbi causas et naturam non agnovisse. Quod vero nomen illius non dixerint, nihil quoque refert. Multae sunt in morborum catalogo aegritudines, nomine et non cura carentes. Nec hic morbus propriam habet nomenclaturam, quam cum sit virginibus peculiaris, virgineus quoque indigitari poterit: quem Brabantinorum matronae, febrem albam, ob faciei pallorem, et amatoriam appellare solent: quum palleat omnis amans, et color hic sit aptus amanti. Quamvis febris admodum raro coincidat. Sed hic morbus virgines frequenter infestat, quum viro iam maturae, ex ephebis excesserint. Nam id temporis, natura duce, sanguis menstruus ad matricis loculos, et venas ab epate defluit: qui quum ob illarum angusta oscula, quae nondum patuerunt, viscosis quoque et crudis humoribus obstructa, et denique ob sanguinis grossitiem, erumpere non possit: tum rursum per venae cavae maiorisque arteriae propagines, ad cor, epar, diaphragma, et praecordiorum venas regurgitat: capite quoque bona pars impartitur, et circa viscera accidentia gravia parit, dispnoeam, tremulum cordis palmum, epatis inflationem, stomachi fastidium, cardialgiam: nec raro cum amentia epilepsiam, et delirium. Quod Hippocrates in libello de Virginum morbis, his testatur verbis: Virgines, inquit, quibus nuptiarum tempus advenit, maturaeque iam viro sunt, spectrorum imaginariis terroribus affliguntur, praesertim quum menses descendunt. Nam ante hoc, non admodum male afficiuntur. Postea vero sanguis in matricis locellos, tanquam effluxurus destillat et descendit. Quum autem oscula exitus obstructa fuerint, sanguisque ob cibaria et corporis incrementum auctus, illic collectus subsistit plurimus, nec unde effluat exitus venarum pateant, prae copia cor, septum transversum, praecordiaque petit. quibus repletis, cor sibi non constat, et torpet, ex torpore vero desipit et delirat. Nil certe mirum, quum epar a feculento mensium sanguine non expurgetur, et eo praecordiorum venae infarctae fuerint, hypocondriorum[3] viscera intumescere, et his diaphragma (ut in hydrope) coarctari, quod difficilem parit anhelitum, teste Gal. in fine tertii de Dispnoea libri, ubi universaliter inquit: Si internus tumor aut dolor circa hypocondria[4] constiterit, tum parva et creba[5] fit spiratio. Deinde quum cor, stomachus et epar, utriusque venae chylis et arteriae ramis, velut communi vinculo connectantur, his sane sanguine grosso, flatuosoque spiritu et vapore refertis et obstructis, ut hos cor extrudat, et deoppilet, ne suffocetur frequenti arteriarum et systoles motu eluctatur, et palmo contremiscit: quo defatigato, quid obstat ἀσφιξίας, καὶ πνευμάτων ἀπολήψεις, καὶ ἀπνοίας id est, pulsus, et spirituum ac anhelitus interceptiones coincidere? quibus aeger obmutescat, et ut deploratus iaceat. Unde mehercle Galen. in Acutorum diaeta scite ait: δύναται δέ καὶ πλῆθος τε καὶ πάχος αἵματος οὐ μόνον τὰς ἀρτηρίας πνευματῶσαι ποτὲ, καὶ δίεξοδον οὐκ ἔχειν, ἀλλὰ καὶ αὐτὰς ἰδίως ὀνομαζομένας φλέβας id est, Potest autem et multitudo et densitas sanguinis non modo arterias inflare, et exitum obstruere, sed et ipsas proprie nominatas venas. Postremo, an filia tua hac affecta aegritudine, nubere debeat, et quae sit huius curatio, en fidum ex Hippocratis divite medicinarum penu consilium communicabo, qui in libello de Morbis virginum ait: Huius morbi liberatio est, venae sectio, si nihil obstiterit. Ego vero, inquit, praecipio, virgines hoc morbo afflictas, ut quamprimum viris cohabitent, et copulentur: si conceperint, convalescent: si vero in pubertate hoc morbo non corripientur, tum paulo post eas invadet, nisi viro nupserint. At vero ex maritatis, steriles magis id patiuntur. Hoc saluberrimo divini Hippocratis consilio, si medicamenta menses provocantia, et obstructionum aperitiva, sanguinis grossi subtiliativa adiunxeris, nihil his praesentius reperire et excogitare poteris: quibus ego in huius virginei morbi cura nunquam falsus, aut spe sui frustratus. Quare bono sis animo, filiam tuam elocato: nuptiis quoque ego libens interero. Vale.

NOTES

Introduction

1 Green (2001: 1) similarly asks, 'Why have different societies, at different times, seen diseases that we no longer see? Why did they interpret physiological processes differently from the way we do?' In the preface to the first edition of his history of epilepsy, Temkin took the approach of writing about what earlier generations had *called* 'epilepsy' (1971: ix); in an epilogue to the second edition, he asked 'Have we then really traced the history of a disease?' and concluded that he had studied the 'human history', as opposed to the 'natural history', of the condition (1971: 383–4). In his recent history of tuberculosis, Dormandy distinguished between the periods before and after the identification of the causative microorganism: before this identification, 'the illness had been known by many names and had undoubtedly been confused with many other conditions' (1999: 1). For the disease of virgins, there was no such watershed in the laboratory.

2 Loudon (1980: 1669) also notes that 'the clinical descriptions (at least up to 1850) were remarkably consistent'.

3 Over the period being studied here, all the labels, except for hypochromic anaemia, were in use throughout. In casebooks, Dr Barker of Shrewsbury used *morbus virgineus* as the equivalent of 'green sickness' in 1596 (Lucinda McCray Beier, personal communication, using BL Sloane MS 663, 3/22) while a few years later, in 1603, Richard Napier used the label 'green sickness' alongside the English translation of this Latin label, 'the disease of virgins' (Sawyer 1986: 491). In de Castro (1603: 128), 'white fever' was the primary term, with 'the disease of virgins' as its equivalent; 'love fever' and 'white jaundice' also feature. The 'disease of virgins', 'white fever' and 'chlorosis' were used interchangeably by Varandal (1619: 4–5; 1620: 1). By the mid-seventeenth century, Johnston (1657: 80) gave as synonyms 'the White, the Virgins, the Pale, the Lovers Feaver'. In Jane Sharp's *The Midwives Book* (1671: 256; Hobby 1999: 194), 'white Feaver' also appeared explicitly as an alternative name for green sickness in a list of 'Maids diseases', based on Sennert (1664: 100). My thanks to Elaine Hobby for drawing my attention to Sharp's reliance on this work. W. Johnson (1849: 30) wrote that 'Chlorosis is the Greek synonyme [*sic*] of that homespun term, familiar to mothers and nurses, the green-sickness' and used 'the white-sickness' as a further equivalent (1849: 46). On the nineteenth-century articulation of hypochromic anaemia, and the role of blood testing, see p. 15–16 and chapter 5.

4 For other European languages, see Uzac (1853: 23). On the equivalence of 'les pâles couleurs' and chlorosis, see Astruc (1761–5: 1–64; vol. 2, ch. 8), headed 'Des pâles couleurs, ou du Chlorosis', and 'chlorosis or the pale colours', in Raciborski (1868: 285).

5 The phrasing of Lange (1554: 74).

6 The date of the first clinical description of anorexia nervosa is commonly given as 1873 or 1874, when William Withey Gull's paper 'firmly marginalized competing nomenclatures' (O'Connor 1995: 535; cf. Loudon 1980: 1674). Skrabanek 1983, however, traces anorexia in young girls back to at least the fifth century AD. As is always the case with attempts at retrospective diagnosis, it all depends on which features one chooses to regard as being 'central' to the condition; furthermore, anorexia as a *symptom* existed many centuries before it was seen as a *disease* while, as Brumberg 1992 has shown, motives for not eating may themselves vary dramatically over time.

7 See p. 22 on how Richard Napier located the boundary between these two conditions in the early seventeenth century.

8 See pp. 21–2 on the shift from 'green sickness' to 'consumption' in diagnoses of Jane Kitson's condition in 1558–60.

9 E.g. Schurig (1730: 117).

10 For these last three possibilities, see the case of Helena, Montanus 1565, *consilium* 307; given in Spach (1597: 325–6) as *consilium* iv, and discussed by King (1999). Dixon (1995: 240) merges all these labels into a single 'mysterious universal ailment of many names'; in this book I will argue that they carry significantly different messages about the body, and different implications for its treatment. See further King (1996b).

11 *quia frequenter virginibus accidere conspicimus*.

12 Compare hysteria: once seen as a physical condition caused by an errant womb, literally 'wandering' around the body in search of moisture, it came under the successive control of gynaecology, psychotherapy, cardiology, and neurology. On hysteria and chlorosis, see pp. 7–9.

13 *La fille pâle demande le mâle* (Raciborski 1868: 332); cf. Rocher (1989: 16) for the same proverb in Laurent Joubert's *Medley* of 1578; also used in Uzac (1853: 14).

14 Schleiner (1995) has drawn attention to a similar medical debate in Renaissance medicine, concerning whether a physician should help a woman with retained seed to expel it, by masturbation. The *locus classicus* is Galen, *On the Affected Parts* 6.5, on the widow with retained seed who expelled it 'feeling both pain and pleasure' after a midwife rubbed her inner thighs. Such rubbing could be done by the woman herself, as in Dubois' treatment for menstrual suppression (1555: 180), where she rubs her genitals (Lat. *fricet muliebria*, Fr. 'qu'elle frotte sa nature') and her inner thighs with a sachet filled with the herb artemisia. The Spaniard Mercado, a Jewish convert to Catholicism, and personal physician to Philip II and Philip III, states that 'we know that the Christian physician is not permitted to do this', *nam scimus non licere medico christiano*. This is not just about religious affiliation: in the seventeenth century the Protestant Daniel Sennert also said that a Christian physician should not recommend this treatment (Schleiner 1995: 126).

15 *Medicinalium epistolarum miscellanea* 1.21 (Lange 1554: 74–7).

16 *Peri parthenión* (L 8.466–71), *Concerning virgins*, *On the disease(s) of virgins* – or, since a more accurate translation of the Greek *parthenoi* may be young unmarried girls, *On the disease(s) of young girls*. The text is discussed in detail in chapter 2 of this volume.

17 See for example Figlio (1978); Loudon (1980; 1984); Starobinski (1981); Siddall (1982); Brumberg (1982).

18 Heath and Patek (1937: 297) insisted, however, that 'the disease has not disappeared but on the contrary in mild form is fairly common, and in the severe form not extremely rare'. In the mid-1980s, there was a further flurry of medical activity with the intention of showing that, in the words of the correspondence in

Journal of the American Medical Association (1987), 'Chlorosis lives!'. See Cahan (1987); Pallangyo (1987); Guggenheim (1995).

19 The letter is given in full on pp. 46–8; the original Latin may be found in the Appendix.

20 It would, however, seem unlikely that a respectable girl in the mid-nineteenth century under medical interrogation would express any enthusiasm for sex.

21 The bloodless appearance of the chlorotic recalls the vampire; the date of the famous stay at the Villa Diodati outside Geneva, during which Mary Shelley started *Frankenstein* and either Percy Bysshe Shelley or his personal physician, John Polidori, started the short story, 'The Vampyre', was 1816; Bram Stoker's *Dracula* was published in 1897. See further Jarrot (1999). For an explicit use of the image of the womb *as* vampire in the female body, see W. Johnson (1849: 24); his father, E. Johnson (1856: 154), used a similar image, writing that the cheeks of the chlorotic 'are sometimes so pallid that one might imagine every particle of red blood to have been sucked out of her body'.

22 On 'Anna O.' (Bertha Pappenheim), and the importance of the doctor's responses to her sexuality, see Appignanesi and Forrester (1993: 72–86).

23 In Anna's case, it is her father who consults Lange, but other descriptions imply that the initial concern for the well-being of sufferers comes from their mothers; e.g. de Baillou (1643: 58) on 'complaining mothers' (*querulae matres*) who are shocked by the speed with which their afflicted daughters appear to be wasting away. Hansen (1931: 182) noted the lack of references to chlorosis in ancient poetry and art, believing that anything adversely affecting the marriage prospects of young girls would surely have been the subject of 'lively and long discussion' by their mothers, and would thereby have entered non-medical literature. See also Hansen (1928). Theriot argues for the mid-nineteenth century as a period when chlorosis peaked, and links this to problems with the transition from girl to woman, leading to mother/daughter conflicts; for her, chlorosis becomes a way of gaining more attention from the mother (1988: 126).

24 It also led some medical practitioners to question the value of the diagnosis in *women*; see for example Strange (2000: 621). The existence of 'male hysteria' was discussed in the First World War, when the label of 'shell-shock' quickly came to be used in preference because of its 'simplicity, alliteration, and military sound' (Showalter 1993: 321).

25 Until the nineteenth century, green sickness or chlorosis in males was seen as a joke; p. 20.

26 Discussed further in chapter 4.

27 Cf. Hansen (1931: 176); Hudson (1977: 449). In a thesis for the Paris Medical Faculty, Boisseul (1828: 11–12) used the presence of chlorosis in young boys as evidence that it was a distinct illness, not a symptom of amenorrhoea. Uzac (1853), another Paris Medical Faculty dissertation, is unusual in supporting the idea of male chlorosis throughout history. Heath and Patek (1937: 299–300) argued for a rare form of chlorosis in adolescent boys with 'excessive blood loss or marked gastro-intestinal abnormality'.

28 The association with solitude also suggests masturbatory activity by the sufferer; see chapter 1. The text of W. Johnson's 1849 book, *An Essay on the Diseases of Young Women*, is identical to that of his 1850 publication, *The Morbid Emotions of Women; their Origin, Tendencies, and treatment*; on the Johnsons, see chapter 5 of this volume.

29 Sharp (1671: 292; Hobby 1999: 218) lists signs distinguishing 'a woman with child, when her courses are stopt, from a maid that hath hers stopt'; compare Sennert (1664: 71).

30 See, for example, the work of Laurent Joubert (1529–82), regent and chancellor of the university of Montpellier and personal physician to several members of the

French royal family; Rocher (1989: 99–102). In support of conception without apparent menstruation, medical writers could cite Aristotle *GA* 727b.

31 For example, Tait (1889: 284): 'A practitioner is told that a girl has not menstruated for sixteen months, and therefore he assumes that she cannot be pregnant. The story is true, but she may be pregnant four or five months all the same', because her ovaries would continue to function.

32 On pica, see chapter 4 of this volume.

33 In a similar vein, Wear (2000: 17) argues that, in 1550, when it was believed that 'the best medical knowledge was to be found in the works of Greek and Roman medical writers', what counted as 'research' lay 'either in the retrieval of that knowledge in its purest form or in its refinement'. The steady stream of inaugural dissertations by medical professors from the seventeenth to the early nineteenth century on the theme of chlorosis demonstrates the longevity of this search for a classical pedigree; see for example nearly thirty dissertations from c.1665–1809 in the BL tract collection, T.543.

34 The four texts printed in sextodecimo format (Calvi 1526) were *Diseases of women* 1–3, and *Nature of woman*. For reactions to these Hippocratic works in the later sixteenth century, see chapter 2 of this volume.

35 Temkin's translation remains the only one available in English; for a critical edition of the text, however, see the Budé edition of Burguière *et al.* (1988–2000).

36 On Soranos' approach to virginity, see chapter 2 of this volume. Green (2001: 20) notes that, because of the significance of the Hippocratic tradition in early medieval medical texts, the absence of menstruation remained 'cause for grave concern'. On the central role of menstruation in Hippocratic/Galenic theory, see chapter 3, p. 68–70.

37 In the introduction to volume 8, which includes *Diseases of women*, Littré made the comparison explicit, writing that 'Ce tableau des affections utérines qui affligeaient les femmes grecques, il y a plus de deux mille ans, est tout à fait semblable à celui que nous avons présentement sous les yeux; et il est évident que rien, dans leur existence, ne les mettait, plus que nos femmes, à l'abri de ces malades si fréquentes et si pénibles' (p. 2). See also Duminil (1979: 154) – 'Until the nineteenth century, medicine nourished itself on Hippocrates – or at least on that which it believed it could find in Hippocrates.'

38 I owe this reference to Vivian Nutton. See also Minghetti (1960: 369–78); Durling (1961: 285); Green (1987: 301 n. 9); Fichtner (1995a: 99–100).

39 For a discussion of debates over the existence and role of 'female seed' in Renaissance medical writers, see Maclean (1980: 35–7).

40 My thanks to Mark Buchan for sharing with me his reading of the letter as a witty account of an entirely imaginary patient.

41 The English Sweat is the subject of *Epistula* 1.20. The 1589 edition of Lange's *Epistulae medicinales* includes *Epistula* 2.13, *De novis morbis*, in which Lange addresses the 'new disease' issue directly. This letter is found only in the later editions, published after Lange's death in 1565. On the Sweat, and the question of new diseases, see further p. 61 of this volume.

42 Meynell (1990: 46, 48) notes that this work was written in Latin, privately printed in 1690, then published in Nuremberg in 1692, and the Latin text printed in the first edition in England in 1693. It was a very popular short work, going into a number of editions in rapid succession.

43 Another translation (Sydenham 1695: 78–9), reads: 'Ill colour of Face, and of the whole Body, Swellings in the Face, Eye-lids and Ankles, Heaviness of the whole Body, a stretching Weariness of the Legs and Feet, difficult Breathing, Feverish Pulse, Sleepiness, *Pica*, or longing for things that ought not to be eaten, and stoppage of the Courses'. For the influence of different translations of Sydenham, see

Wear (2000: 451 n. 46). The Latin, quoted here from Kühn's edition of 1827, reads: *Adsunt vultus et totius corporis decoloratio; intumescentia in facie, palpebris et malleolis; gravitas totius corporis; crurum ac pedum tensiva lassitudo; respiratio difficilis; cordis palpatio; capitis dolor; pulsus febrilis; somnolentia; pica, et mensium suppressio.* A very similar list is given in Maubray (1724: 43).

44 As Irvine Loudon (personal communication, 25 November 2002) has pointed out to me, the emergence of the concept of anaemia – of having too little blood, rather than too much or the wrong sort – occurring around 1850, constituted a radical departure from humoral medicine. 'Once the anaemia label had been invented it scooped up a whole collection of more of less vague conditions.'

45 Even for the Victorian period, W. Johnson (1849: 5) is unusual in seeing both chlorosis and hysteria as disorders of puberty.

46 Hobby (1999: 218, based on Sennert 1664: 71).

1 The nature of green sickness

1 For Lange's Latin text, see Appendix. 'On account of the pale face', Latin *ob faciei pallorem*, could equally well be 'on account of the pale appearance'.

2 Varandal (1619: 4–5; 1620: 1): *quem vulgus pallidos colores sive foedus, icterum album, febrem amatoriam, morbum virgineum appellant, nos ex Hipp. chlorosim quia est species cachexiae comitata pravo quodam colore ex albo plus minus virescente.* Fissell (1991: 103) notes that, at least in British medicine, the more general shift to Latinate medical terms did not occur until the late eighteenth century.

3 Uzac (1853: 13) dates the naming of chlorosis to around 1600.

4 On Napier and the sixty volumes of his medical notes, dated from 1597–1634, see also MacDonald (1981).

5 See note 3 in the Introduction to this volume.

6 Based on Aristotle, women were thought to be the colder sex. See further p. 95.

7 Other Shakespearean references to green sickness include *Romeo and Juliet* III.v.156 (c.1595), on which see Potter (2002).

8 Cited in Wear (2000: 75); although the juxtaposition with jaundice suggests that this is a 'digestive', non-sex-specific reference rather than being seen as a disease exclusive to young women, Wear comments that this passage 'does give the reader the sense that this is a humdrum condition' (personal communication, 2 April 2001). It also gives the sense that jaundice and green sickness are already seen as *separate* conditions. On the emergence of green sickness from jaundice in Boorde, see p. 22 and 25.

9 Elaine Hobby drew this example to my attention. The symptoms listed by Cary all appear on Sydenham's list (p. 14).

10 I owe this reference to John Appleby. Margaret became ill soon after her brother Edward's death, which occurred in or after 1573 (DNB). Her reflections on her treatment by her brother John, 'to whom the Lordship fell to' (Williamson 1920: 285) recall Johnson (1856: 153) on the sufferer from chlorosis: 'If she be a novel reader, she fancies herself the victim of domestic tyranny.'

11 CUL, Hengrave Hall MS 88, 1: f.115 (1558). My thanks to James Daybell for bringing this example to my attention and for discussing it with me. On Pagett (1505–63), a privy councillor and Secretary of State under Henry VIII, and involved in the international dealings to set up a marriage for Mary in March 1553–4, see DNB.

12 Although conception was thought possible in a girl who had not visibly menstruated (see p. 10), consummation may have been delayed until the obvious establishment of the menstrual function. Thomas Lorkyn's copy of the 1566 edition of Caspar Wolf's *Gynaeciorum* collection (CUL N*.9.50) was annotated at

the end of the sixteenth century; the only text in this collection which shows the signs of Lorkyn's interest is Jacques Dubois, *De mensibus mulierum, et hominis genera-tione*, first published in 1555. Lorkyn has underlined the points that virgins not yet menstruating can conceive, and that conception can occur even while the menses are flowing. Peter Murray Jones (personal communication) suggests that Lorkyn's interest in these matters stems from the fact that he had just married a very young wife!

13 CUL, Hengrave Hall MS 88, 1: f.83 (1559).

14 On Boorde's life and works, see Furnivall (1870); Henry (1991: 206); the text was written by 1542 (Furnivall 1870: 14). In de Castro (1603: 128), the equivalent of the virgins' disease is not green, but white, jaundice (*alba ictericia*). Boorde (1547: 73^v–74^r used *Hictericia* ('the latyn worde') or *Ictericia* ('The barbarous worde') for the generic 'jaundice', and then went on to divide it into three kinds.

15 Earlier in the book, Boorde writes that 'Agriaca is no greke worde, nor no latyn word, but a terme in phisicke signifienge a sicknes named the grene sicknes or the grene Jawnes, some Arabies doth use this worde' (1547: 11r). It involves corruption of the blood, weakness and a faintness around the heart. Discussions with Remke Kruk and Emilie Savage-Smith have failed to solve the problem of what was meant here. There is no 'g' in Arabic, nor is there a 'c'. 'Agriaca' sounds as if it should come from the Greek *agrios*, meaning savage or harsh. It is possible that the word in mind was 'agaric' (Arabic *aghāriqa*); however, this would be the remedy rather than the disease. Agaric was a word used for various fungi on trees and also for mushrooms; in the sixteenth century it was considered a powerful purgative, particularly against phlegm (e.g. da Monte, in Spach 1597: 325), and was used for failure to menstruate (e.g. Wirsung 1605: 483, where it is used as a purge after letting blood for suppressed menstruation; Johnston 1657: 75).

16 Galen took this model from the Hippocratic *On the nature of man*.

17 Good summaries of the humoral system are given by Sawyer (1986: 212–20); Dobson (1997: 262–82); Wear (2000: 37–40).

18 Stewart 2001: 43 links this 'new language of organs' to the rise of endocrinology, but emphasises how such a language remained gendered. On digestion in the humoral system, see further chapter 3 of this volume.

19 Aristotle, *PA* 650a8 ff.; *GA* 774a14–20.

20 For a detailed discussion of the sixteenth-century debates on the question of whether women are colder than men, and whether this necessarily implies their imperfection, see Maclean (1980: 33–5).

21 On the uses of *Aphorisms*, see Beccaria (1961); Kibre (1976); Müller-Rohlfsen (1980).

22 Bleeding from the male body could also be classified as 'menstrual', although the label would be modified by the addition of terms such as 'supernatural'. In the fourteenth-century commentary on pseudo-Albertus Magnus, three types of menses are listed: natural (women's menstrual periods), supernatural (the bleeding of the Jews, on which see Biller (1992); Pomata (1992: 62–5), and against nature; 'for example, some Christians of melancholy disposition bleed through the anus and not through the penis' (tr. Lemay 1992: 71). Seventeenth-century European learned societies reported cases of 'male menstruation' (Pomata 1992), which was regarded as a beneficial release of otherwise dangerous blood from various parts of the body caused by the healing powers of Nature; see further Schurig (1729: 118–25).

23 On Bullein see Mitchell (1959); Mambretti (1974); DNB. The DNB entry states that he does not appear on the roll of the College of Physicians, and he is certainly not listed in *Munk's Roll*; *contra* Copeman (1960: 94). The DNB suggests that William Pagett was supported by members of the Boleyn family when he was at

Cambridge: biographical materials on Bullein suggest that he was related to Anne Boleyn. There is therefore a possibility that Bullein knew the Pagetts, and even that he was one of the 'best learned' physicians on whom Sir William relied to treat Jane Kitson.

24 The Oxford English Dictionary expands on 'peraccidentes' as 'by accident', 'by virtue of some accessory or non-essential circumstance', 'contingently' or 'indirectly'. This could suggest that visual 'greenness' was not seen as essential to the condition in 1558.

25 The 1558 edition held by the Wellcome Institute for the History of Medicine has three owners' names on the title page: Henry Dinelye 1558 (i.e. Dingley, probably the compiler of the 1564 collection of medical recipes WMS 244), John Wallis and Robert Roberts. A further owner, Charles Bernard, appears on the fly leaf and another, George Dyngley 1599, on the final page. On the connections between green sickness and obstruction of the spleen, see section on Richard Napier in this volume, p. 22.

26 On p. 237 of this manuscript, another recipe for green sickness is included in a section on disorders of the stomach.

27 See further chapter 4.

28 On the history of theriac, see Watson (1966).

29 Ruel's edition of Dioscorides was printed in 1550, followed by the commentaries of Amatus Lusitanus in 1553 and Mattioli in 1558; Mattioli's aim was to retrieve the plants used in antiquity, using information from travellers in the eastern Mediterranean (Wear 2000: 67–8).

30 The Galenic passage used is from *On simple medicines* 58 (K 12.48–9); this does not mention menstrual suppression, but describes its powers to disperse thick humours. Compare Ruel (1550: 278); Amatus Lusitanus (1553), *humores crassos et lentos extenuat*.

31 Elaine Hobby has brought to my attention the appearance of this remedy in T.P. (perhaps Hannah Woolley), *The Accomplish'd Lady's Delight* (1677: 128), with the replacement of 'red Mynts' by 'red Fennel'.

32 Schenck von Grafenberg (1600: IV case 256). This is the complete edition; the section in which Lange's letter appears was first printed in 1596.

33 As I shall discuss in the next chapter, virginity, too, can have its (disputed) external signs.

34 *Velut exsanguinea pallescere*, Lange (1554: 74).

35 It was Loudon (1980: 1672) who suggested this chronological divide; I would add that, at all stages of the conditions being studied here, paleness of some kind is more important than greenness.

36 *plumbeus vel subalbidus efficitur*.

37 For the Latin, see p. 148 note 2.

38 '[C]ouleur de cire ou de suif, & quelquefois même d'un jaune feuille morte, ou d'un jaune tyrant sur le verd ou sur le noir'. There is no equivalent description in the (much shorter) account of chlorosis in the earliest English version, (Astruc 1743), but Astruc (1762–7, vol. 1: 172) reads 'Moreover, the colour of the face fades; and the freshness of the skin goes off. The patients become pale, of a leaden hue, with a colour like wax or tallow, and sometimes even of a yellow brown, or of a yellow, verging towards green or black.' The 'tallow' imagery also features in *Romeo and Juliet* III.v.156–7, where Capulet calls Juliet 'green-sickness carrion' and 'You tallow-face'; see further Potter (2002: 272).

39 Purple features in Mercado (1579: 204), but compare also W. Johnson (1849: 31) on a servant girl whose 'lips exchanged the tint of the cherry for that of the lilac blossom'. The floral imagery was taken even further by his father E. Johnson, (1856: 155), who told of sudden onset in 'a hale and buxom country lass': 'in one night a blight came, the roses [in her cheeks] were all withered'.

40 The distinction between internal and external was also used in the rhetoric of women's exclusion from medical practice in sixteenth-century Germany, their work being officially limited to 'external' conditions. This in turn meant that the status of barber-surgeons remained low, because their work was seen as undifferentiated from that of women; see Wiesner (1986: 49–51, 190).

41 On bloodletting in the disease of virgins, see pp. 73–9.

42 BL C.112.f.9.(44) and BL C.112.f.9.(47). On medical advertisements, see further chapter 5.

43 Compare the proverbial saying, 'Like a leek, he has a white head and a green tail', (Tilley 1950: 375), applied to an old but lusty man.

44 For *Enfield Common, or the young damsel cured of the green sickness by a lusty gallant who happen'd to meet her in the Mid'st of Enfield Common*, see the collection of Osterley Park Ballads, BL C.39.k6. The young damsel so enjoys her cure that she asks her 'Physician' to repeat the treatment, because she longs 'to be a Mother'. In a similar vein, in *The Practical Part of Love* (1660) and its 1662 version, *Venus Undrest*, Helena develops green sickness in Croydon and takes the cure, many times, in London; see Thompson (1979: 39–40).

45 The first printed edition of Trotula's *Cum auctor* (the *Liber de sinthomatibus mulierum*), drastically edited by Georg Kraut, was published in Strasbourg in 1544. The text was also included in the compendium of thirteen ancient medical texts published by Paulus Manutius in 1547 under the title *Medici Antiqui Omnes*. See Green (1996; 2001). Monica Green is also producing a monograph, *Women and Literate Medicine in Medieval Europe: Trota and the Trotula*.

46 This is the translation given in Green (2001: 75); the Latin is *Unde quandoque in viriditatem vel lividitatem aut in colorem qualis est color graminis facies earum mutatur* (Green 2001: 74). The version given in the *Gynaeciorum* collection (Wolf 1566a: 220–1; Spach 1597: 42) reads *humiditatem* for *lividitatem* here. See Lemay (1978: 393), however, which suggests here a 'grey face'.

47 *Palleat omnis amans, color hic est aptus amanti.* This is also cited, without attribution, by Luis Mercado, in his 1579 discussion of the 'white fever' which draws heavily on Lange's 1554 description of the 'disease of virgins'. Mercado (1579: 201) uses the Ovid lines to support the identity of 'love fever', 'white fever' and the 'disease of virgins'. See also the use of Ovid in Varandal (1619: 5; 1620: 2); Stengel (1896: 329).

48 Ferrand (1623: ch. 15), in Beecher and Ciavolella (1990: 274–5, 448 n. 5); the Galenic passage is from the commentary on Hippocrates, *Diet in acute diseases*, CMG V.9, 1, p. 182.

49 See p. 6–7 for the nineteenth-century image of the erotic chlorotic.

50 BL, C.40.m.10.(161). On the English proverbial use of 'as green as grass', see Whiting and Whiting (1968: 250–1).

51 Ferrand (1623: ch. 14) – see edition of Beecher and Ciavolella (1990: 41, 271–2), with Beecher (1988) on Ferrand and other physicians of his time who wrote treatises on love sickness.

52 Weinberg (1950) notes that several manuscripts of pseudo-Longinus are known from the period 1450–1500; Sappho's poem is also preserved in a papyrus fragment from the third century BC, for which see *Omaggio all'xi congr. internaz. di papirologia*, Pubblicazioni della Società italiana per la ricerca dei papiri greci e latini in Egitto, Florence 1965, p. 165. Kenneth Kitchell states that the poem was 'extremely popular in England, translated early and often' (personal communication).

53 For example, *Iliad* 7.479, where the Greek troops waiting outside the city of Troy are affected by *chloron deos*, 'green fear' (Irwin 1974: 62–4; Cyrino 1995: 164 n. 69). Compare Euripides, *Suppliant women* 598–9, 'pale fear perturbs me below my liver'.

54 Other echoes can be found in the third-century BC Theocritos, *Idylls* 2.106–10, and the description of Medea's love sickness in Apollonius Rhodius, *Argonautica* 3.960–5; in the latter, however, blushing replaces pallor.

55 This sense of the fleeting moment is also found in classical Greek literature: see Carson (1990: 145–7). My thanks to Ross Wordie for discussing hay-making practice with me. Other translations of Sappho's phrase, which try to account for the juxtaposition of green, grass and emotional response, include 'I am paler than [dried] grass', 'paler I am than dried grass in autumn', and 'grassy pale I grow' (Cox 1925: 70–2).

56 Sennert (1664: 100) locates the condition 'in Virgins fit for a Man', but lacks Sharp's interest in 'love'. Drysdale (1875: 168–9) proposed that chlorosis was caused by the lack of healthy sexual outlets for single women; on his attitudes to sexuality and birth control, see Benn (1992: 56), demonstrating that his chlorosis sections were based on the work of Samuel Ashwell.

57 On Bienville, see Rousseau (1982) with the criticisms of Groneman (1994: 346–7). Despite his interest in the connections between scientific discourse and artistic narrative (e.g. 1982: 111), Rousseau does not discuss the novelistic quality of the extended case histories in Bienville.

58 On further fears by English commentators of the late eighteenth century that novels would not only corrupt individuals, but also damage society, because people from different classes would be reading the same books, see Levy (1999: 51–2).

59 The 1777 edition of Buffon's *Histoire naturelle, générale et particulière* similarly included in its study of 'erotomania' a detailed letter from a priest, 'Monsieur x', outlining his personal difficulties with this condition (Buffon 1971: 102–7).

2 A new disease? The classical sources for the disease of virgins

1 On da Monte's Galenism, see Wear (2000: 36, 118–19). The work on women's diseases was reprinted in a sextodecimo format in Paris in 1556, see p. 11 of this volume.

2 'Le divin Hippocrates soigneux de ceste santé et foecundité de la femme et stimulé d'un esprit charitable à la secourir, a escript quatre livres à part en sa saveur' (Liébault 1582). This work is listed in the catalogues of the British Library and the Wellcome Institute for the History of Medicine as having been compiled from Giovanni Marinello's *Infirmità delle Donne* (1563). The same comment recurs for Liébault's *Trois livres de l'embellissement et ornement du corps humain* and Marinello's *Ornamenti delle donne*. However, as Lonie (1985: 321 n. 23) has pointed out, the originality of Liébault's work is defended in Bayle's *Dictionary*, and my own comparison of Marinello with the French edition of Liébault (*Trois livres aux infirmitez et maladies des femmes*, 1582) shows that, although the material inevitably overlaps, it is very differently organised and handled, with Liébault using and citing his sources (including Galen, Aristotle and Hippocrates). On Marinello, see Bell (1999: 25).

3 Uzac (1853: 12) argued that Lange's treatment of Anna dates from the period 1520–30; however, his use of Calvi puts the case after 1525.

4 My thanks to Vivian Nutton and Frans Schlesinger for their advice on this translation. The full Latin text of Lange's letter is given in the Appendix. The letter is also translated in Major (1932).

5 Achates was the loyal companion of the hero Aeneas.

6 '*Sed hic morbus virgines infestat, quum viro iam maturae, ex ephebis excesserint. Nam id temporis, natura duce, sanguis menstruus ad matricis loculos, et venas ab epate defluit.*' Almost identical wording is given by de Castro (1603: 128).

7 In both translations given by Calvi, and also in Cornarius, there is only a single 'mouth' of exit here, suggesting the vaginal exit. Lange's plural shifts the focus to

the 'mouths' of the channels supplying blood to the womb. See further chapter 2, pp. 57–8.

8 Galen, *De difficultate respirationis/De spirande difficultate* 3.12; Vassès (1533: 74/ lines 28–30) gives '*In totum siquidem, ut diximus, cum vel tumor, vel dolor in hypochondriis fuerit, parva de necessitate et frequens adest respiratio, ut nihil mirum sit, si in sequentibus, ubi hypochondrium hypolaparou, id est, subinane dixit, adiecerit spirituosum autem non valde*'; see also Cornarius (1536: 96). K 7.954 gives '*In universum enim ut diximus, quum aut tumor, aut dolor quispiam in partibus hypochondriorum constiterit, parvus et densus necessario sit spiritus.*'

9 In Galenic medical theory, this channel collects blood from the liver and delivers it to the right side of the heart.

10 The Greek Lange gives here recalls the discussion of *pneumatôn apolêpsis* in Galen's commentary on Hippocrates' *Regimen in acute diseases* 4.26–7 (CMG V.9, 1 p. 294.7 and p. 295.29). Here, Galen discusses a Hippocratic passage in which an excess of black bile or sharp and bitter humours causes internal pain; the blood is corrupted, and the breaths cannot reach their natural channels; if the bad humours reach the heart, liver or great vein, the result will be fits or madness.

11 Here Lange gives in Greek the text of Galen's commentary on Hippocrates' *Regimen in acute diseases* 4.78 (CMG V.9, 1 p. 336.11–13).

12 'Hippocratis de virginum natura liber' (Calvi 1525: 133).

13 'Hippocratis de virginalibus, virginumve morbis, liber' (Calvi 1525: 47). In the 1526 edition, the contents list gives the text only once, coming in the traditional position after *Eighth month child* and before *Nature of woman* as Book 17, but Book 23 is the second translation, placed after the third volume of *Diseases of women*. An early owner of the British Library copy (541.f.1) has noticed this duplication, and altered the contents list to take it into account. According to L 10.61, Calvi's own codex, Vatican 278, combined the late twelfth-century Vatican 276 with the fourteenth-century Vatican 277, being based on 277 but giving the readings of 276 in the margins. The translation given as book 17 is in better Latin, and makes more use of 'doubling', giving two Latin words for one Greek word; that given as book 23 tends to omit words and phrases which the translator is unable to understand. Both translators also seem to have access to the tenth-century manuscript Marcianus Graecus 269 (M), which refers to 'wandering' fevers (Greek *planêtas*).

14 Ranchin (1627: 372) usefully summarises the two sides of the debate up to his own time.

15 See for example Lefkowitz (1981: 13–15); King 1983; Andò (1990); Catonné (1994); Dean-Jones (1994: 48); Demand (1994: 95–9); King (1998: ch. 4); Flemming and Hanson (1998). A full translation is given by Flemming and Hanson; a partial one appears in Lefkowitz and Fant (1992: 242–3).

16 E.g. Trotula, *Quoniam ergo mulieres viris sunt debiliores natura*; Green (2001: 70); Baillou (1648: 63); Maclean (1980: 57); Pomata (1992: 74).

17 The symptom of seeing ghosts or demons was mentioned in Catholic commentators on the text, for example Mercado (1579: 182–3).

18 Maubray (1724: 48) claims that Lange's letter specifies that conception cures the condition because the blood which has been retained 'contrary to nature' is used up in forming the foetus, while the bad humours accumulated in the womb are evacuated after childbirth.

19 Kibre (1945; 1980: 347 n. 1) criticised the long-dominant opinion that Hippocratic writings were virtually unknown in the West before the fifteenth century, listing all surviving manuscripts then known which included sections of Hippocratic works.

20 On the Ravenna translations, see Müller-Rohlfsen 1980; Mazzini 1985; on Paris BN 11219, Beccaria (1959: 36, 38–9); Agrimi (1985: 391–2). On Leningrad

Lat.F.v.VI.3, see also Egert (1936); Diepgen (1933: 228–9); Walter 1935. The *editio princeps* is Vázquez Buján (1986).

21 Greek *physis*, one of many Greek terms for menstruation. On others, see King (1998: 60).

22 On the absence of Arabic translations of the text (as opposed to the title), see Ullmann (1977: 248), *contra* Sezgin (1970: 40–1 no. 17, 45 no. 3). On Galen's plans, see Ullmann (1977: 254); Green (1987: 303 n. 15).

23 On Basil of Ancyra, *On the true purity of virginity*, see Shaw (1998); on John Chrysostom, Shore (1983: 115, cited in Kelly 2000: 4).

24 Sennert (1664: 96–7) notes that 'Some say … if a membrane be there, it is preternatural, and a Disease in the Organ.' So too was the clitoris, or *nympha*, described as *hic morbus*, 'this disease', by Mercuriale (in Bauhin 1586–8, vol. 2: 159; 1591: 192), and identified with the Hippocratic *kiôn* which may be more accurately seen as a vulval wart (see *NW* 65; L 7.400; *DW* 2.212; L 8.406; and discussion in King 1998: 18). Mercuriale, despite locating the organ he describes at the mouth of the womb, elides it with descriptions of a female organ which can grow so large in some women that they are taken to have changed sex. See further chapter 3, p. 89 on Buffon's views on the hymen.

25 Compare Sennert (1664: 96–7). As Bicks (2003: 77) notes, Sharp concentrates on how the belief in the hymen as a certain sign of virginity acts against women; for example, she warns women not to marry near the time of menstruation, to avoid any confusion between types of bleeding. By the late nineteenth century, for some the hymen was a far more certain organ, believed to exist in the foetus as early as the fifth month of pregnancy (e.g. Oliver 1893: 13). At this time, sex with a virgin was thought to cure venereal disease (Spongberg 1997: 110); the age of consent was raised from 13 to 16 by the Criminal Law Amendment Bill of 1885, and, as Spongberg (1997: 122–3) demonstrated, other writers of this period, concerned with issues of child prostitution, continued to doubt the reliability of the hymen as evidence of prior sexual behaviour.

26 Compare Sennert (1664: 98), who tries to solve the problem by proposing that young virgins bleed, but older ones do not. Similar ambivalence may be found in Maubray (1724: 39) – bleeding at first intercourse is 'a certain sign of Virginity, when it does appear; yet, if it don't, the Virgin is not therefore to be suspected'.

27 Paster (1993: 43) discusses the urine of a virgin. Joubert (Rocher 1989: 210–11) gives some tests which he rejects, but he still thinks that a virgin can 'piss straight and far' in an 'unfettered and clear' manner, and describes this style as 'this beautiful mark of maidenhood' (Rocher 1989: 216, 220; Paster 1993: 44; Bell 1999: 211–12; cf. Ranchin 1627: 354). Kelly (2000: 29) describes urine tests for virginity which focus on the sound of urination, the speed of urination after the administration of the test, or the clarity of the end product. See also Lemay (1978: 396; 1981: 175–6; 1992: 128). On stories in which virginity is made apparent – or not – in Greek literature, see Sissa (1990b: 343–6).

28 One of the Trotula texts, *On treatments for women*, includes a set of recipes including 'A constrictive for the vagina so that they may appear as if they were virgins', and the use of leeches in the vagina on the night before the wedding; see Green (2001: 144–6). This interest in restoring virginity existed alongside proverbs such as 'Maidenhead once lost can never be found' (Whiting and Whiting 1968: 365). Other restoratives were more general, such as a bath in comfrey roots (Sennert 1664: 99).

29 In the eighteenth century Buffon, whose ideas about female puberty will be discussed in chapter 3, also thought that such a relationship existed, and as evidence cited the breaking of the voice at puberty and the high-pitched voices of eunuchs (Roger 1997: 167). In the sixteenth century, however, Joubert (Rocher

1989: 210) had criticised what he presented as the popular misconception that the neck thickened and the voice correspondingly altered at the loss of virginity.

30 Munich (1993: 144), writing on late Victorian literature, suggests that 'A virgin cannot know herself as virginal, for that would give her the unvirginal knowledge she cannot have to retain her flowery sweetness.'

31 Wolf (1566b: 5); Minghetti (1960); Fravega (1962); Manuli (1982: 39–40); Pinault (1992: 123); Hanson and Green (1994: 1046–7).

32 *autem oscula exitus obstructa fuerint.* The reading '*oscula*' was also followed in Donati's commentary on the Hippocratic text (Donati 1582: 18).

33 Cornarius collated three ancient manuscripts, including Munich gr. 71, a copy of BN gr. 2140. On his editorial activities, see Mondrain (1997).

34 Sharp's source here, Sennert (1664: 105), had also cited Lange, so this does not mean that Sharp had read the text for herself.

35 *coloremque crebro variat et mutat.* Cornarius (1546: 286), however, prefers a manuscript giving *chreios* rather than *chroia*, translating as *et omnem vitae utilitatem excedentia.*

36 *quidam varios trahit colores.*

37 Hirsch (1885: 493–4) also suggested that, although the term 'chlorosis' was not used in antiquity and the middle ages, references to pallor and a yellow tint in earlier texts may point to the condition's existence.

38 Syphilis arrived in Europe in 1495. The English Sweat appeared in 1485, with further outbreaks in 1508, 1517, 1528 and 1551. Discussions include the very full and useful article by Shaw (1933, which covers in detail the alternative names for the condition); recent contributions, focused on identifying the disease agent, include Dyer (1997) (using parish registers); Taviner *et al.* (1998); Carlson and Hammond (1999).

39 Lange, *Medicinalium epistolarum miscellanea* 2.13. The quotation is taken from Pliny, *Natural history* 26.6.9, a discussion of the emperor Tiberius contracting the new disease of *colum*: 'What should we say this means, what anger of the gods? Were the recognised kinds of human disease, more than three hundred, too few, that new ones too should add to man's fear?'

40 It was used by many subsequent classical writers (Longrigg 1992: 27), including Crepereius Calpurnianus who followed it slavishly when describing the effects of the so-called 'plague of Galen' on Nisibis in 166 AD (Gilliam 1961: 228 n. 16). This last plague is supposed to have started in Seleucia, when a Roman soldier accidentally allowed an unhealthy vapour to escape from a golden casket in a temple of Apollo. This story, found in the *Scriptores Historiae Augustae* (*Life of Verus* 8, 1–2), neatly links the Homeric explanation for new diseases – the whim of the gods (since it occurs in the temple of Apollo) – with the Hesiodic explanation – they all escaped from Pandora's jar.

41 The belief in locally specific diseases is supported by the approach of *Airs, Waters, Places* and also lies behind the Hippocratic comment that it is useful to move to another country in a long-standing illness (*Epidemics* 6.5.13; L 5.318; Loeb VII, 258).

42 This view is echoed in the words of a gay physician talking about AIDS in the 1980s: 'A disease which killed only gay white men? It seemed unbelievable … I used to teach epidemiology, and I had never heard of a disease that selective' (cited in Treichler 1988: 201).

3 The menstruating virgin

1 In modern editions, the section Lange is using is not in Book 4, but Book 3; the confusion arises by counting what is now listed as *On the causes of diseases* (*De causis*

morborum) as the first book of *On the causes of symptoms* (*De symptomatum causis*). In the Renaissance, *On the causes of symptoms* was translated into Latin by Thomas Linacre (1524) and Niccoló Leoniceno (1528).

2 On the details of Galen's views of the heart and of the role of breathing, and on those of his predecessors, see Debru (1996).

3 Sydenham (1695: 53; 1753: 658) states, in contrast, that the normal amount of blood lost in menstruation should be enough 'to fill the shell of a goose's egg'. However, in the copy held at the Wellcome Library, someone has crossed this out, perhaps wishing to retain the higher levels of loss expected in the Hippocratic/Galenic tradition.

4 '*Aliquando accidit dyarria propter nimiam frigiditatem matricis, vel quia vene eius sunt multum graciles, ut in extenuatis mulieribus, quia tunc humores spissi et superflui non habent liberos meatus per quos possint erumpere, vel quia humores sunt spissi et viscosi, et propter conglutinationem eorum exitus impeditur, vel quia deliciose comedunt, vel quia ex aliquo labore multum sudant*' (Green 2001: 72).

5 There is a strong contrast between this medical interest in establishing the limits of normality, and the relaxed approach of the female Physical Education instructors (between 1900 and 1940) studied by Verbrugge; 'some doctors continued to problematize menstrual phenomena that physical educators regarded as natural variations' (2000: 72). Verbrugge argues that the instructors continued to operate with an 'ancient plethora model' (2000: 74), because this allowed them to establish their own professional authority over that of the supposed experts.

6 On the imagery of wounding in relation to the female body, see Fowler (1987).

7 It was possible to regard the process of menstruation as pathological, a belief reflected in terminology such as 'being unwell', but the blood itself as entirely normal. Strange (2000: 615) argues that the notion of menstruation as 'being unwell' was partly the result of medical research being based on those women who did indeed experience severe discomfort or pain, and partly due to the idea that the normal state of a woman consisted in the amenorrhoea of pregnancy and breast-feeding. See also Strange (2001).

8 Oudshoorn (1994) discusses the role of studies of the sex hormones in this process from the 1920s onwards.

9 '*viris cohabitent, et copulentur*'.

10 The Greek Aldine text was published in 1526; *On the disease of virgins* appears on p. 92^{v}.

11 In his two separate translations of *On the disease of virgins*, Calvi gives '*cum viris coniungi et commisceri: nam si concipient, sanescent*' (1525: 67–8) and '*cum viris misceri, et cohabitare, quae si concipiant, sanescunt*' (1525: 196).

12 Lange, '*Huius morbi liberatio est, venae sectio, si nihil obstiterit*'; Calvi gives '*sed huius liberatio, et medela est (nisi quid vetet) sanguinis missio*' (1525: 67–8) and '*sed huius mali, sanguinis missio, nisi quid impedit, medela est*' (1525: 196). In the copy of the 1526 printing of Calvi held by the British Library it is this advice – rather than the section on marriage – which has been highlighted by a sixteenth-century reader.

13 It is retained in Donati's commentary on the text (1582: 40).

14 Calvi (1526: 46): '*Sed huius liberatio, et medela est (nisi quid vetet) sanguinis missio.*' The alternative translation of this text in Calvi uses the same term.

15 Cornarius (1546: 286): '*Caeterum curatio ut hinc liberentur, est sanguinis detractio, si nihil fuerit quod impediat.*' The wording was followed by Mercado (1579: 183).

16 '*Huius morbi liberatio est, venae sectio, si nihil obstiterit.*'

17 '*Et ego saepe paellas defectis menstruis tabe prope correptas ad pristinam valetudinem revocari copiosiori sanguinis detractione.*'

18 This is much stronger in Sharp than in her source, Sennert 1664: 105, and it is worth noting that she is here making a claim to authority based on direct personal experience.

19 Discussed in Lewis (1980: 112); cf. King (1998: 5). Newman (1965: 42), working on the Gururumba of New Guinea, suggests that they see artificially induced male nosebleeds as the equivalent of female menstruation.

20 Galen, *On treatment by bloodletting* 18; K 11.283, 11.302–3; Brain (1986: 93); cf. Rivière (1655: 404).

21 As Brain (1986: 145–8) shows, Celsus (4.27.1d) suppressed the menses by bleeding at the elbow, while Aretaeus (6.10.3) – a contemporary of Galen – bled from the lower limbs for all disorders of the womb. The saphena vein was also the one used in Arabic medicine; see Bos (1997: 264), where Ibn al-Jazzār explains that bleeding from the foot, 'although it attracts the menstrual blood in a direction opposite to the one it [naturally] tends to take, helps to let it flow copiously'. Sharp (1671: 294; Hobby 1999: 220) noted that 'Authors agree not what veins must be opened to move the Terms' (following Sennert 1664: 77). Brain (1986: 130 n. 83) also cites Trousseau (1872: 218), who claimed – *contra* Galen – that 'Bleeding from the arm … is a measure of immense potency and it is not unusual for the uterine flux to appear an hour after the bloodletting'. However, Wiltshire (1885: 514) cites examples where bleeding from the arm was being used in the nineteenth century to *stop* menstruation.

22 Galen, *On treatment by bloodletting* 9; K 11.278–9; (Brain 1986: 81, 13, 11.290); Brain (1986: 87); cf. Culpeper (1651: 86).

23 The notion of menses as 'fruit' is of interest, since the normal metaphor from the medieval period onwards presents them as 'flowers' because the flowers precede the fruit; cf. the post-eleventh-century treatise, *Tractatus de egritudinibus mulierum*, Green (1996: 128); Trotula, *Cum auctor* in Green (2001: 73, 21–2); Paré (1575: 787–8); Sharp (1671: 288). See also Demaitre (2001: 22) on adaptations in Flemish gynaecologies. Fissell (1995: 436) cites Culpeper (1651: 19), repeated by Sennert (1664: 97) and Sharp (1671: 48) Hobby 1999: 43); loss of virginity is called deflowering because of the floral appearance of the vaginal entrance, like 'the bud of a rose half-blown'. The imagery of menses as flowers was used in the mid-seventeenth century by An Collins' *Divine Songs and Meditacions* (1653), which described how her failure to have her 'flowers', marriage or children was replaced by poetry. See in particular 'Another Song' (Graham *et al.* 1989: 67–9). I owe this reference to Elaine Hobby.

24 Montanus (1565, *consilium* 307; given in Spach 1597: 325–6 as *consilium* iv).

25 '*phlebotomiê rhuetai*' (Littré 2.468); the Greek used by Vassès (1543: 125) gives '*phlebotomia luetai*' here.

26 'Marriage is a Sovereign Cure for those that cannot abstain' (Sharp 1671: 263; Hobby 1999: 199). Sharp's source, Sennert (1664: 105), puts this rather differently: 'It is probable, and agreable [*sic*] to Reason and Experience, that Venery is good.'

27 Klairmont-Lingo (1999: 341) translates these terms even more violently; for example, 'the neck of the womb split, the edge of labia peeled or flayed … and the clitoris flayed and skinned'.

28 On the parallels between the exploration of the body through anatomy, and travel writing at the time of the 'discovery' of the New World, see Montrose (1993); Bicks (2003: 72).

29 BL Stowe Mss vol. 28, 5, cited in Falkiner (1904: 349–50). I owe this reference to John McGurk. See also Cullingford (1993: 55–72) on the political uses of female imagery for Ireland.

30 E.g. Carol (1995: 51–60).

31 Raciborski's work predates the main period of the French eugenics movement in the final decade of the nineteenth and the beginning of the twentieth century; Schneider (1986) has demonstrated how this movement grew out of 'puericulture', the idea of preparing the body to bear healthy children in order to improve the species. This would ideally include medical examination before marriage. Raciborski wrote not only within the context of puericulture (a word coined by Charles Alfred Caron in 1865; see Carol 1995: 40), but also within a broader context of 'pre-eugenicist' ideas about degeneration and 'hygiene'; Carol (1995: 43–5) further links these to the appropriation by médecins-accoucheurs of the traditional role of the midwife in not only delivering, but also advising, women. On the role played by nubility 'in the triumph of gynaecology' in late nineteenth-century British medicine, see Strange (2000: 611–12).

32 In a different expression of the link between sexuality and the onset of menstruation, Sennert (1664: 69) claimed that girls who start to menstruate too early are 'for the most part very lecherous, and short lived'.

33 '...owing to the reading of obscene Books, unchaste Touching, &c for hereby the Subject becomes as it were a Woman before her due Time'. On the theological and moral problems raised in discussions of manual removal of the seed, by the patient, the midwife or the physician, in Renaissance writing, see p. 145 of this volume, n. 14.

34 '*At vero ex maritatis, steriles magis id patiuntur.*'

35 '*mulieres iam adultae*', and '*mulieres iam grandes*'.

36 '*ex maritatis*'.

37 '*ex mulieribus viro iunctis*' (Cornarius 1546: 286). This use of Calvi could also provide internal evidence that Lange's letter was written after 1546.

38 Particularly influential here was Isidore of Seville's model of six ages of life; see for example Taddei (2002: 19–20). Here, adolescence was situated between the ages of 14 and 28, and was characterised as a 'period of growth and concupiscence'. The model was applied to herself by Margaret, Countess of Cumberland, writing in the 1590s; see Williamson (1920: 285).

39 On the conduct, or advice, books, see for example Davies (1977); Eales (1998).

40 *Contra* Theriot (1988: 120), who tries to restrict chlorosis to 'provid[ing] information about the struggles of adolescent girls' only in the 1870s and 1880s.

41 Here, bizarrely, Buffon repeats the late antique Christian view that there is a 'virginity of the soul'; see p. 55 of this volume.

42 In writings on chlorosis, this voyeurism is more apparent in French medicine, but English and American writers give a less florid version. In broad terms, French medicine embraces the erotic chlorotic at the beginning of the nineteenth century, English-language medicine towards the end of the century. Munich 1993: 143 suggests that the period from 1892–8 saw 'a heightened interest in *jeunes filles en fleur*', centred on Freud's 'virginal anxiety'.

43 Compare the German proverb, given in Schurig (1730: 117), 'Garstige Jungfern, Schöne Weiber' ('Ugly maidens, pretty wives').

44 See also Drysdale (1875: 169). On early modern imagery of the countryside in medicine, 'as a place either of wisdom or of ignorance', see Wear (2000: 56).

45 Galenic medicine held that, menstruation being due to a plethora, those women who worked hard would use up their excess blood and so menstruate less heavily. As noted earlier (chapter 1), this meant that country women were thought to have only scanty menstrual loss. Seventeenth-century writers believed that 'savages' never menstruated, because their bodies were too hot; e.g. Sennert (1664: 68).

46 The idea that moving from the country to the city was dangerous to health was found from at least the seventeenth century onwards; see Whorton (2000: 30).

47 Strange (2000: 617–20) discusses how, in the period from 1850–1930, subsequent amenorrhoea was thought to be linked to the onset of insanity.

4 Dietary factors

1 E.g. Mercado (1579: 201); Fontanus (1652: 5); Tanner (1659: 314–7); Fraundorffer (1696: 11); Sydenham (1753: 658); Manning (1771: 90 ff). The picture given by Stengel, cited in Siddall (1982: 255) links the morbid appetite to oedema; the patient appears well-fed, despite her dietary problems, because of the swelling. Sydenham's description (1753: 658; cf. Hudson 1977: 450) has swelling of the face, eyelids and ankles, with lassitude of the feet and legs.

2 The story also features in Aulus Gellius, *Attic nights* 15.10, where it was attributed to a section on disorders of the mind in Plutarch's lost work, *On the soul*. It is summarised in Polyaenus, *Stratagems* 8.63.

3 '*at noster auctor idem antiquissimus,ac prudentissimus horum malorum culpam omnem in menstruorum detentionem, ac suppressionem referendam semper censuit*'. Cf. Stephanus (1635: 32); Le Loyer (1605: 110r–v).

4 *Disease of virgins* (L 8.466), '*dia te ta sitia kai tên auxêsin tou sômatos*'; Lange (1554), '*ob cibaria et corporis incrementum*'; Calvi (1526: 133), '*ob cibaria, corporisque incrementum*'; Calvi (1526: 47), '*ob cibaria, corporisque incrementum*'; Cornarius (1546: 286), '*propter cibos et corporis augmentum*'.

5 Homer, *Iliad* 5.341–2; cf. Aristotle, *PA* 650a34–5, 651a14–15; Byl 1980: 41.

6 In some (undated) nineteenth-century editions of the *Masterpiece*, this is misprinted as 'such as the green weasel colonet, short-breathing, trembling of the heart, etc.'.

7 '*stomachum cibum, ac praecipue carnem fastidire*'.

8 See chapter 3.

9 Examples of such fasting behaviour include the seventeenth-century Martha Taylor, who supposedly lived without food for a year (Reynolds 1669) and Mollie Fancher, whose survival on nothing at all for over twelve years enthralled 1870s, Brooklyn (Stacey 2002).

10 'Il n'est pas rare de rencontrer des jeunes filles chlorotiques de quinze et seize ans qui ne soient pas encore réglées, même parmi les enfants appartenant à des familles aisées, et habitant les grandes villes' (Raciborski 1868: 379).

11 E.g. *Diseases of women* 1.1 (L 8.14); Galen, *On bloodletting against Erasistratus* 5; K 11.164–5; Brain (1986: 25–6).

12 In ps-Xenophon, *Oikonomikos*, a classical Greek text popular in the early modern period, men are associated with 'active' and 'outside', women with 'passive' and 'inside'. See further p. 129, on the influence of the polarities used for male/female in this text.

13 '*virgines et mulierculae istae innuptae*'; discussed also by Vandereycken and Van Deth (1994: 141), who suggest that Varandal may have had cosmetics rather than pica in mind here.

14 Boarding schools for girls were seen as a breeding-ground for chlorosis; for example, Raciborski (1868: 287, 289) regarded them as damaging because diet was not individually tailored to the needs of different girls. Education away from the home contributed to the creation of 'adolescence', in which girls were held in limbo between childhood and adulthood; see p. 83–8 of this volume.

15 Latin *grossus*; cf. Mercado (1579: 203) which uses *crassus* here.

16 In Sennert (1664: 101), green-sick girls 'desire to eat absurd things'.

17 Sennert (1664: 105) adds that keeping a pregnant woman away from the food she craves may also cause a birthmark on her child. On beliefs about the need to

placate pregnant women's food cravings in medieval Arabic culture, see Kruk (1987/8: 425–6).

18 On the metaphor see p. 157, n. 23.

19 He is listed as a navy surgeon in the 1805 *List of the Members of the Royal College of Surgeons of London* (List 1805: 39).

20 Compare Fogo (1803: 7–11) with Fox (1839: 13–18). Fogo, despite using Cullen's *First Lines of the Practice of Physic* (1786) and the *Edinburgh Practice of Physic* (1803), gives the impression he is citing Cullen when in fact he is citing Hamilton's commentary sections.

21 Wellcome Institute for the History of Medicine accession no. 66244; Ms notes on p. 86f.

22 I owe much here to the combined efforts of John Symons and Chris Hilton.

23 My thanks to Lucinda McCray Beier for this reference, 3/22 in her numbering of BL Sloane MS 663.

24 Sharp (1671: 292; Hobby 1999: 218) includes 'Costiveness' as a symptom of menstrual suppression.

25 Clark (1887); Taylor (1896: 720); Jones (1897: 42).

26 Ptomaine was a term coined from the Greek for 'corpse', to describe the compounds produced by matter decaying in the large intestine (Whorton 2000: 24).

27 Lettsom also believed that the trend for wearing long hair up on the head made the head too hot (1795: 27).

5 'The laboratory came to the rescue': technology and chlorosis

1 The case was widely discussed, for example in de Baillou (1648: 63); Ferrand chs. 13 and 14 (Beecher and Ciavolella 1990: 266 and 272); Wack (1990: 9). Beecher and Ciavolella (1990: 119, 272) note the early-seventeenth-century debate over the existence of a 'lover's pulse'. A further ancient example of the diagnosis of love by a physician is the story of Hippocrates' diagnosis of King Perdiccas' love for his father's concubine.

2 The noises 'caused by acts of breathing, speaking, and coughing' (Flint 1883: 14) as opposed to percussion, the sounds caused by striking the chest wall.

3 This argument is supported by Brain (1986: 160), who points out that bacteria need iron in order to multiply. An even more blatant allegation of iatrogenic chlorosis occurs in the attribution by the mid-eighteenth-century doctor John Rutherford of a case of chlorosis to an 'unskillfull Midwife' who lacerated the patient's vagina during childbirth (WMS 6888).

4 '*et cum toto corpore pallida esset, ac mollitiem contraxisset, ob menses retentos*'.

5 Sharp's source here, Sennert (1664: 76), merely noted that pessaries should not be used in virgins.

6 Based on Sharp (1671: 260; Hobby 1999: 197).

7 Compare the recipe in W.M. 1655: 85. Other green sickness remedies attached to 'famous names' include 'Lady Worcester's Medicine for the Green Sickness' (W.M. 1655: 69–70) and the Countess of Kent's remedy (Grey 1653: 46). I owe these references to Elaine Hobby.

8 Rubbing the thighs continued to be recommended into the nineteenth century; see Maubray (1724: 47); Trabuc (1818: 15).

9 See Pomeroy (1994); Hutson (1994) provides a useful discussion of the uses of ps-Xenophon in the early modern period.

10 Nashe, *Choice of Valentines* III.407 (c.1593) and Stubbes, *Anatomy* I.154 (1583), cited in Williams (1994: 364–6).

11 Todd (1998) discusses the role of dance as a form of exercise in American women's education from 1800 to 1875; see especially pp. 19, 99 and 109.

12 On Wood-Allen see Morantz-Sanchez (1985: 218–20); Wood-Allen did not approve of married women working outside the home – unless their wages were needed for the family – and saw motherhood as woman's profession. However, she also wanted to make motherhood 'scientific'. It was also specifically the round dance that was condemned as a 'lewd dance of pleasure' carrying the risk of miscarriage in Roesslin's *Rosegarten*, a midwifery manual first published in Germany in 1513 but subsequently translated into many European languages; Arons (1994: 84).

13 BL C.112.f.9, 2, 9 and 11.

14 BL C.112.f.9, 44 and 47.

15 BL C.112.f.9, 24. Green sickness is also described as an 'obstruction' in BL C.112.f.9, 53.

16 BL C.112.f.9, 125.

17 BL C.112.f.9, 131.

18 BL C.112.f.9, 8; Harley 5931, 79/114; and BL C.112.f.9, 61.

19 This pattern of family practice is also found in Harley 5931, 76, 89, 111, 123 and 188, and BL C.112.f.9, 78, 97, 140, 142 and 150; the latter is by an Italian doctor whose wife can cure 'hanging down of the Matrix' (prolapse of the womb) in half an hour.

20 Harley 5931, 111.

21 BL C.112.f.9, 26.

22 BL C.112.f.9, 67.

23 BL 551.a.32.199. On the classical sources for Agnodike as 'the first midwife', and the popularity of this story in later medical history, see King (1998: 181–7).

24 See p. 158, n. 45.

25 Because the competition for which Jacobi entered this essay was marked blind, it was not realised that this had been written by a woman doctor; see Morantz-Sanchez (1985: 55).

26 For the relationship between anaemia and chlorosis, see Introduction, pp. 15–16.

27 Not all women bought into Hall's message. The President of Bryn Mawr College responded furiously to Hall's book as an attack on her womanhood; see further Dyhouse (1981: 121). As Dyhouse (1981: 122) notes, Hall's 'descriptions of adolescent girls are generally couched in a particularly glutinous, leery prose'.

28 Strange (2000: 624–5) has suggested that research by the Medical Women's Federation, which published a statement on menstruation in 1925 arguing that 'it is not an illness', was criticised by the male establishment on the grounds that the MWF was trying to prove this in order to support members' own professional position.

Appendix

1 talos, 1556: 490 Lyons edition.

2 pathognomonicis, Lyons.

3 hypochondriorum, Lyons.

4 hypochondria, Lyons.

5 crebra, Lyons.

BIBLIOGRAPHY

Agrimi, Jole (1985) 'L'*Hippocrates Latinus* nella tradizione manoscritta e nella cultura altomedievali', in Innocenzo Mazzini and Franca Fusco, *I Testi di Medicina Latini Antichi: Problemi Filologici e Storici*, Atti del I Convegno Internazionale, 26–28 aprile, Università di Macerata: G. Bretschneider, pp. 388–98.

Akakia, Martinus (1597) *De morbis muliebribus*, in Israel Spach, *Gynaeciorum, sive de mulierum tum communibus, tum gravidarum, parientium, et puerperarum affectibus et morbis, libri Graecorum, Arabum, Latinorum veterum et recentium quotquot extant ...*, Strasbourg: Zetzner, pp. 745–801.

Altomare, Donato Antonio (1559) *De medendis humani corporis malis: ars medica*, Lyons: A. Vincenti.

Aly, Amou Abou (1992) 'The medical writings of Rufus of Ephesus', PhD thesis, University of London.

Amatus Lusitanus (1553) *In Dioscoridis Anazarbei de materia medica libros quinque enarrationes*, Venice.

—— (1556) *Curationum medicinalium centuriae quatuor*, Basel: H. Froben and N. Episcopius.

Amundsen, Darrel W. and Diers, Carol J. (1969) 'The age of menarche in classical Greece and Rome', *Human Biology* 41: 125–32.

Andò, Valeria (1990) 'La verginità come follia: il *Peri Parthenion* ippocratico', *Quaderni Storici* 75: 715–37.

Andral, Gabriel (1829) *A Treatise on Pathological Anatomy* I (trans. R. Townsend and W. West), Dublin: Hodges and Smith.

Angeleri, Carlo (ed.) (1955) *Pietro Crinito, De honesta disciplina*, Edizione nazionale dei classici del pensiero italiano, Serie II, 2, Rome: Fratelli Bocca.

Anon. (1694) *Aristotle's Masterpiece, or, the Secrets of Generation Displayed in all the Parts Thereof*, London: printed for W.B.

Appignanesi, Lisa and Forrester, John (1993) *Freud's Women*, London: Virago Press.

Arons, Wendy (1994) *When Midwifery Became the Male Physician's Province: the Sixteenth-Century Handbook 'The Rose Garden for Pregnant Women and Midwives', Newly Englished*, Jefferson, NC and London: McFarland.

Ashwell, Samuel (1836) 'Observations on chlorosis, and its complications', *Guy's Hospital Reports* 1: 529–79.

Astruc, Jean (1743) *A Treatise on all the Diseases incident to Women*, London: M. Cooper; facsimile reprint, New York: Garland, 1985.

—— (1761–5) *Traité des maladies des Femmes*, Paris: Cavelier.

—— (1762–7) *A Treatise on the Diseases of Women*, 3 vols, London: J. Nourse.

Baader, Gerhard and Winau, Rolf (eds) (1989) *Die hippokratischen Epidemien: theorie, praxis, tradition* (Proceedings of the Colloque hippocratique, Berlin 10–15 September 1984), *Sudhoffs Archiv* Heft 27, Stuttgart: Franz Steiner.

Baillou, Guillaume de (1640) *Epidemiorum et Ephemeridum libri duo*, Paris: J. Quesnel.

—— (1643) *De Virginum et Mulierum Morbis liber, in quo multa ad mentem Hippocratis explicantur*, Paris: J. Quesnel.

—— (1648) *Paradigmata et Historiae Morborum*, in J. Thévart (ed.), *Opera omnia*, Paris: J. Quesnel.

Bartels, Else (1982) 'Biological sex differences and sex stereotyping', in Elizabeth Whitelegg *et al.*, *The Changing Experience of Women*, Oxford: Martin Robertson, pp. 254–66.

Bates, Don (ed.) (1995) *Knowledge and the Scholarly Medical Traditions*, Cambridge: Cambridge University Press.

Bauda, Abraham (1672) *Discours curieux contre l'abus des saignées*, Sedan: G. de Meerbec.

Bauhin, Caspar (1586–8) *Gynaeciorum sive mulierum affectibus commentarii Graecorum, Latinorum, Barbarorum, iam olim et nunc recens editorum …*, Basel: Conrad Waldkirch.

Beard, Mary (1980) 'The sexual status of Vestal Virgins', *Journal of Roman Studies* 70: 12–27.

—— (1995) 'Re-reading (Vestal) virginity', in Richard Hawley and Barbara Levick (eds), *Women in Antiquity: New Assessments*, London: Routledge, pp. 166–77.

Beccaria, Augusto (1959) 'Sulle tracce di un antico canone latino di Ippocrate e de Galeno I. Le prime traduzioni latine di Ippocrate', *Italia Medioevale e Umanistica* 2: 1–56.

—— (1961) 'Sulle tracce di un antico canone latino di Ippocrate e de Galeno II. Gli Aforismi di Ippocrate nella versione e nei commenti del primo medioevo', *Italia Medioevale e Umanistica* 4: 1–75.

Beecher, Donald A. (1988) 'The lover's body: the somatogenesis of love in Renaissance medical treatises', *Renaissance and Reformation* 24: 1–11.

Beecher, Donald A. and Ciavolella, Massimo (eds) (1990) *Jacques Ferrand; A Treatise on Lovesickness*, Syracuse, NY: Syracuse University Press.

Beier, Lucinda McCray (1987) *Sufferers and Healers: The Experience of Illness in Seventeenth-Century England*, London and New York: Routledge and Kegan Paul.

Bell, Rudolph M. (1999) *How to Do It: Guides to Good Living for Renaissance Italians*, Chicago, IL and London: University of Chicago Press.

Ben-Amos, Ilana Krausman (1994) *Youth and Adolescence in Early Modern England*, New Haven, CT and London: Yale University Press.

Bender, S. (1953) 'Symptoms of menstruation', *Nursing Mirror*, 17 April: 159–60.

Benn, J. Miriam (1992) *The Predicaments of Love*, London: Pluto Press.

Berger, Margret (ed.) (1999) *Hildegard of Bingen, On Natural Philosophy and Medicine: Selections from* Cause et cure, Cambridge: D.S. Brewer.

Berriot-Salvadore, Evelyne (1993) *Un corps, un destin: la femme dans la médecine de la Renaissance*, Paris: Champion.

Biagi, Maria Luisa Altieri *et al.* (1992) *Medicina per le donne nel Cinquecento: Testi di Giovanni Marinello e di Girolamo Mercurio*, Turin: Utet.

Bicks, Caroline (2003) *Midwiving Subjects in Shakespeare's England*, Burlington, VT: Ashgate.

Bienville, D.T. de (1775) *Nymphomania, or a Dissertation Concerning the Furor Uterinus*, London: J. Bew (French *La Nymphomanie, ou Traité de la fureur utérine*, Amsterdam: M.-M. Rey, 1771, trans. Edward Sloane Wilmot).

Biller, Peter (1992) 'Views of Jews from Paris around 1300: Christian or "scientific"?', in Diana Wood (ed.) *Christianity and Judaism*, Woodbridge; Boydell (*Studies in Church History 29*)

Bird, David T. (1982) *A Catalogue of Sixteenth-Century Medical Books in Edinburgh Libraries*, Edinburgh: Royal College of Physicians of Edinburgh.

Blackwell, Elizabeth (1882) *The Moral Education of the Young in Relation to Sex*, 6th edition, London: Hatchards; reprinted in Elizabeth Blackwell (1902), *Essays in Medical Sociology*, vol. I, London: Ernest Bell, pp. 175–309.

—— (1902) 'The Human Element', reprinted in *Sex Essays in Medical Sociology*, vol. I, London: Ernest Bell, pp. 1–82 (first published in 1894).

Boisseul, Jean (1828) *De la puberté chez la femme*, Paris: Didot le Jeune.

Bonnet-Cadilhac, Christine (1993) 'Traduction et commentaire du traité hippocratique "Des maladies des jeunes filles" ', *History and Philosophy of the Life Sciences* 15: 147–63.

Boorde, Andrew (1547) *The Breviary of Helthe*, London: W. Middleton.

Bos, Gerrit (ed. and trans.) (1997) *Ibn al-Jazzar on Sexual Diseases and their Treatment*, London and New York: Kegan Paul International.

Boucé, Paul-Gabriel (1982) 'Some sexual beliefs and myths in eighteenth-century Britain', in Paul-Gabriel Boucé (ed.), *Sexuality in Eighteenth-century Britain*, Manchester: Manchester University Press, pp. 28–46.

Bradley, James and Dupree, Marguerite (2001) 'Opportunity on the edge of orthodoxy: medically qualified hydropathists in the era of reform, 1840–60', *Social History of Medicine* 14: 417–37.

Brain, Peter (1986) *Galen on Bloodletting*, Cambridge: Cambridge University Press.

Bramwell, Byrom (1899) *Anaemia and Some of the Diseases of the Blood-Forming Organs and Ductless Glands*, Edinburgh: Oliver and Boyd; London: Simpkin, Marshall and Co. Ltd.

Bretheau, A.-J.-A. James (1865) *De la puberté chez la femme*, Paris: A. Parent.

Bright, Timothie (1580) *A Treatise Wherein is Declared the Sufficiencie of English Medicines, for Cure of all Diseases, Cured with Medicine*, London: H. Middleton for T. Man.

Brumberg, Joan Jacobs (1982) 'Chlorotic girls, 1870–1920: a historical perspective on female adolescence', *Child Development* 53: 1468–77.

—— (1988) *Fasting Girls: The Emergence of Anorexia Nervosa as a Modern Disease*, Cambridge, MA and London: Harvard University Press.

—— (1992) 'From psychiatric syndrome to "communicable" disease: the case of anorexia nervosa', in Charles E. Rosenberg and Janet Golden (eds), *Framing Disease: Studies in Cultural History*, New Brunswick, NJ: Rutgers University Press, pp. 134–54.

—— (1993) ' "Something happens to girls": menarche and the emergence of the modern American hygienic imperative', *Journal of the History of Sexuality* 4: 99–127.

Buffon, Comte de [George-Louis Leclerc] (1971) *De l'homme: Présentation et notes de Michèle Duchet*, Paris: Maspero.

Bullein, William (1558) *A Newe Booke Entituled the Gouernement of Healthe*, London: John Day.

—— (1559) *A Newe Boke of Phisicke called ye Government of Health*, London: John Day.

—— (1562) *Bullein's Bulwarke of Defence againste all sicknes, sorres and wundes*, London: Jhon Kyngston.

Bullough, Vern L. (1972–3) 'An early American sex manual, or, Aristotle who?', *Early American Literature* 7: 236–46.

Burguière, Paul, Gourevitch, Danielle and Malinas, Yves (1988–2000) *Soranos d'Éphèse, Maladies des Femmes*, 4 vols, Paris: Les Belles Lettres.

Burne, John (1840) *A Treatise on the Causes and Consequences of Habitual Constipation*, London: Longman, Orme, Brown, Green and Longmans.

Burq, Victor (1852) *Note sur une application nouvelle des métaux à l'étude et au traitement de la chlorose*, pamphlet extracted from *La Gazette Médicale de Paris*.

Byl, Simon (1980) *Recherches sur les grands traités biologiques d'Aristote: sources écrites et préjugés*, Brussels: Palais des Académies.

Bylebyl, Jerome J. (1971) 'Galen on the non-natural causes of variation in the pulse', *Bulletin of the History of Medicine* 45: 482–5.

Bynum, Caroline Walker (1987) *Holy Feast and Holy Fast: The Religious Significance of Food to Medieval Women*, Berkeley and London: University of California Press.

Bynum, William (2001) 'Discarded diagnoses: chlorosis', *The Lancet* 358 (9275): 78.

Bynum, William and Roy Porter (eds) (1993) *Medicine and the Five Senses*, Cambridge: Cambridge University Press.

Cabot, Richard Clarke (1908) 'Pernicious and secondary anaemia, chlorosis, and leukaemia', in William Osler and Thomas McCrae (eds), *Modern Medicine: Its Theory and Practice*, vol. IV, Philadelphia, PA: Lea and Febiger.

Cadden, Joan (1993) *Meanings of Sex Difference in the Middle Ages*, Cambridge and New York: Cambridge University Press.

Cahan, Mitchell A. (1987) 'Chlorosis lives! – and slips through MeSH', *Journal of the American Medical Association* 258: 1174.

Calvi, Marco Fabio (1525) *Hippocratis Coi medicorum omnium longe principis, Octoginta volumina ...*, Rome: Franciscus Minitius.

—— (1526) *Hippocrates de foemina natura*, Paris: Claudius Chevallonius.

Campbell, J.M.H. (1923) 'Chlorosis: a study of the Guy's Hospital cases during the last thirty years, with some remarks on its etiology and the causes of its diminished frequency', *Guy's Hospital Reports* 73: 247–97.

Carlson, James R. and Hammond, Peter W. (1999) 'The English sweating sickness (1485–c.1551): a new perspective on disease etiology', *Journal of the History of Medicine* 54: 23–54.

Carol, Anne (1995) *Histoire de l'eugénisme en France: les médecins et la procreation XIXe–XXe siècle*, Paris: Éds du Seuil.

Carson, Anne (1990) 'Putting her in her place: woman, dirt, and desire', in David M. Halperin, John J. Winkler and Froma I. Zeitlin (eds), *Before Sexuality: The Construction of Erotic Experience in the Ancient Greek World*, Princeton, NJ: Princeton University Press, pp. 135–69.

Cary, Walter (1583) *A Briefe Treatise, called Caries Farewell to Physicke: Wherein thou shalt find Rare and Speciall Helpe for Manie Common Diseases*, London: Henry Denham.

Castro, Rodrigues de (1603) *De universa mulierum medicina*, Hamburg: Froben.

Catonné, Jean-Philippe (1994) 'A nosological reflection on the Peri Parthenion: elucidating the origin of hysterical insanity', *History of Psychiatry* 5: 361–86.

Celli, Blas Bruni (1984) *Bibliografía Hipocrática*, Venezuela: Ediciones del Rectorado, Universidad Central de Venezuela.

Chapple, Harold (1918) 'The gynaecological aspect of intestinal stasis', in Sir William Arbuthnot Lane, *The Operative Treatment of Chronic Intestinal Stasis*, 4th edition, London: Henry Frowde and Hodder & Stoughton, pp. 318–26.

Chevallier, Paul (1955) 'De la maladie "des pales couleurs" à l'anémie hypochrome chronique', *Histoire de la Médecine* 5 (8): 3–16.

Churchill, Fleetwood (1864) *On the Diseases of Women*, 5th edition, Dublin: Fannin and Co.; London: Longman.

Ciavolella, Massimo (1988) 'Métamorphoses sexuelles et sexualité féminine durant la Renaissance', *Renaissance and Reformation* 24: 13–20.

Clark, Sir Andrew (1887) 'Observations on the anaemia or chlorosis of girls, occurring more commonly between the advent of menstruation and the consummation of womanhood', *Proceedings of the Medical Society of London* 11: 55–66 (reprinted as 'Anaemia or chlorosis of girls, occurring more commonly between the advent of menstruation and the consummation of womanhood', *The Lancet*, 19 November, pp. 1003–5).

Clologe, Charles H.T. (1905) *Essai sur l'histoire de la gynécologie dans l'antiquité grècque jusqu'à la collection hippocratique*, Bordeaux: Arnaud.

Cogan, Thomas (1584) *The Haven of Health: Chiefely Gathered for the Comfort of Students, and Consequently of all Those that have a Care of their Health …*, London: printed by Henrie Midleton, for William Norton.

Coley, Frederic C. (1894) 'On the physical signs of chlorosis', *The Practitioner* 52: 264–8.

Collins, An (1653) *Divine Songs and Meditacions* (ed. Sidney Gottlieb), Tempe, AZ: Medieval and Renaissance Texts and Studies, vol. 161, 1996.

Cooper, Kate (1996) *The Virgin and the Bride: Idealised Womanhood in Late Antiquity*, Cambridge, MA and London: Harvard University Press.

Copeman, William S.C. (1960) *Doctors and Disease in Tudor Times*, London: Dawson's.

Corde, Maurice de la (1574) *Hippocrates Coi libellus Peri Parthenion, hoc est, De iis quae virginibus accidunt*, Paris: Gabriel Buon.

—— (1585) *Hippocratis Coi, Medicorum Principis, liber prior de morbis mulierum*, Paris: Dionysius Duvallius (also in Bauhin 1586–8, vol. 3: 1–514; Spach 1597: 492–744).

Cornarius, Janus (1536) *Claudii Galeni libri novem, nunc primum Latini facti* (includes *Libri V iam primum in Latinam linguam conversi: De causis respirationis. De utilitate respirationis. De difficultate respirationis libri III* and *De uteri dissectione, de foetus formatione et de semine libri*), Basel: Froben.

—— (1538) *Hippocratis Coi Medici vetustissimi, et omnium aliorum principis, libri omnes, ad vetustos codices summo studio collati et restaurati* (*Greek*), Basel: Froben.

—— (1546) *Hippocratis Coi medicorum omnium longe principis, opera quae ad nos extant omnia*, Basel: Froben.

Coturri, E. (1968) 'Il ritrovamento di antichi testi di medicina nel primo secolo del Rinascimento', *Episteme* 2: 91–110.

Cox, Edwin Marion (1925) *The Poems of Sappho, with Historical and Critical Notes, Translations, and a Bibliography*, London: Williams and Norgate; New York: Scribners.

Crawford, Patricia (1981) 'Attitudes to menstruation in seventeenth-century England', *Past and Present* 91: 47–73.

—— (1984) 'Printed advertisements for women medical practitioners in London, 1670–1710', *Society for the Social History of Medicine Bulletin* 35: 66–70.

Cressy, David (1997) *Birth, Marriage and Death: Ritual, Religion, and the Life-cycle in Tudor and Stuart England*, Oxford: Oxford University Press.

Crinito, Pietro (1504) *De honesta disciplina*, Florence: P. da Giunta.

Crosby, William C. (1987) 'Whatever became of chlorosis?', *Journal of the American Medical Association* 257: 2799–80.

Cullen, William (1786) *First Lines of the Practice of Physic*, 4 vols, Edinburgh: C. Elliot.

—— (1803) *The Edinburgh Practice of Physic, Surgery and Midwifery*, London: G. Kearsley.

Cullingford, Elizabeth Butler (1993) *Gender and History in Yeats's Love Poetry*, Cambridge: Cambridge University Press.

Culpeper, Nicholas (1650) *A Physical Directory*, London: Peter Cole.

—— (1651) *A Directory for Midwives*, London: Peter Cole.

—— (1676) *The English Physitian Enlarged*, London: G. Sawbridge.

Cunningham, Andrew (1997) *The Anatomical Renaissance: The Resurrection of the Anatomical Projects of the Ancients*, Aldershot: Scolar Press; Brookfield, VT: Ashfield.

Cyrino, Monica Silviera (1995) *In Pandora's Jar: Lovesickness in Early Greek Poetry*, Lanham, MD and London: University Press of America.

Daremberg, Charles (ed.and trans.) (1862) *Oeuvres d'Oribase*, III, Paris: Imprimerie Nationale.

Davies, Kathleen (1977) 'The sacred condition of equality – how original were puritan doctrines of marriage?', *Social History* 2: 563–80.

Dean-Jones, Lesley (1994) *Women's Bodies in Classical Greek Science*, Oxford: Clarendon Press.

Debru, Armelle (1996) *Le corps respirant: la pensée physiologique chez Galien*, Leiden: E.J. Brill.

Demaitre, Luke (2001) 'Domesticity in Middle Dutch "Secrets of Men and Women"', *Social History of Medicine* 14: 1–25.

Demand, Nancy (1994) *Birth, Death, and Motherhood in Classical Greece*, Baltimore, MD: Johns Hopkins University Press.

Denman, Thomas (1788) *An Introduction to the Practice of Midwifery*, London: J. Johnson.

—— (1832) *An Introduction to the Practice of Midwifery*, 7th edition, London: E. Cox.

Devereux, George (1970) 'The nature of Sappho's seizure in fr. 31 LP as evidence of her inversion', *Classical Quarterly* 20: 17–31.

Diepgen, Paul (1933) 'Reste antiker Gynäkologie im frühen Mittelalter', *Quellen und Studien zur Geschichte der Naturwissenschaften* 3: 226–42.

—— (1937) *Die Frauenheilkunde der Alten Welt. Handbuch der Gynäkologie XII, 1*, Munich: Bergmann.

D'Irsay, Stephen (1926) 'Notes to the origin of the expression: Atra mors', *Isis* 8: 328–32.

Dixon, Laurinda S. (1995) *Perilous Chastity: Women and Illness in pre-Enlightenment Art and Medicine*, New York and London: Cornell University Press.

Dobson, Mary (1997) *Contours of Death and Disease in Early Modern England*, Cambridge: Cambridge University Press.

Dodoens, Rembert (1578) *A Niewe Herball or Historie of Plantes*, Antwerp: H. Loë for G. Dewes (French, *Histoire des plantes*, Antwerp, 1557, trans. Henry Lyte).

Donati, Giovanni Battista (1582) *Commentarius in magni Hippocratis Coi librum de morbis virginum*, Lucca: J. Guidobonius.

Dormandy, Thomas (1999) *The White Death: A History of Tuberculosis*, London and Rio Grande: Hambledon Press.

Drysdale, George (1875) *The Elements of Social Science, or, Physical, Sexual, and Natural Religion: An Exposition of the True Cause and Only Cure of the Three Primary Social Evils: Poverty, Prostitution, and Celibacy*, 13th edition, London: E. Truelove.

Dubois, Jacques (1555) *De mensibus mulierum, et hominis generatione, Iacobi Silvii medicae rei apud Parrhisios interpretis Regii, commentarius*, Paris: I. Hulpeau (also in Wolf 1566a: 771–868; Bauhin 1586–8, vol. 1: 304–40; Spach 1597: 148–66).

—— (1559) *Livre de la nature et utilité des moys des femmes, et de la curation des maladies qui surviennent, composé en Latin par Jacques Sylvius* (trans. Guillaume Chrestien), Paris: Morel.

Ducatillon, Jeanne (1977) *Polémiques dans la collection hippocratique*, Univ. de Lille III: Thesis, Univ. de Paris IV.

Duden, Barbara (1987) *Geschichte unter der Haut: Ein Eisenacher Arzt und seine Patientinnen um 1730*, Stuttgart: Klett-Cotta (*The Woman Beneath the Skin: A Doctor's Patients in Eighteenth-Century Germany*, trans. Thomas Dunlap, Cambridge, MA and London: Harvard University Press, 1991).

Duminil, Marie-Paule (1979) 'La recherche hippocratique aujourd'hui', *History and Philosophy of the Life Sciences* 1: 153–81.

—— (1983) *Le sang, les vaisseaux, le coeur dans la collection hippocratique*, Paris: Eds Belles Lettres.

Duncan, James Matthews (1889) 'Clinical lecture on hysteria, neurasthenia and anorexia nervosa', *The Lancet* 18 May: 973–4.

Dupleix, Scipion (1626) *La curiosité naturelle redigée en questions selon l'ordre Alphabetique*, Rouen: Manassez de Preavix.

Dupouy, Edmond (1892) *Médecine et moeurs de l'ancienne Rome d'après les poètes latins*, Paris: Baillière.

Durling, Richard J. (1961) 'A chronological census of Renaissance editions and translations of Galen', *Journal of the Warburg and Courtauld Institutes* 24: 230–305.

Dyer, Alan (1997) 'The English sweating sickness of 1551: an epidemic anatomized', *Medical History* 41: 362–84.

Dyhouse, Carol (1981) *Girls Growing Up in Late Victorian and Edwardian England*, London: Routledge and Kegan Paul.

Eales, Jacqueline (1998) 'Gender construction in early modern England and the conduct books of William Whately (1583–1639)', in Robert N. Swanson (ed.), *Gender and Christian Religion: Papers Read at the 1996 Summer Meeting and the 1997 Winter Meeting of the Ecclesiastical History Society*, Woodbridge: Boydell (*Studies in Church History* 34).

Edwards, Lilas G. (1999) 'Joan of Arc: gender and authority in the text of the *Trial of Condemnation*', in Katherine J. Lewis, Noël James Menuge and Kim M. Phillips (eds), *Young Medieval Women*, Stroud: Sutton Publishing, pp. 133–52.

Egert, Ferdinand P. (1936) *Gynäkologischen Fragmente aus dem frühen Mittelalter nach einer Petersburger Handschrift aus dem VII–IX Jahrhundert*, Berlin: Emil Ebering.

Eisenbichler, Konrad (ed.) (2002) *The Premodern Teenager: Youth in Society 1150–1650*, Toronto: Centre for Reformation and Renaissance Studies.

Erickson, Robert A. (1982) ' "The books of generation": some observations on the style of the British midwife books, 1671–1764', in Paul-Gabriel Boucé (ed.), *Sexuality in Eighteenth-Century Britain*, Manchester: Manchester University Press, pp. 74–94.

Evans, Cadwallader (1757) 'A relation of a cure performed by Electricity, from Mr Cadwallader Evans, student in physic at Philadelphia, communicated Oct. 21, 1754', *Medical Observations and Inquiries* 1: 83–6.

Evans, Hughes (1993) 'Losing touch: the controversy over the introduction of blood pressure instruments into medicine', *Technology and Culture* 34: 784–807.

Ewaldt, Joannes Nicolaus (1665) 'De ΧΛΩΡΩΣΕΙ, seu foedis virginum coloribus', Doctoral thesis, Jena.

Falkiner, C. Litton (1904) *Illustrations of Irish History and Topography*, London: Longmans, Green and Co.

Fernel, Jean (1547) *De naturali parte medicinae libri septem*, Venice: Joannes Gryphius.

—— (1648 [1547]) *Les Sept Livres de la therapeutique universelle de Messire Jean Fernel*, Paris: Jean le Bouc.

Fichtner, Gerhard (1995a) *Corpus Galenicum. Verzeichnis der galenischen und pseudo-galenischen Schriften*, Tübingen: Institut für Geschichte der Medizin.

—— (1995b) *Corpus Hippocraticum. Verzeichnis der hippokratischen und pseudohip-pokratischen Schriften*, Tübingen: Institut für Geschichte der Medizin.

Figlio, Karl (1978) 'Chlorosis and chronic disease in nineteenth century Britain: the social construction of somatic illness in a capitalist society', *Social History* 3: 167–97.

Findlay, Miss M.E. (1905–7) 'The education of girls', *The Paidologist* 7: 83–93.

Fissell, Mary (1991) 'The disappearance of the patient: narrative and the invention of hospital medicine', in Roger French and Andrew Wear (eds), *British Medicine in an Age of Reform*, London: Routledge, pp. 92–109.

—— (1995) 'Gender and generation: representing reproduction in early modern England', *Gender and History* 7: 433–56.

Flemming, Rebecca (2000) *Medicine and the Making of Roman Women: Gender, Nature, and Authority from Celsus to Galen*, Oxford: Oxford University Press.

Flemming, Rebecca and Hanson, Ann Ellis (1998) 'Hippocrates' *"Peri partheniôn"* (*Diseases of young girls*): text and translation', *Early Science and Medicine* 3: 241–52.

Flint, Austin (1883) *A Manual of Auscultation and Percussion: embracing the physical diagnosis of diseases of the lungs and heart, and of thoracic aneurism*, 3rd edition, Philadelphia, PA: Henry C. Lea's Son.

Floyer, Sir John (1707) *The Physician's Pulse-watch; or, an Essay to Explain the Old Art of Feeling the Pulse, and to Improve it by the Help of a Pulse-watch …*, London: S. Smith and B. Walford.

Fogo, Andrew (1803) *Observations on the Opinions of Ancient and Modern Physicians, Including those of the Late Dr Cullen on Amenorrhea, or Green-sickness*, Newcastle: D. Akenhead.

Föllinger, Sabine (1996) *Differenz und Gleichheit. Das Geschlechterverhältnis in der Sicht griechischer Philosophen des 4. bis 1. Jahrhunderts v. Chr.*, Stuttgart: F. Steiner (*Hermes* Einzelschriften, Heft 74).

Fontanus, Nicholas (1652) *The Womans Doctour*, London: J. Blague and S. Howes.

Forbes, Thomas Rogers (1971) *Chronicle from Aldgate: Life and Death in Shakespeare's London*, New Haven, CT and London: Yale University Press.

Foreest, Pieter van (1595) *Observationum et curationum medicinalium*, Lyons: Ex Officino Plantiniana.

Fossel, Viktor (1914) 'Aus den medizinischen Briefen des pfalzgräflichen Leibarztes Johannes Lange (1485–1565)', *Sudhoffs Archiv für Geschichte der Medizin* 7: 238–52.

Fowler, Don (1987) 'Vergil on killing virgins', in Michael Whitby, Philip Hardie and Mary Whitby (eds), *Homo Viator: Classical Essays for John Bramble*, Bristol: Bristol Classical Press; Oak Park, IL: Bolchazy-Carducci Publishers, pp. 185–98.

Fowler, W.M. (1936) 'Chlorosis: an obituary', *Annals of Medical History* 8: 168–76.

Fox, Samuel (1839) *Observations on the Disorder of the General Health of Females called Chlorosis: Shewing the True Cause to be Entirely Independent of Peculiarities of Sex*, London: S. Highley.

Fraundorffer, Philippus (1696) *Opusculum de morbis mulierum*, Norimbergae: Impensis Johannis Ziegeri.

Fravega, Gina (1962) *Harmoniae gynaeciorum, epitome di Gaspare Wolf su Moschione, Cleopatra e Teodoro Prisciano*, Genova: Scientia Veterum 30.

Fuchs, Leonhart (1539) *De medendi methodo libri quatuor*, Paris: Conrad Neobarius.

—— (1542) *De historia stirpium*, Basel: Michael Isingrin.

—— (1555) *De usitata huius temporis componendorum miscendorumque medicamentorum ratione libri quatuor*, Basel: per Ioannem Oporinum.

Furley, David J. and Wilkie, James S. (1984) *Galen on Respiration and the Arteries*, Princeton, NJ: Princeton University Press.

Furnivall, Frederick James (ed.) (1870) *Andrew Boorde's Introduction and Dyetary*, Early English Text Society Extra Series, 10 (reprinted 1975), Millwood, NY: Kraus Reprint Co.

Gaisser, Julia Haig (1993) *Catullus and his Renaissance Readers*, Oxford: Clarendon Press.

Garofalo, Ivan (ed.) (1988) *Erasistrati Fragmenti*, Pisa: Giardini.

Gibbs, Denis D. (1971) 'The physician's pulse watch', *Medical History* 15: 187–90.

Gibson, Thomas (1682) *The Anatomy of Human Bodies Epitomized*, London: M. Flesher for T. Flesher.

Gilliam, J.F. (1961) 'The plague under Marcus Aurelius', *American Journal of Philology* 82: 225–51.

Good, Byron J. (1994) *Medicine, Rationality, and Experience: An Anthropological Perspective*, Cambridge: Cambridge University Press.

Goodall, E.W. (1935) 'A French epidemiologist of the sixteenth century', *Annals of Medical History* 7: 409–27.

Goss, Charles Mayo (1962) 'On the anatomy of the uterus', *The Anatomical Record* 144: 77–83.

Gove, Mary S. (1846) *Lectures to Women on Anatomy and Physiology*, New York: Harper and Brothers.

Gowers, Sir William R. (1877) 'On the numeration of blood-corpuscles', *The Lancet* 2 (1 December): 797–8.

—— (1878) 'On a case of anaemia, observed with the haemacytometer', *The Lancet* 1 (11 May): 675–7.

Gowing, Laura (1996) *Domestic Dangers: Women, Words and Sex in Early Modern London*, Oxford: Clarendon Press.

Grafton, Anthony (1991) *Defenders of the Text: The Traditions of Scholarship in an Age of Science, 1450–1800*, Cambridge, MA: Harvard University Press.

Grafton, Anthony and Jardine, Lisa (1986) *From Humanism to the Humanities. Education and the Liberal Arts in Fifteenth- and Sixteenth-century Europe*, London: Duckworth.

Graham, Elspeth *et al.* (eds) (1989) *Her Own Life: Autobiographical Writings by Seventeenth-Century Englishwomen*, London: Routledge.

Green, Monica H. (1987) 'The *De genecia* attributed to Constantine the African', *Speculum* 62: 299–323 (reprinted in Green, *Women's Healthcare in the Medieval West*, Aldershot: Ashgate, 2000, III).

—— (1996) 'The development of the *Trotula*', *Revue d'Histoire des Textes* 26: 119–203 (reprinted in Green, *Women's Healthcare in the Medieval West*, Aldershot: Ashgate, 2000, V).

—— (ed. and trans.) (2001) *The* Trotula: *A Medieval Compendium of Women's Medicine*, Penn: University of Pennsylvania Press.

Greene, Robert (1583) *Mamillia. A Mirrour or Looking-glasse for the Ladies of Englande*, London: T. Woodcocke.

Grey, Elizabeth (1653) *A Choice Manual of Rare and Select Secrets in Physick*, London: G. Dawson for W. Shears.

Griffiths, Paul (1996) *Youth and Authority: Formative Experiences in England 1560–1640*, Oxford: Clarendon Press.

Grmek, Mirko D. (1989) 'La dénomination latine des maladies considérées commes nouvelles par les auteurs antiques', in Guy Sabbah (ed.), Centre Jean-Palerne Memoires X, *Le latin médical: la constitution d'un langage scientifique*, Université de Saint-Etienne, pp. 195–214.

Groneman, Carol (1994) 'Nymphomania: the historical construction of female sexuality', *Signs* 19: 337–67.

Grosart, Alexander B. (1881–3) *The Life and Works of Robert Greene, M.A.*, vol. 2, *Mamillia: Parts I and II and Anatomie of Flatterie, 1583–1593*, printed for private circulation.

Gruner, Christian Gottfried (1772) *Censura librorum Hippocrateorum qua veri a falsis integri a suppositis segregantur*, Vratislavia: J.F. Korn, Snr.

Guerrini, Anita (2000) *Obesity and Depression in the Enlightenment: The Life and Times of George Cheyne*, Norman: University of Oklahoma Press.

Guggenheim, Karl Y. (1995) 'Chlorosis: the rise and disappearance of a nutritional disease', *Journal of Nutrition* 7: 1822–5.

Habershon, Samuel Osborne (1863) 'On idiopathic anaemia', *The Lancet* 1 (9 May): 518–19; (16 May): 551–2.

Hale, John (1994) *The Civilization of Europe in the Renaissance*, New York: Atheneum.

Hall, Granville Stanley (1904) *Adolescence: Its Psychology and its Relations to Physiology, Anthropology, Sociology, Sex, Crime, Religion and Education*, vol. 1, London: Sidney Appleton.

Halperin, David M., Winkler, John J. and Zeitlin, Froma I. (eds) (1990) *Before Sexuality: The Construction of Erotic Experience in the Ancient Greek World*, Princeton, NJ: Princeton University Press.

171

Halpern, Richard (1986) 'Puritanism and Maenadism in *A Mask*', in Margaret W. Ferguson, Maureen Quilligan and Nancy J. Vickers (eds), *Rewriting the Renaissance: The Discourses of Sexual Difference in Early Modern Europe*, Chicago, IL and London: University of Chicago Press, pp. 88–105.

Hamilton, Alexander (1787) *Outlines of the Theory and Practice of Midwifery*, Edinburgh: C. Elliot (first published 1784).

Hamilton, James (1805) *Observations on the Utility and Administration of Purgative Medicines in Several Diseases*, Edinburgh: C. Stewart.

Hanawalt, Barbara A. (1992) 'Historical descriptions and prescriptions for adolescence', *Journal of Family History* 17: 341–51.

—— (1996) ' "The Childe of Bristowe" and the making of middle-class adolescence', in Barbara A. Hanawalt and David Wallace (eds), *Bodies and Disciplines: Intersections of Literature and History in Fifteenth-Century England*, Minneapolis and London: University of Minnesota Press, pp. 155–78.

Hansen, Axel (1928) *Om chlorosens, der aegte blegsots, optraeden: Europa gennem tiderne: en medico-historisk undersøgelse*, Kolding: V. Schoeffers Forlag.

—— (1931) 'Die Chlorose im Altertum', *Sudhoffs Archiv für Geschichte der Medizin* 24: 175–84.

Hanson, Ann Ellis (1992) 'The origin of female nature', *Helios* 19: 31–71.

Hanson, Ann Ellis and Armstrong, David (1986) 'Vox virginis', *Bulletin of the Institute of Classical Studies* 33: 97–100.

Hanson, Ann Ellis and Green, Monica H. (1994) 'Soranus of Ephesus: *Methodicorum princeps*', *Aufstieg und Niedergang der Römischen Welt* 37.2, Berlin and New York: Walter de Gruyter, pp. 968–1075.

Haraway, Donna (1991) *Simians, Cyborgs, and Women: The Reinvention of Nature*, New York: Routledge.

Harris, Barbara J. (2001) 'Space, time, and the power of aristocratic wives in Yorkist and early Tudor England, 1450–1550', in Thomas Kuehn, Anne Jacobson Schutte and Silvana Seidel Menchi (eds), *Time, Space, and Women's Lives*, Kirksville, MO: Truman State University Press, pp. 245–64 (first published as *Tempi e spazi di vita femminile tra Medioevo ed età moderna*, Annali dell'Istituto storico italo-germanico Quaderno 51, Bologna: Il Mulino, 1999).

Harris, Charles Reginald Schiller (1973) *The Heart and the Vascular System in Ancient Greek Medicine from Alcmaeon to Galen*, Oxford: Clarendon Press.

Harris, Jonathan Gil (1998) *Foreign Bodies and the Body Politic: Discourses of Social Pathology in Early Modern England*, Cambridge: Cambridge University Press.

Heath, Clark W. and Patek, Arthur J. (1937) 'The anemia of iron deficiency', *Medicine* 16: 267–350.

Henry, John (1991) 'Doctors and healers: popular culture and the medical profession', in Stephen Pumfrey, Paolo L. Rossi and Maurice Slawinski (eds), *Science, Culture and Popular Belief in Renaissance Europe*, Manchester and New York: Manchester University Press, pp. 191–221.

Heywood, Thomas (1624) *Gynaikeion: or, nine bookes of various history concerning women*, London: Adam Islip.

Hibbott, Yvonne (1990) 'Medical books of the sixteenth century', in Alain Besson (ed.), *Thornton's Medical Books, Libraries and Collectors*, 3rd edition, Aldershot: Gower Publishing, pp. 43–82.

Hirsch, August (1885) *Handbook of Geographical and Historical Pathology*, vol. 2, London: New Sydenham Society, vol. CXII (German, *Handbuch der historisch-geographisch Pathologie*, 1881–6).

Hobby, Elaine (ed.) (1999) Jane Sharp, *The Midwives Book, or the Whole Art of Midwifry Discovered*, New York and Oxford: Oxford University Press.

Hollick, Frederick (1852) *The Diseases of Women: Their Causes and Cure Familiarly Explained with Practical Hints for their Prevention and for the Preservation of Female Health*, 50th edition, New York: T.W. Strong.

Hudson, Robert P. (1977) 'The biography of disease: lessons from chlorosis', *Bulletin of the History of Medicine* 51: 448–63.

Humphreys, Margaret (1997) 'Chlorosis: "the virgin's disease"', in Kenneth A. Kiple (ed.), *Plague, Pox and Pestilence: Disease in History*, London: Weidenfeld and Nicolson, pp. 160–5.

Hurst, Arthur F. (1919) *Constipation and Allied Intestinal Disorders*, London: Henry Frowde and Hodder & Stoughton.

Hutson, Lorna (1994) *The Usurer's Daughter: Male Friendship and Fictions of Women in Sixteenth-century England*, London: Routledge.

Irigoin, Jean (1973) 'Tradition manuscrite et histoire du texte. Quelques problèmes relatifs à la Collection Hippocratique', *Revue d'histoire des textes* 3: 1–13.

Irwin, Eleanor (1974) *Colour Terms in Greek Poetry*, Toronto: Hakkert.

Jacobi, Mary Putnam (1877) *The Question of Rest for Women during Menstruation*, Boylston Prize Essay, 1876, New York: G.P. Putnam's Sons.

Jacobi, Mary Putnam and Victoria A. White (1880) *On the Use of the Cold Pack Followed by Massage in the Treatment of Anaemia*, New York: G.P. Putnam's Sons.

James, Robert (1743–5) *A Medical Dictionary*, London: T. Osborne.

Jardine, Lisa and Grafton, Anthony (1990) ' "Studied for action": how Gabriel Harvey read his Livy', *Past and Present* 129: 30–78.

Jarrot, Sabine (1999) *Le vampire dans la literature du XIXe au siècle. De l'Autre à un autre soi-même*, Paris and Montreal: L'Harmattan.

Johnson, Edward (1856) *The Domestic Practice of Hydropathy*, London: Simpkin, Marshall & Co.

Johnson, Walter (1849) *An Essay on the Diseases of Young Women*, London: Simpkin, Marshall & Co.

—— (1850) *The Morbid Emotions of Women: Their Origin, Tendencies, and Treatment*, London: Simpkin, Marshall & Co.

—— (1852) *Principles of Homeopathy*, London: Simpkin, Marshall & Co.

Johnston, John (1657) *The Idea of Practical Physick in Twelve Books* (trans. Nicholas Culpeper), London: Peter Cole.

Jones, Ernest Lloyd (1897) *Chlorosis: The Special Anaemia of Young Women*, London: Baillière Tindall and Cox.

Jouanna, Jacques (1983) 'Littré, éditeur et traducteur d'Hippocrate', in *Actes du Colloque Émile Littré, 1801–1881, Paris, 7–9 octobre 1981*, Centre international de Synthèse, Paris: Éds Albin Michel, pp. 285–301.

—— (1992) *Hippocrate*, Paris: Fayard.

Kelly, Kathleen Coyne (2000) *Performing Virginity and Testing Chastity in the Middle Ages*, London: Routledge.

Kibre, Pearl (1945) 'Hippocratic writings in the Middle Ages', *Bulletin of the History of Medicine* 18: 371–412.

—— (1976) 'Hippocrates latinus: repertorium of Hippocratic writings in the Latin Middle Ages: II', *Traditio* 32: 257–92.

—— (1979) 'Hippocrates latinus: repertorium of Hippocratic writings in the Latin Middle Ages: V', *Traditio* 35: 273–302.

—— (1980) 'Hippocrates latinus: repertorium of Hippocratic writings in the Latin Middle Ages: VI', *Traditio* 36: 347–72.

King, Helen (1983) 'Bound to bleed: Artemis and Greek women', in A. Cameron and A. Kuhrt (eds), *Images of Women in Antiquity*, London: Croom Helm, pp. 109–27; reprinted in Laura K. McClure (ed.), *Sexuality and Gender in the Classical World*, Oxford: Blackwell, 2002, pp. 77–97.

—— (1985) 'From parthenos to gynê: the dynamics of category', PhD thesis, University of London.

—— (1989) 'The daughter of Leonides: reading the Hippocratic corpus', in Averil Cameron (ed.), *History as Text*, London: Duckworth, pp. 13–32.

—— (1993) 'Once upon a text: hysteria from Hippocrates', in Sander Gilman, Helen King, Roy Porter, George S. Rousseau and Elaine Showalter, *Hysteria Beyond Freud*, Berkeley: University of California Press, pp. 3–90.

—— (1994) 'Producing woman: Hippocratic gynaecology', in Leonie Archer, Susan Fischler and Maria Lyke (eds), *Women in Ancient Societies: An Illusion of the Night*, London: Macmillan, pp. 102–14.

—— (1996a) 'Hippocrates, Galen and the origins of the "disease of virgins" ', *International Journal of the Classical Tradition* 2: 372–87.

—— (1996b) Review of Laurinda Dixon, *Perilous Chastity*, *Medical History* 40: 505–6.

—— (1998) *Hippocrates' Woman: Reading the Female Body in Ancient Greece*, London: Routledge.

—— (1999) 'Hippocratic gynaecological therapy in the sixteenth and seventeenth centuries', in Ivan Garofolo *et al.* (eds), *Aspetti della Terapia nel Corpus Hippocraticum (Atti del IXe Colloque hippocratique, Pisa, 25–29 settembre 1996)*, Florence: Leo Olschki, pp. 499–515.

Kjennerud, R. (1948) 'Black death', *Journal of the History of Medicine* 3: 359–60.

Klairmont-Lingo, Alison (1999) 'The fate of popular terms for female anatomy in the age of print', *French Historical Studies* 22: 335–49.

Kneipp, Sebastian (1893; reprinted 1979) *My Water-Cure, as Tested Through More than Thirty Years*, Wellingborough: Thorsons Publishers.

Kritzman, Lawrence K. (1991) *The Rhetoric of Sexuality and the Literature of the French Renaissance*, Cambridge and New York: Cambridge University Press.

Kruk, Remke (1987/8) 'Pregnancy and its social consequences in mediaeval and traditional Arab society', *Quaderni di Studi Arabi* 5/6: 418–30.

Lackey, Carolyn J. (1978) 'Pica: a nutritional anthropology concern', in E.E. Bauwens (ed.), *The Anthropology of Health*, St Louis, MO: C.V. Mosby, pp. 121–9.

Laín Entralgo, Pedro (1970) *The Therapy of the Word in Classical Antiquity* (ed. and trans. Lelland J. Rather and John M. Sharp), New Haven, CT: Yale University Press.

Lane, Sir William Arbuthnot (1909) *The Operative Treatment of Chronic Constipation*, London: James Nisbet & Co.

Lane-Poole, Stanley (1878a and b) *The People of Turkey: Twenty Years' Residence among Bulgarians, Greeks, Albanians, Turks, and Armenians by a Consul's Daughter and Wife*, 2 vols, London: John Murray.

Lange, Johannes (1554) *Medicinalium epistolarum miscellanea*, Basel: J. Oporinus.

Langham, William (1597) *The Garden of Health*, London: deputies of C. Barker.

Langholf, Volker (1990) *Medical Theories in Hippocrates: Early Texts and the 'Epidemics'*, Berlin and New York: de Gruyter.

Lansing, Carol (2002) 'Girls in trouble in late medieval Bologna', in Konrad Eisenbichler (ed.), *The Premodern Teenager: Youth in Society 1150–1650*, Toronto: Centre for Reformation and Renaissance Studies, pp. 293–309.

Le Clerc, Daniel (1699) *The History of Physick*, London: D. Brown, A. Roper and J. Leigh (French, *Histoire de la Médecine*, Geneva: J.A. Chouët and D. Ritter, 1696).

Le Loyer, Pierre (1586) *III Livres des Spectres*, Angers: G. Nepueu.

—— (1605) *A Treatise of Specters or Strange Sights, Visions and Apparitions*, London: M. Lownes.

Lefkowitz, Mary R. (1981) *Heroines and Hysterics*, London: Duckworth.

Lefkowitz, Mary R. and Maureen B. Fant (1992) *Women's Lives in Greece and Rome: A Source Book in Translation*, 2nd edition, London: Duckworth.

Lemay, Helen Rodnite (1978) 'Some thirteenth and fourteenth century lectures on female sexuality', *International Journal of Women's Studies* 1: 391–400.

—— (1981) 'William of Saliceto on human sexuality', *Viator* 12: 165–81.

—— (1992) *Women's Secrets: A Translation of Pseudo-Albertus Magnus'* De Secretis Mulierum *with Commentaries*, New York: SUNY Press.

Leoniceno, Niccolò (1497) *Libellus de Epidemia, quam vulgo morbum Gallicum vocant*, Venice: Aldus Manutius.

Lettsom, John Coakley (1795) *Hints Respecting the Chlorosis of Boarding-schools*, London: C. Dilly.

Levey, Martin and Souryal, Safwat S. (1968) 'Galen's *On the secrets of women* and *On the secrets of men*', *Janus* 55: 208–19.

Levy, Anita (1999) *Reproductive Urges: Popular Novel-reading, Sexuality, and the English Nation*, Philadelphia: University of Pennsylvania Press.

Lewis, Gilbert (1980) *Day of Shining Red: An Essay in Understanding Ritual*, Cambridge: Cambridge University Press.

Liébault, Jean (1582) *Trois Livres appartenant aux infirmitez et maladies des femmes, pris du Latin de M. Jean Liebaut, Docteur Medecin à Paris, et faicts François*, Paris: Jacques de Puys.

—— (1585) *Thrésor des rèmedes secrets pour les maladies des femmes*, Paris: Robert Jacques de Puys.

—— (1597) *Thrésor des rèmedes secrets pour les maladies des femmes*, Paris: Robert Foüet.

Lippi, Donatella and Arieti, Stefano (1985) 'La ricezione del *Corpus hippocraticum* nell'Islam', in Innocenzo Mazzini and Franca Fusco, *I Testi di Medicina Latini Antichi: Problemi Filologici e Storici*, Atti del I Convegno Internazionale, 26–28 aprile, Università di Macerata: G. Bretschneider, pp. 399–402.

List (1805) *A List of the Members of the Royal College of Surgeons of London, July the 11th, 1805*, London: J. Adlord.

Lloyd, Geoffrey E.R. (1979) *Magic, Reason and Experience*, Cambridge: Cambridge University Press.

—— (1983) *Science, Folklore and Ideology*, Cambridge: Cambridge University Press.

Longrigg, James (1985) 'A "seminal" debate in the fifth century BC?', in Allan Gotthelf (ed.), *Aristotle on Nature and Living Things: Philosophical and Historical Studies presented to David M. Balme*, Pittsburgh, PA: Mathesis Publications; Bristol: Bristol Classical Press, pp. 277–87.

—— (1992) 'Epidemic, ideas and classical Athenian society', in Terence Ranger and Paul Slack (eds), *Epidemics and Ideas: Essays on the Historical Perception of Pestilence*, Cambridge: Cambridge University Press, pp. 21–44.

Lonie, Iain M. (1981) *The Hippocratic Treatises 'On Generation', 'On the Nature of the Child', 'Diseases IV'*, Berlin: de Gruyter.

—— (1985) 'The "Paris Hippocratics": teaching and research in Paris in the second half of the sixteenth century', in Andrew Wear, Roger K. French and Iain M. Lonie (eds), *The Medical Renaissance of the Sixteenth Century*, Cambridge: Cambridge University Press, pp. 155–74.

Loraux, Nicole (1993) *The Children of Athena: Athenian Ideas about Citizenship and the Division between the Sexes* (trans. Caroline Levine), Princeton, NJ: Princeton University Press (first published as *Les enfants d'Athéna: idées athéniennes sur la citoyenneté et la division des sexes*, Paris: Maspero, 1981 and Editions La Découverte, 1984).

Lord, Alexandra (1999) ' "The great *arcana* of the deity": menstruation and menstrual disorders in eighteenth-century British thought', *Bulletin of the History of Medicine* 73: 38–63.

Loudon, Irvine S.L. (1980) 'Chlorosis, anaemia and anorexia nervosa', *British Medical Journal* 281: 1669–75.

—— (1984) 'The diseases called chlorosis', *Psychological Medicine* 14: 27–36.

Loughlin, Marie H. (1997) *Hymeneutics: Interpreting Virginity on the Early Modern Stage*, Lewisburg, TN: Bucknell University Press; London: Associated University Presses.

MacDonald, Michael (1981) *Mystical Bedlam: Madness, Anxiety, and Healing in Seventeenth-century England*, Cambridge: Cambridge University Press.

McFarland, Ronald E. (1975) 'The rhetoric of medicine: Lord Herbert's and Thomas Carew's poems of green-sickness', *Journal of the History of Medicine* 30: 250–8.

Maclean, Ian (1980) *The Renaissance Notion of Woman: A Study in the Fortunes of Scholasticism and Medical Science in European Intellectual Life*, Cambridge: Cambridge University Press.

McMurtrie, Henry (1871) *The Woman's Medical Companion and Nursery-Adviser*, Philadelphia, PA: T. Ellwood Zell.

Major, Ralph H. (1932) *Classic Descriptions of Disease: With Biographical Sketches of the Authors*, Springfield, IL: C.C. Thomas.

Mambretti, Catherine Cole (1974) 'William Bullein and the "lively fashions" in Tudor medical literature', *Clio Medica* 9: 285–97.

Manning, Henry (1771) *A Treatise on Female Diseases: In which are also Comprehended those Most Incident to Pregnant and Child-bed Women*, London: Printed for R. Baldwin.

Manuli, Paola (1980) 'Fisiologia e patologia del femminile negli scritti ippocratici dell'antica ginecologia greca', in Mirko D. Grmek (ed.), *Hippocratica. Actes du Colloque hippocratique de Paris 1978*, Paris: Eds de CNRS, pp. 393–408.

—— (1982) 'Elogia della castità: La *Ginecologia* di Sorano', *Memoria* 3: 39–49.

—— (1983) 'Donne mascoline, femmine sterili, vergini perpetue. La ginecologia greca tra Ippocrate e Sorano', in Silvia Campese, Paola Manuli and Giulia Sissa, *Madre Materia. Sociologia e biologia della donna greca*, Turin: Boringhieri, pp. 147–92.

Marcovich, M. (1972) 'Sappho fr. 31: anxiety attack or love declaration?', *Classical Quarterly* 22: 19–32.

Marinello, Giovanni (1563) *Le medicine partenenti alle infermità delle donne*, Venice: Francesco de Franceschi Senese.

Martinez, David (1995) ' "May she neither eat nor drink": love magic and vows of abstinence', in Marvin Meyer and Paul Mirecki (eds), *Ancient Magic and Ritual Power*, Leiden: E.J. Brill, pp. 335–59.

Mattioli, Pier-Andrea (1558) *Commentarii in Libros Sex Pedacii Dioscoridis Anazarbei de Materia Medica*, Venice: Ex Officina Erasmiana, Vincentii Valgrisii.

Maubray, John (1724) *The Female Physician, Containing All the Diseases Incident to that Sex*, London: J. Holland.

Mazzini, Innocenzo (1985) 'Ippocrate latino dei secolo V–VI: tecnica di traduzione', in Innocenzo Mazzini and Franca Fusco, *I Testi di Medicina Latini Antichi: Problemi Filologici e Storici*, Atti del I Convegno Internazionale, 26–28 aprile, Università di Macerata: G. Bretschneider, pp. 383–7.

Mazzini, Innocenzo and Fusco, Franca (1985) *I Testi di Medicina Latini Antichi: Problemi Filologici e Storici*, Atti del I Convegno Internazionale, 26–28 aprile, Università di Macerata: G. Bretschneider.

Mercado, Luis (1579) *De mulierum affectionibus*, Vallesoleti: D. Fernandez a Corduba (also in Bauhin 1586–8, vol. 4: 1–567; Spach 1597: 803–1080).

Mercuriale, Girolamo (1587) *De morbis muliebribus praelectiones*, Venice: F. Valgrisus (also in Bauhin 1586–8, vol. 2: 1–194; Spach 1597: 209–303).

—— (1591) *De morbis muliebribus praelectiones*, Venice: apud Juntas.

Meyerhof, Max (1931) ''Ali at-Tabari's "Paradise of Wisdom", one of the oldest Arabic compendiums of medicine', *Isis* 16: 6–54.

Meynell, Geoffrey Guy (1990) *A Bibliography of Dr. Thomas Sydenham (1624–1689)*, Folkestone: Winterdown Books.

Mezière, Victor (1846) *De la puberté dans les deux sexes*, Paris: Rignoux.

Minghetti, Renato (1960) 'Studio comparativo tra il "De gynaeceis" ascritto a Galeno, il "Gynaecia" di Teodoro Prisciano e l'"Harmoniae gynaeciorum" del Wolff', in *Atti del XVI Congresso Nazionale di Storia della Medicina*, Bologna: Società Italiana di Storia della Medicina.

Mitchell, William S. (1959) 'William Bullein, Elizabethan physician and author', *Medical History* 3: 188–200.

Mondrain, Brigitte (1997) 'Éditer et traduire les médecins grecs au XVIe siècle. L'exemple de Janus Cornarius', in Danielle Jacquart (ed.), *Les Voies de la science grecque. Études sur la transmission des texts de l'Antiquité au dix-neuvième siècle*, Geneva: Librairie Droz, pp. 391–417.

Monte, Giambattista da (1554) *Opusculum de uterinis affectibus*, Venice: apud Balthassarem Constantinum (also in Bauhin 1586–8, vol.2: 197–251; Spach 1597: 303–30).

—— (1556) *Opusculum de uterinis affectibus maxime utile*, Paris: apud Aegidium Gourbinum.

—— (1565) *Consultationum Medicarum Opus absolutissimum*. Basel: [Per Henricum Petri, et Petrum Pernam].

—— (1587) *Medicina Universa*, Frankfurt: Apud Andreae Wecheli heredes, Claud. Marnium & Ioann. Aubrium.

Montrose, Louis A. (1986) '*A Midsummer Night's Dream* and the shaping fantasies of Elizabethan culture: gender, power, form', in Margaret W. Ferguson, Maureen Quilligan and Nancy J. Vickers (eds), *Rewriting the Renaissance: The Discourses of Sexual Difference in Early Modern Europe*, Chicago, IL and London: University of Chicago Press, pp. 65–87.

—— (1993) 'The work of gender in the discourse of discovery', in Stephen Greenblatt (ed.), *New World Encounters*, Berkeley and London: University of California Press, pp. 177–217.

Morantz-Sanchez, Regina Markell (1985) *Sympathy and Science: Women Physicians in American Medicine*, New York and Oxford: Oxford University Press.

Moutard-Martin, Eugène (1846) *Des accidents qui accompagnent l'établissement de la menstruation, de la chlorose en particulier*, Paris: Rignoux.

Müller-Rohlfsen, I. (1980) *Die Lateinische Ravennatische Übersetzung der hippokratischen Aphorismen aus dem 5./6. Jahrhundert n. chr.*, Geistes- und socialwissenschaftliche Dissertation 55, Hamburg: Hartmut Lüdke.

Munich, Adrienne Auslander (1993) 'What Lily knew: virginity in the 1890s', in Lloyd Davis (ed.), *Virginal Sexuality and Textuality in Victorian Literature*, New York: SUNY Press, pp. 143–57.

Munkhoff, Richelle (1999) 'Searchers of the dead: authority, marginality, and the interpretation of plague in England, 1574–1665', *Gender and History* 11: 1–29.

Muret, Marc-Antoine de (1554), *Catullus et in eum commentarius*, Venice: Aldine.

Myrepsus, Nicolaus (1541) *Liber de compositione medicamentorum secundum loca*, Ingolstadt: In officina Alexandri Vueissenhorn.

Nathanson, Constance (1991) *Dangerous Passages: The Social Control of Sexuality in Women's Adolescence*, Philadelphia, PA: Temple University Press.

Newcomb, Lori Humphrey (2002) *Reading Popular Romance in Early Modern England*, New York: Columbia University Press.

Newman, Philip L. (1965) *Knowing the Gururumba*, New York and London: Holt, Rinehart and Winston.

Nicolson, Malcolm (1993) 'The introduction of percussion and stethoscopy to early nineteenth-century Edinburgh', in William F. Bynum and Roy Porter (eds), *Medicine and the Five Senses*, Cambridge: Cambridge University Press, pp. 134–53.

Norri, Juhani (1992) *Names of Sicknesses in English, 1400–1550: An Exploration of the Lexical Field*, Helsinki: Suomalainen Tiedeakatemia.

Nutton, Vivian (ed.) (1979) Galen, *On Prognosis*, CMG V.8.1, Berlin: Akademie-Verlag.

—— (1984) 'John Caius und Johannes Lange: medizinischer Humanismus zur Zeit Vesals', *NTM – Schriftenreihe für Geschichte der Naturwissenschafte, Technik und Medizin* 21: 81–7.

—— (1985) 'Humanist surgery', in Andrew Wear, Roger K. French and Iain M. Lonie (eds), *The Medical Renaissance of the Sixteenth Century*, Cambridge: Cambridge University Press, pp. 75–99.

—— (1988) ' "Prisci dissectionum professores": Greek texts and Renaissance anatomists', in A. Carlotta Dionisotti, Anthony Grafton and Jill Kraye (eds), *The*

Uses of Greek and Latin: Historical Essays, Warburg Institute Surveys and Texts XVI, London: Warburg Institute, pp. 111–26.

—— (1989) 'Hippocrates and the Renaissance', in Gerhard Baader and Rolf Winau (eds), *Die hippokratischen Epidemien: theorie, praxis, tradition* (Proceedings of the Colloque hippocratique, Berlin 10–15 September 1984), *Sudhoffs Archiv* Heft 27, Stuttgart: Franz Steiner, pp. 420–39.

Nye, Robert A. (1999) 'Sex and sexuality in France since 1900', in Franz X. Eder, Lesley A. Hall and Gert Hekma (eds), *Sexual Cultures in Europe: National Histories*, Manchester and New York: Manchester University Press, pp. 91–113.

O'Connor, Erin (1995) 'Pictures of health: medical photography and the emergence of anorexia nervosa', *Journal of the History of Sexuality* 5: 535–72.

Olive, Antoine Alexandre (1819) 'Dissertation inaugurale sur la première menstruation, l'age critique et les soins hygiéniques que réclament les femmes à ces deux époques', Paris Medical Faculty, 1 May.

Oliver, James (1893) *Manual of the Diseases Peculiar to Women*, London: J. & A. Churchill.

Otten, Charlotte F. (1992) *English Women's Voices 1540–1700*, Miami: Florida International University Press.

Oudshoorn, Nelly (1994) *Beyond the Natural Body: An Archeology of Sex Hormones*, London and New York: Routledge.

Pagel, Walter (1982) *Joan Baptista van Helmont*, Cambridge: Cambridge University Press.

Pallangyo, Kisali J. (1987) 'Chlorosis lives! – and slips through MeSH', *Journal of the American Medical Association* 258: 1174.

Pallister, Janis L. (trans.) (1982) *Ambroise Paré, On Monsters and Marvels*, Chicago, IL: University of Chicago Press.

Paré, Ambroise (1575) *Les Oeuvres en vingt-six livres*, Paris: Buon (gynaecological material also in Bauhin 1586–8, vol. 2: 404–84; Spach 1597: 403–42).

Parsons, John Carmi (2002) 'The medieval aristocratic teenaged female: adolescent or adult?', in Konrad Eisenbichler (ed.), *The Premodern Teenager: Youth in Society 1150–1650*, Toronto: Centre for Reformation and Renaissance Studies, pp. 311–21.

Paster, Gail Kern (1993) *The Body Embarrassed: Drama and the Disciplines of Shame in Early Modern England*, Ithaca, NY: Cornell University Press.

Patek, Arthur J. and Heath, Clark W. (1936) 'Chlorosis', *Journal of the American Medical Association* 17: 1463–6.

[Pechey, John] (1694) *Some Observations Made upon the Bermudas Berries Imported from the Indies: Shewing their Admirable Virtues in Curing the Green-sickness*, London.

Phillips, Kim M. (1999) 'Maidenhood as the perfect age of woman's life', in Katherine J. Lewis, Noël James Menuge and Kim M. Phillips (eds), *Young Medieval Women*, Stroud: Sutton Publishing, pp. 1–24.

Pierce, Robert (1697) *Bath Memoirs: Or, Observations in Three and Forty Years Practice at the Bath*, Bristol: Printed for H. Hammond, Bath.

Pinault, Jody Rubin (1992) 'The medical case for virginity in the early second century C.E.: Soranus of Ephesus, *Gynecology* 1.32', *Helios* 19: 123–39.

Platter, Felix (1586–8) *De mulierum partibus generationi dicatis tabulae*, in Caspar Bauhin, *Gynaeciorum sive mulierum affectibus commentarii Graecorum, Latinorum,*

Barbarorum, iam olim et nunc recens editorum ..., Basel: Conrad Waldkirch (extracted from his *De corporis humani structura et usu*, first published 1583).

Pollock, Linda A. (1989) 'Embarking on a rough passage: the experience of pregnancy in early-modern England', in Valerie Fildes (ed.), *Women as Mothers in Pre-Industrial England: Essays in Memory of Dorothy McLaren*, London and New York: Routledge, pp. 39–67.

Pomata, Gianna (1992) 'Uomini mestruanti. Somiglianza e differenza fra i sessi in Europa in età moderna', *Quaderni Storici* 79: 51–103.

Pomeroy, Sarah B. (1994) *Xenophon, Oeconomicus: a social and historical commentary, with a new English translation*, Oxford: Clarendon Press.

Pontano, Giovanni (1490) *De fortitudine bellica et heroica*, Naples: per M. Moranum.

Porta, Giovan Battista della (1601) *De humana physiognomonia libri IV*, Ursellis: Cornelii Sutorii.

Porter, Roy (1985) ' "The Secrets of generation display'd": *Aristotle's Masterpiece* in eighteenth century England', in *Eighteenth Century Life*, special issue, Robert P. Maccubbin (ed.), *Unauthorized Sexual Behaviour during the Enlightenment* 9: 1–21, Williamsburg, VA: College of William and Mary.

—— (1990) 'Female quacks in the consumer society', *History of Nursing Society Journal* 3: 1–25.

Porter, Roy and George S. Rousseau (1998) *Gout: The Patrician Malady*, New Haven, CT and London: Yale University Press.

Potter, Ursula (2002) 'Greensickness in *Romeo and Juliet*: considerations on a sixteenth-century disease of virgins', in Konrad Eisenbichler (ed.), *The Premodern Teenager: Youth in Society 1150–1650*, Toronto: Centre for Reformation and Renaissance Studies, pp. 271–91.

Prescott, Heather Munro (1998) *A Doctor of Their Own: The History of Adolescent Medicine*, Cambridge, MA and London: Harvard University Press.

Raciborski, Adam (1868) *Traité de la menstruation: ses rapports avec l'ovulation, la fécondation, l'hygiène de la puberté et de l'age critique, son role dans les différentes maladies, ses troubles et leur traitement*, Paris: Baillière.

Ralegh, Sir Walter (1596) *The Discovery of the Large, Rich, and Beautiful Empire of Guiana* (ed. Sir Robert H. Schomburgk), Hakluyt Society, 1st series, no. 3, 1848.

Ranchin, François (1627) *Tractatus de morbis virginum*, in *Opuscula Medica*, Lyons: Pierre Ravaud.

Rebello, Pedro Julião (1550) *The Treasuri of Helth: Contaynynge Many Profytable Medicines*, London: W. Coplande.

Reece, Richard (1826) *On the Means of Obviating and Treating Costiveness*, London: Longman, Rees, Orme, Brown and Green.

Reiser, Stanley Joel (1993) 'The science of diagnosis: diagnostic technology', in William F. Bynum and Roy Porter (eds), *Companion Encyclopedia of the History of Medicine*, vol. 2, London and New York: Routledge, pp. 824–51.

Reynolds, John (1669) *A Discourse upon Prodigious Abstinence: Occasioned by the Twelve Moneths Fasting of Martha Taylor, the Famed Derbyshire Demosell ...*, London: R.W. for Nevill Simmons and Dorman Newman.

Rhazes (1505) *Continens Rasis ordinatus et correctus ...* (al-Ḥāwī), Venice: Bon. Locatellum.

Rhodes, Peter J. (1988) *Thucydides: History II*, Warminster: Aris & Phillips.

Richardson, Adolphus J. (1891) 'On *bruit de diable* in chlorosis', *The Lancet* I: 1426–7.

Rigler, Lorenz (1852) *Die Türkei und deren Bewohner*, vol. 1, Vienna: C. Gerold.

Risse, Guenter (1986) *Hospital Life in Enlightenment Scotland: Care and Teaching at the Royal Infirmary of Edinburgh*, Cambridge: Cambridge University Press.

Rivière, Lazare (1655) *The Practice of Physick*, London: P. Cole.

Rocher, Gregory David de (trans.) (1989) *Laurent Joubert: Popular Errors*, Tuscaloosa: University of Alabama Press.

Roe, Shirley A. (1981a) *Matter, Life, and Generation: 18th-century Embryology and the Haller–Wolff Debate*, Cambridge: Cambridge University Press.

—— (ed.) (1981b) *The Natural Philosophy of Albrecht von Haller*, New York: Arno Press.

Roger, Jacques (1997) *Buffon: A Life in Natural History*, Ithaca, NY and London: Cornell University Press (original published in French, *Buffon, un philosophe au Jardin du Roi*, Librairie Arthème Fayard, trans. Sarah Lucille Bonnefoi, 1989).

Rorarius, Nicolaus (1566) *Contradictiones, dubia et paradoxa, in libros Hippocratis, Celsi, Galeni, Aetii, Aeginetae, Avicennae, cum eorundem conciliationibus*, Venice: D. & J.B. Guerreus.

Rosenberg, Charles E. (1992) 'Framing disease: illness, society, and history', in Charles E. Rosenberg and Janet Golden (eds), *Framing Disease: Studies in Cultural History*, New Brunswick, NJ: Rutgers University Press, pp. xiii–xxvi.

Rosenberg, Charles E. and Golden, Janet (eds) (1992) *Framing Disease: Studies in Cultural History*, New Brunswick, NJ: Rutgers University Press.

Rosin, Heinrich (1907) 'Diseases of the blood in relation to marriage', in Hermann Senator and Siegfried Kaminer (eds), *Marriage and Disease, Being an Abridged Version of 'Health and Disease in Relation to Marriage and the Married State'* (trans. Joseph Dulberg), London: Rebman Ltd, ch. 9.

Rousseau, George S. (1982) 'Nymphomania, Bienville and the rise of erotic sensibility', in Paul-Gabriel Boucé (ed.), *Sexuality in Eighteenth-century Britain*, Manchester: Manchester University Press, pp. 95–119.

Rousseau, Jean-Jacques (1768) *Emilius: Or, a Treatise of Education*, 3 vols, Edinburgh: A. Donaldson.

Rowbottom, Margaret and Susskind, Charles (1984) *Electricity and Medicine: History of their Interaction*, San Francisco, CA: San Francisco Press; London: Macmillan.

Ruddock, Edward Harris (1892) *The Lady's Manual of Homoeopathic Treatment in the Various Derangements Incident to her Sex*, London: The Homoeopathic Publishing Co.

Rue, Ambroise Joseph (1819) 'Essai sur la première menstruation, précédé de quelques considerations sur la chlorose', Paris Medical Faculty, 4 May.

Ruel, Joannes (1550) *Pedanii Dioscoridis Anazarbei, de Medicinali materia, Libri sex, Ioanne Ruellio suessionensi interprete*, Lyons: Apud Balthazarem Arnolletum.

Ruhräh, John (1934) 'Johannes Lange, 1485–1565: a note on the history of chlorosis', *American Journal of Diseases of Children* 48: 393–6.

Rütten, Thomas (1993) 'Pseudohippokrates, Marco Fabio Calvo und Robert Burton: zur Rezeptiongeschichte eines antiken Textes', in R. Kinsky (ed.), *Offenheit und Interesse: Studien zum 65. Geburtstag von Gerhard Wirth*, Amsterdam: Hakkert, pp. 31–43.

Sadler, John (1636) *The Sick Womans Private Looking-glasse*, London: Printed by Anne Griffin for Philemon Stephens and Christopher Meridith.

Said, Edward W. (1978) *Orientalism*, London: Routledge and Kegan Paul.

Salih, Sarah (1999) 'Performing virginity: sex and violence in the *Katherine* group', in Cindy L. Carlson and Angela Jane Weisl (eds), *Constructions of Widowhood and Virginity in the Middle Ages*, New York: St Martin's Press, pp. 95–112.

Sarrazin, Pierre (1921) *La Ginécologie dans les écrits hippocratiques*, Paris: Arnette.

Sawyer, Ronald C. (1986) 'Patients, healers, and disease in the Southeast Midlands, 1597–1634', PhD thesis, University of Wisconsin-Madison.

Schenck, Johann Georg (1606) *ΠΙΝΑΞ Auctorum in re medica, graecorum, latinorum priscorum, Arabum, Latinobarbarorum, Latinorum recentorium ... qui Gynaecia, sive Muliebria pleno argumento ...*, Strasbourg: Zetzner.

Schenck von Grafenberg, Joannes (1600) *Observationum medicarum, rararum, novarum, admirabilium, et monstrorum libri*, Frankfurt: E. Paltheniana, sumt. J. Rhodius.

Schleiner, Winfried (1995) *Medical Ethics in the Renaissance*, Washington, DC: Georgetown University Press.

Schneider, William H. (1986) 'Puericulture, and the style of French eugenics', *History and Philosophy of the Life Sciences* 8: 265–77.

Schoenfeldt, Michael C. (1999) *Bodies and Selves in Early Modern England: Physiology and Inwardness in Spenser, Shakespeare, Herbert, and Milton*, Cambridge: Cambridge University Press.

Schultz, James A. (1991) 'Medieval adolescence: the claims of history and the silence of German narrative', *Speculum* 66: 519–39.

Schurig, Martin (1729) *Parthenologia Historico-Medica, hoc est, Virginitatis Consideratio*, Dresden and Leipzig: C. Hekel.

—— (1730) *Gynaecologia historico-medica, hoc est, congressus muliebris consideratio*, Dresden and Leipzig: Hekel.

Schwarz, Emil (1951) *Chlorosis: A Retrospective Investigation*, Supplementum *Acta Medica Belgica*, Brussels: Presses imprimerie médicale et scientifique.

Sedgwick, Catharine Maria (1845) *Means and Ends, or Self-training*, New York: Harper and Brothers.

Sennert, Daniel (1664) *Practical Physick; the Fourth Book in Three Parts* (trans. Nicholas Culpeper and Abdiah Cole), London: Peter Cole.

Sezgin, Fuat (1970) *Geschichte des arabischen Schriftums*, Band 3, Leiden: E.J. Brill.

Sharp, Jane (1671) *The Midwives Book, or the Whole Art of Midwifry Discovered*, London: S. Miller (ed. Elaine Hobby, New York and Oxford: Oxford University Press, 1999).

Shaw, Manley Bradford (1933) 'A short history of the sweating sickness', *Annals of Medical History* 5: 246–74.

Shaw, Teresa M. (1998) 'Creation, virginity and diet in fourth-century Christianity: Basil of Ancyra's *On the true purity of virginity*', in Maria Wyke (ed.), *Gender and the Body in the Ancient Mediterranean*, Oxford: Blackwell, pp. 155–72.

Shore, Sally Rieger (trans.) (1983) *John Chrysostom, On Virginity; Against Remarriage*, Lewiston: Edwin Mellen Press.

Shorter, Edward (1983) *A History of Women's Bodies*, London: Allen Lane.

—— (1986) 'Paralysis: the rise and fall of a "hysterical" symptom', *Journal of Social History* 19: 549–82.

Showalter, Elaine (1987) *The Female Malady: Women, Madness and English Culture 1830–1980*, London: Virago (first publication, New York: Pantheon Books, 1985).

—— (1993) 'Hysteria, feminism, and gender', in Sander Gilman, Helen King, Roy Porter, George S. Rousseau and Elaine Showalter, *Hysteria Beyond Freud*, Berkeley: University of California Press, pp. 286–344.

Siddall, A. Clair (1982) 'Chlorosis: aetiology reconsidered', *Bulletin of the History of Medicine* 56: 254–60.

Sigerist, Henry E. (1928) 'Kultur und Krankheit', *Kyklos* 1: 60–3.

Siggel, Alfred (1941) 'Gynäkologie, Embryologie und Frauenhygiene aus dem "Paradies der Weisheit über die Medizin" des Abu Hana Ali b. Sahl Rabban at-Tabari nach der Ausgabe von Dr. Zubair as-Siddiqi', *Quellen und Studien zur Geschichte der Naturwissenschaften und der Medizin* 8: 216–72.

Simmer, Hans H. (1977) 'Pflüger's nerve reflex theory of menstruation: the product of analogy, teleology and neurophysiology', *Clio Medica* 12: 57–90.

Simon, Bennett (1978) *Mind and Madness in Ancient Greece*, Ithaca, NY: Cornell University Press.

Sissa, Giulia (1990a) *Greek Virginity* (trans. Arthur Goldhammer), Cambridge, MA: Harvard University Press (French, *Le Corps virginal: la virginité féminine en Grèce ancienne*, Paris: Hachette, 1987).

—— (1990b) 'Maidenhood without maidenhead: the female body in ancient Greece', in David M. Halperin, John J. Winkler and Froma I. Zeitlin (eds), *Before Sexuality: The Construction of Erotic Experience in the Ancient Greek World*, Princeton NJ: Princeton University Press, pp. 339–64.

Skene, Alexander J.C. (1895) *Medical Gynecology: A Treatise on the Diseases of Women from the Standpoint of the Physician*, Edinburgh and London: Young J. Pentland.

Skrabanek, Petr (1983) 'Notes towards the history of anorexia nervosa', *Janus* 70: 109–28.

Slack, Paul (1979) 'Mirrors of health and treasures of poor men: the uses of the vernacular medical literature of Tudor England', in Charles Webster (ed.), *Health, Medicine and Mortality in the Sixteenth Century*, Cambridge: Cambridge University Press, pp. 237–73.

Smith, Francis Barrymore (1982) *Florence Nightingale: Reputation and Power*, London: Croom Helm.

Smith, Hilda (1976) 'Gynaecology and ideology in seventeenth-century England', in B.A. Carroll (ed.), *Liberating Women's History*, Urbana, IL: University of Illinois Press, pp. 97–114.

Smith, Wesley D. (1979) *The Hippocratic Tradition*, Ithaca, NY: Cornell University Press.

Snyder, Jane McIntosh (1991) 'Public occasion and private passion in the lyrics of Sappho of Lesbos', in Sarah B. Pomeroy (ed.), *Women's History and Ancient History*, Chapel Hill: University of North Carolina Press, pp. 1–19.

Spach, Israel (1591) *Nomenclator scriptorum medicorum. Hoc est, Elenchus eorem, qui artem medicam suis scriptis illustrarunt*, Frankfurt: ex officina typographica Nicolai Bassæi, et Lazari Zetzneri.

—— (1597) *Gynaeciorum, sive de mulierum tum communibus, tum gravidarum, parientium, et puerperarum affectibus et morbis, libri Graecorum, Arabum, Latinorum veterum et recentium quotquot extant …*, Strasbourg: Zetzner.

Spongberg, Mary (1997) *Feminizing Venereal Disease: The Body of the Prostitute in Nineteenth-century Medical Discourse*, New York: New York University Press.

Stacey, Michelle (2002) *The Fasting Girl: A True Victorian Medical Mystery*, New York: Jeremy P. Tarcher/Putnam.

Starobinski, Jean (1981) 'Chlorosis: the "green sickness"', *Psychological Medicine* 11: 459–98.

Stengel, Alfred (1896) *Twentieth Century Practice* (ed. Thomas L. Stedman), vol. 7: *Diseases of the Respiratory Organs and Blood, and Functional Sexual Disorders*, London: Sampson Low, Marston and Co.

Stephanus, Joannes (1635) *In Hippocratis Coi libellum De virginum morbis commentarius*, Venice: Brogiollum.

Stewart, Mary Lynn (2001) *For Health and Beauty: Physical Culture for Frenchwomen, 1880s–1930s*, Baltimore, MD: Johns Hopkins University Press.

Stockman, Ralph (1895a) 'A summary of sixty-three cases of chlorosis', *Edinburgh Medical Journal* 41 (1): 413–17.

—— (1895b) 'Observations on the causes and treatment of chlorosis', *British Medical Journal* 2 (14 December): 1473–6; (reprinted in *Nutrition* 7 (1991): 12–15).

Stoertz, Fiona Harris (2002) 'Sex and the medieval adolescent', in Konrad Eisenbichler (ed.), *The Premodern Teenager: Youth in Society 1150–1650*, Toronto: Centre for Reformation and Renaissance Studies, pp. 225–43.

Strange, Julie-Marie (2000) 'Menstrual fictions: languages of medicine and menstruation, c. 1850–1930', *Women's History Review* 9: 607–28.

—— (2001) 'The assault on ignorance: teaching menstrual etiquette in England, c. 1920s to 1960s', *Social History of Medicine* 14: 247–65.

Stransky, Eugene (1974) 'On the history of chlorosis', *Episteme* 8: 26–45.

Sudell, Nicholas (1666) *Mulierum amicus*, London: J. Hancock.

Sydenham, Thomas (1695) *Compleat Method of Curing Almost All Diseases*, 2nd edition, London: H. Newman & R. Parker.

—— (1753) *The Entire Works*, London: E. Cave.

—— (1827) *Processus Integri in Morbis fere Omnibus Curandis*, in Carl Gottlob Kühn (ed.), *Opera Universa Medica*, Leipzig: Voss.

T.P. (1677) *The Accomplish'd Lady's Delight in Preserving, Physick, Beautifying, and Cookery*, London: B. Harris.

Taddei, Ilaria (2002) '*Puerizia, adolescenza* and *giovinezza*: images and conceptions of youth in Florentine society during the Renaissance', in Konrad Eisenbichler (ed.), *The Premodern Teenager: Youth in Society 1150–1650*, Toronto: Centre for Reformation and Renaissance Studies, pp. 15–26.

Tait, Lawson (1889) *Diseases of Women and Abdominal Surgery*, vol. 1, Leicester: Richardson and Co.; Philadelphia, PA: Lea Brothers.

Tanner, John (1659) *The Hidden Treasures of the Art of Physick*, London: G. Sawbridge (first published 1656).

Tardy, Claude (1648) *In libellum Hippocratis de virginum morbis: commentario paraphrastica*, Paris: apud Jacobum de Senlecque, et apud Carolum du Mesnil.

Taviner, Mark, Thwaites, Guy and Gant, Vanya (1998) 'The English sweating sickness, 1485–1551: a viral pulmonary disease?', *Medical History* 42: 96–8.

Taylor, Frederick (1896) 'A discussion on anaemia: its causation, varieties, assorted pathology, and treatment', *British Medical Journal* 2 (19 September): 719–25.

Temkin, Owsei (1956; reprinted 1991) *Soranus' Gynecology*, Baltimore, MD: Johns Hopkins University Press.

—— (1971) *The Falling Sickness: A History of Epilepsy from the Greeks to the Beginnings of Modern Neurology*, 2nd edition, Baltimore, MD: Johns Hopkins University Press.

Theriot, Nancy M. (1988) *The Biosocial Construction of Femininity: Mothers and Daughters in Nineteenth-century America*, New York and London: Greenwood Press.

Thompson, Roger (1979) *Unfit for Modest Ears*, London: Macmillan.

Tilley, Morris Palmer (1950) *A Dictionary of the Proverbs in England in the Sixteenth and Seventeenth Centuries*, Ann Arbor: University of Michigan Press.

Tilt, Edward John (1853) *On Diseases of Women and Ovarian Inflammation, in Relation to Morbid Menstruation, Sterility, Pelvic Tumours, and Affections of the Womb*, 2nd edition, London: John Churchill.

Todd, Jan (1998) *Physical Culture and the Body Beautiful: Purposive Exercise in the Lives of American Women, 1800–1875*, Macon, GA: Mercer University Press.

Trabuc, C.-C. Marius (1818) 'Quelques mots sur la chlorose qui attaque les filles à l'époque de la puberté', Montpellier Medical Faculty, 19 January.

Traister, Barbara H. (1991) ' "Matrix and the pain thereof": a sixteenth-century gynaecological essay', *Medical History* 35: 436–51.

Trapp, Helga (1967) 'Die hippokratische Schrift De natura muliebri: Ausgabe und textkritischer Kommentar', dissertation, University of Hamburg.

Treichler, Paula A. (1988) 'AIDS, gender, and biomedical discourse', in Elizabeth Fee and Daniel M. Fox (eds), *AIDS: The Burdens of History*, Berkeley: University of California Press, pp. 190–266.

Trotula (1544) *Trotulae curandarum Aegritudinum Muliebrium, ante, in et post partum liber unicus, nusquam antea editus* (ed. Georg Kraut), Strasbourg: Joannes Schottus.

Trousseau, Armand (1872) *Lectures on Clinical Medicine* vol. 5, London: New Sydenham Society.

Turner, Daniel (1714) *De morbis cutaneis, A Treatise of Diseases incident to the Skin*, London: R. Bonwicke *et al.*

Ullmann, Manfred (1970) *Die Medizin in Islam*, Leiden: E.J. Brill.

—— (1977) 'Zwei spätantike Kommentare zu der hippokratischen Schrift De morbis muliebribus', *Medizinhistorisches Journal* 12: 245–62.

—— (1978) *Islamic Medicine*, Edinburgh: Edinburgh University Press.

Uzac, J. (1853) *De la chlorose chez l'homme*, Paris: Baillière.

van Straten, Folkert T. (1981) 'Gifts for the gods', in Henk S. Versnel (ed.), *Faith, Hope and Worship: Aspects of Religious Mentality in the Ancient World*, Leiden: Brill, pp. 65–151.

Vance, Ap Morgan (1908) 'Hysteria as the surgeon sees it', *American Journal of Obstetrics and Diseases of Women and Children* 58: 757–67.

Vandereycken, Walter and Van Deth, Ron (1994) *From Fasting Saints to Anorexic Girls: The History of Self-Starvation*, London: Athlone Press (first published as *Van vastenwonder tot magerzucht: anorexia nervosa in historisch perspectief*, Amsterdam: Boom, 1988; adapted as *Hungerkünstler, Fastenwunder, Magersucht: eine Kulturgeschichte der Ess-störungen*, Zülpich: Biermann Verlag).

Varandal, Jean (1619) *De morbis et affectibus mulierum*, Lyons: B. Vincent.

—— (1620) *Ioannis Varandaei celeberrimorum Academiae Monspeliensis Medicorum, etc, De Morbis Mulierum Lib III*, Montpellier: Francis Chouët.

—— (1666) *Traité des Maladies des Femmes*, Paris: Robert de Ninville.

Vassès, Jean (1533) *De causis respirationis libellus. De usu respirationis liber unus. De spirandi difficultate libri tres*, Paris: Simon de Colines.

—— (1543) *Galen, In Hippocratis de victus ratione in morbis acutis, Ioanne Vassaeo interprete*, Paris: Ioannem Roigny.

Vázquez Buján, Manuel E. (1986) *El De mulierum affectibus del Corpus Hippocraticum*, Santiago del Compostela: Universidad de Santiago del Compostela.

Verbrugge, Martha H. (2000) 'Gym periods and monthly periods: concepts of menstruation in American physical education, 1900–1940', in Mary M. Lay *et al.*, *Body Talk: Rhetoric, Technology, Reproduction*, Wisconsin: University of Wisconsin Press, pp. 67–97.

Vernant, Jean-Pierre (1974) 'Le mythe prométhéen chez Hésiode', in *Mythe et société en Grèce ancienne*, Paris: Maspero, pp. 177–94.

—— (1983) 'Hestia-Hermes: the religious expression of space and movement in ancient Greece', in *Myth and Thought among the Greeks*, London: Routledge and Kegan Paul, pp. 127–75 (first published as *Mythe et pensée chez les Grecs*, Paris: Maspero, 1965).

Verso, M.L. (1964) 'The evolution of blood-counting techniques', *Medical History* 8: 149–58.

—— (1971) 'Some nineteenth-century pioneers of haematology', *Medical History* 15: 55–67.

—— (1981) *The Evolution of Haemoglobinometry and Other Essays in the History of Haematology*, Melbourne: Trefusis Publications.

Vertue, H. St H. (1955) 'Chlorosis and stenosis', *Guy's Hospital Reports* 104: 329–48.

von Noorden, Karl (1905) 'Chlorosis', in Paul Ehrlich, Adolph Lazarus, Karl von Noorden and Felix Pinkus, *Diseases of the Blood* (ed. Alfred Stengel), Philadelphia, PA and London: W.B. Saunders and Co., pp. 229–536.

von Staden, Heinrich (1989) *Herophilus: The Art of Medicine in Early Alexandria*, Cambridge: Cambridge University Press.

W.M. (1655) *The Queens Closet Opened*, London: N. Brook.

Wack, Mary F. (1990) *Lovesickness in the Middle Ages: The Viaticum and its Commentaries*, Philadelphia: University of Pennsylvania Press.

Wailoo, Keith (1997) *Drawing Blood: Technology and Disease Identity in Twentieth-century America*, Baltimore, MD: Johns Hopkins University Press.

Walter, George (1935) 'Peri Gynaikeion A of the Corpus Hippocraticum in a mediaeval translation', *Bulletin of the Institute of the History of Medicine* 3: 599–606.

Ward, Gordon (1914) *Bedside Haematology: An Introduction to the Clinical Study of the So-called Blood Diseases and Allied Disorders*, Philadelphia, PA and London: W.B. Saunders.

Watson, Gilbert (1966) *Theriac and Mithridatium: A Study in Therapeutics*, London: Wellcome Historical Medical Library.

Wear, Andrew (1989) 'Medical practice in late seventeenth- and early eighteenth-century England: continuity and union', in Roger French and Andrew Wear (eds), *The Medical Revolution of the Seventeenth Century*, Cambridge: Cambridge University Press, pp. 294–320.

—— (1992) 'The popularization of medicine in early modern England', in Roy Porter (ed.), *The Popularization of Medicine, 1650–1850*, London: Routledge, pp. 17–41.

—— (1995) 'Medicine in early modern Europe, 1500–1700', in Lawrence I. Conrad *et al.* (eds), *The Western Medical Tradition, 800 BC to AD 1800*, Cambridge: Cambridge University Press, pp. 215–361.

—— (2000) *Knowledge and Practice in English Medicine, 1550–1680*, Cambridge: Cambridge University Press.

Weinberg, Bernard (1950) 'Translations and commentaries of Longinus, *On the Sublime*, to 1600: a bibliography', *Modern Philology* 47: 145–51.

Weisser, Ursula (1984) 'Das Corpus Hippocraticum in der arabischen Medizin', in Gerhard Baader and Rolf Winau (eds), *Die hippokratischen Epidemien: theorie, praxis, tradition* (Proceedings of the Colloque hippocratique, Berlin 10–15 September 1984), *Sudhoffs Archiv* Heft 27, Stuttgart: Franz Steiner, pp. 377–408.

Whiting, Bartlett Jere and Helen Wescott Whiting (1968) *Proverbs, Sentences and Proverbial Phrases from English Writings Mainly before 1500*, Cambridge, MA: The Belknap Press for Harvard University Press; London: Oxford University Press.

Whitteridge, Gweneth (1971) *William Harvey and the Circulation of the Blood*, London: Macdonald.

Whorton, James C. (2000) *Inner Hygiene: Constipation and the Pursuit of Health in Modern Society*, New York: Oxford University Press.

Wiesner, Merry (1986) *Working Women in Renaissance Germany*, New Brunswick, NJ: Rutgers University Press.

—— (1993) *Women and Gender in Early Modern Europe*, Cambridge: Cambridge University Press.

Williams, David (1996) *Deformed Discourse: The Function of the Monster in Mediaeval Thought and Literature*, Exeter: University of Exeter Press.

Williams, Gordon (1994) *A Dictionary of Sexual Language and Imagery in Shakespearean and Stuart Literature*, vol. II (G–P), London: Athlone Press.

Williamson, George C. (1920) *George, Third Earl of Cumberland (1558–1605): His Life and his Voyages*, Cambridge: Cambridge University Press.

Wilson, Philip K. (1999) *Surgery, Skin and Syphilis. Daniel Turner's London (1667–1741)*, Amsterdam and Atlanta, GA: Rodopi.

Wiltshire, Alfred (1885) 'Clinical lecture on vicarious or ectopic menstruation, or menses devii', *The Lancet*, 19 September, pp. 513–17.

Wirsung, Christof (1605) *The General Practise of Physicke* (trans. Jacob Mosan), London: R. Field for G. Bishop.

Wolf, Caspar (1566a) *Gynaeciorum, hoc est, de mulierum tum aliis, tum gravidarum, parientium et puerperarum affectibus et morbis, libri veterum ac recentiorum aliquot, partim nunc primum editi, partim multo quam antea castigatiores*, Basel: Thomas Guarinus.

—— (1566b) *Harmonia Gynaeciorum*, in *Gynaeciorum, hoc est, de mulierum tum aliis, tum gravidarum, parientium et puerperarum affectibus et morbis, libri veterum ac recentiorum aliquot, partim nunc primum editi, partim multo quam antea castigatiores*, Basel: Thomas Guarinus, pp. 6–186 (also in Bauhin 1586–8, vol.1: 1–88; Spach 1597: 1–41).

Wood, Gordon R. (1914) *Bedside Haematology: An Introduction to the Clinical Study of the So-called Blood Diseases and Allied Disorders*, Philadelphia, PA and London: W.B. Saunders.

Wood-Allen, Mary (1898) *What a Young Woman Ought to Know*, London and Toronto: Vir Publishing Co.

Yealland, Lewis R. (1918) *Hysterical Disorders of Warfare*, London: Macmillan.

Youngson, Alexander John (1979) *The Scientific Revolution in Victorian Medicine*, London: Croom Helm.

INDEX

abortion 9, 28, 107
adolescence 66, 68, 83–8, 105, 135, 158, 159, 161; chlorosis and 15; comparison between male and female 88; emergence of idea of 84–8
advertisements 17, 34, 128, 131–3
advice manuals 86, 119, 130; *see* conduct books
Aetius of Amida 98, 106, 129
Agnodice: classical myth 161; quack healer 133
agriaca 22, 149
agricultural imagery 20–1, 36, 39, 137, 150
AIDS 155
Albertus Magnus 55, 149
Allbutt, Clifford 96, 102
Amatus Lusitanus 33, 77, 106, 150
Amazons 54
Ambrose of Milan 54
amenorrhoea 9–10, 12, 14, 21, 22, 27, 30, 35–6, 67, 69–70, 95, 102, 109, 127, 128, 132, 137; situations in which normal 27, 133
anaemia 6, 15–16, 33–4, 137, 148; hypochromic 15, 33, 116, 123,131, 144; pernicious 15; *see* iron deficiency
Andral, Gabriel 82, 123
anger 36, 92
ankles: bloodletting from 33, 75, 76–7, 126–7; swelling, as symptom 14, 46, 95, 97
Anna, Lange's patient 7, 13, 46, 51, 57–9, 66, 69, 77, 83, 100–2, 106, 107, 129
Anna O 7, 146
anorexia nervosa 2, 104, 139, 144

aorta 69
apoplexy 36
appetite: lack of 26, 133
apprenticeship 86, 87
Arabic medicine 22, 23, 25, 36, 46, 52, 55–6, 149, 157, 160
Aretaeus 157
Aristotle 23, 49, 99
Aristotle's *Masterpiece* 76, 100, 102, 103–4, 159
arm, bloodletting from 75, 77, 126
Artemis 50, 54, 95
asceticism 58
ash tree 28
ashes, eating 10, 98, 104, 106, 108
Ashwell, Samuel 8, 12, 24, 41, 91, 116, 120, 125–6
astrological medicine 29, 86
Astruc, Jean 9, 31, 77, 81, 82, 98
Athena 54
Athenian plague 63, 64, 65, 95, 127
auto-intoxication 113
Avicenna 78

Baillou, Guillaume de 60, 62, 75, 78, 84, 96, 100, 102, 103, 107, 146
ballads 1, 35, 37
Barker, Dr 19–20, 112, 144
Basil of Ancyra 55, 101
baths: cold 95–6, 109, 127, 129, 133–4, 137; mineral 78, 134
Bauda, Abraham 75
beauty 6, 8, 38, 41, 81, 87, 90, 105
beef-tea 131
Beier, Lucinda McCray 19–20, 160
Ben-Amos, Ilana Krausman 86
Bicks, Caroline 154
Bienville, D.T. de 41

bile: *see* humoral medicine
bile duct 33–4
birth rate 81
black bile: *see* humoral medicine
Black Death 34
Blackwell, Elizabeth 85,135–6
Blaud's pills 128
blood: as seat of disease 116; chemical
    structure of 82, 122–3, 127, 130;
    circulation of 68, 119; collection in
    womb 47; in formation of foetus 11,
    51, 73, 83, 89, 106, 153;
    manufacture of 23, 67, 97, 99, 101,
    108, 123; purification of 134; sex
    differences 122; sufferers as
    'bloodless' 2, 7, 30, 46, 60, 77, 124,
    146; thick and sticky 4, 29, 47, 52,
    70, 78, 106, 116; vomiting 24, 27,
    49; *see also* defloration, humoral
    medicine
blood testing 3, 15, 24, 33,
    116–7,121–4,138
bloodletting 48, 58, 73–9, 94, 112,
    118, 124, 125, 127,128; and
    menstruation 75; as cause of disease
    79; as last resort 75–6, 78;
    restrictions on 77–8, 128; *see also*
    ankles, arm, elbow
blushing, 7, 51, 90, 152
Boorde, Andrew 22, 25, 149
brain 116, 132; and logical faculty 69;
    as seat of love sickness 36, 40; use in
    women 85, 135, 138
Brain, Peter 12, 75, 157, 160
Bramwell, Byrom 7, 15, 91, 122–3,128
breast cysts 24, 115
breath, bad 28, 113
breathing, difficulties 14, 20, 22, 60,
    72, 76, 77, 94, 100, 108, 110–11,
    115, 121, 129, 131, 132; rapid 61,
    96
Bright, Timothie 20
brothels 129
bruit de diable 120–1, 123, 137, 138
Brumberg, Joan Jacobs 1, 15, 16, 85,
    101, 102, 105, 114, 116, 144
Buffon, Comte de 88, 89, 152, 154
Bullein, William 25–7, 28, 30–1, 43,
    66, 67, 105,139, 149–50
Burq, Victor 12
Bynum, Caroline Walker 101

Cabot, Richard Clarke 30, 31, 102, 117
Caelius Aurelianus 57
Calvi, Marco Fabio 11, 17, 45, 49, 52,
    58, 59, 74, 83, 153, 156
Campbell, J.M.H. 13, 15, 30, 82, 90,
    117, 123
Cary, Walter 21, 35, 105, 108
case notes 1, 19–20, 29–30
Castro, Rodrigues de 6, 144
Catholicism 4, 61, 80, 82, 145, 153
Catullus 38, 39, 40, 140
celibacy 138
Celsus 65, 74, 157
chalk: eating 98, 104–5, 108, 109, 125,
    133; as treatment 109, 125; *see* pica
chastity 86
    spiritual 55
Chevallier, Paul 67
Cheyne, George 133
childbirth 34, 51, 75, 83, 109, 160
chloro-anaemia 136
chlorosis: coining of name 19, 31; and
    pregnancy 107; disappearance of 5,
    7, 145–6; late 8, 84, 98; male 8, 20,
    61, 98, 108, 109, 111, 116, 146;
    origins 44–5, 59
Chrestien, Guillaume 128
Christianity 4, 54–5, 57, 58, 61, 72,
    86, 101–2, 135, 140, 149
Churchill, Fleetwood 24
chyle 67, 69
Clark, Sir Andrew 3, 30, 31, 32, 83, 87,
    91, 100, 113–4, 120–1, 130
Clarke, Edward 137
climate 64, 85, 89, 136–7
clitoris 154, 157
clothing, women's 5, 58, 72, 88, 114,
    130
coal eating: *see* pica
coffee 90, 105
Coley, Frederick 83, 111, 121, 125
colic 28
colon 4, 113; removal of 114–5
colour 2, 9, 26, 31, 35, 37, 39, 107,
    150
conception 10, 11, 48, 73, 75, 79, 83,
    85, 133, 148
conduct books 129: *see* advice books
Constantine the African 36
constipation 67, 97, 102, 112–5, 125,
    128
consumption 2, 21–2: *see* tuberculosis

Cooper, Kate 54–5
Corde, Maurice de la 49, 50–1, 52
Cornarius, Janus 58, 74, 83, 155, 156
corsets 114
cosmetics 28, 159
countrywomen 27, 91, 158; see also town
    and country
Cressy, David 35
Cullen, William 9, 36, 108–11, 141
Cunningham, Andrew 71
Cyrino, Monica Silveira 40

dancing 46, 92, 94–5, 98, 129–30, 131,
    133, 161
Dean-Jones, Lesley 75
death 75; and paleness 38–9; causes of
    20; desire for 50, 66, 95; sudden 28
deception 9, 50, 90, 112, 119–20, 130
defloration 53, 56, 89, 124; imagery of
    80, 156; see also hymen
Denman, Thomas 24
diagnosis by letter 13
diagnosis, retrospective 1, 65, 144
diaphragm, 47, 50, 96, 99
diarrhoea 71
diet: as cause of disease 9, 63, 65, 102;
    dietary disturbance 14, 28, 46, 67,
    94–115
digestion, in Galen 68–9, 73
Dioscorides 26, 150
disease: and age/gender categories 8, 16,
    36–7, 40, 42, 60, 66, 67,
    110–11,140–1; 'disappearing' 5;
    iatrogenic 2–3, 5, 33; imaginary
    2–3, 33, 110; labels 2–3, 4, 7, 13,
    19, 22, 29, 30, 33, 36, 43, 44, 47,
    78, 116, 117, 127, 144, 148; nature
    of vii, 1, 2, 13–14, 62–3, 141, 144;
    'new' 13, 25, 26, 27, 60, 61–6, 155;
    overlap between categories 14, 15,
    117, 121, 140
disease of virgins 53, 137; claims for
    classical origins 4–5, 43, 59–61, 66,
    139, 147; earliest description 4,
    46–8, 59
dissection 11, 12, 56, 71
Dixon, Laurinda 145
Donati, Giovanni Battista 53, 74–5, 95,
    155
Dormandy, Thomas 144
drug treatment 124–8; see also
    emmenagogues

Drysdale, George 82, 125
Dubois, Jacques 9, 36, 126, 127, 128,
    145, 149
Duden, Barbara 23, 32–3
Dyhouse, Carol 161
dyspepsia 15, 102, 108, 110, 114

earth, eating see pica
education: boarding schools 85, 105,
    141, 159; medical 11, 36, 46, 51,
    61; women's 85, 122, 135, 138, 161
eggs: avoidance of 101; in treatment
    131
Egypt 65
Eisenbichler, Konrad 86
ejaculation 65
elbow, bloodletting from 77
electric shock 8, 109, 124–5, 137
Elizabeth I 80,140
emmenagogues 9, 26, 67, 74, 97, 107,
    111, 124, 125–8
emotion 86; as a cause of disease 36, 37,
    59, 130
English Sweat 13, 61, 147, 155
epilepsy 36, 47, 144: see also sacred
    disease
Erasistratos 38, 76
erotic chlorotic 6–7, 90, 158
eugenics 81, 135
Evans, Cadwallader 124
Eve 72
exercise 91, 112; as treatment 124, 128,
    130–1, 133; excess 70, 71, 92; lack
    of 57, 88, 92, 132, 136; see also
    dancing
exploration 63,80, 157

factories 91, 113, 119
faeces 31, 49, 112, 125: see constipation
family of patient 6, 7, 9, 15, 42, 46, 85,
    101, 107, 124, 125–6, 136, 141, 146
fashion 91, 105, 113, 123, 160
fasting: thickens blood 106; as
    treatment 76; fasting girls 72, 101,
    102, 159
fermentation 72, 98, 119
Ferrand, Jacques 37, 38
fertility 44, 136; of sufferers 90, 127
Figlio, Karl 44, 92
Findlay, M.E. 137–8
Fissell, Mary 148

flowers, synonym for menses 2, 36, 110, 157

Floyer, Sir John 119

Fogo, Andrew 2, 104, 109–12

Fontanus, Nicholas 129

Forman, Simon 29, 34

Fowler, Don 44

Fox, Samuel 8, 111–12

fresh air: see ventilation

Freud, Sigmund 7, 15, 158

fright 36, 127

fruit, dangers of 63; in diet of sufferer 35, 98, 105; in imagery of disease 77, 157; in imagery of pregnancy 36, 110; see also ripeness

Fuchs, Leonhart 26–7

Galen 5, 10–11, 12, 37, 44, 57, 78, 118, 136; *Commentary on On Prognosis* 97; *Commentary on Regimen in acute diseases* 45, 48, 68, 79, 151, 153; *De passionibus mulierum*12; *On the affected parts* 145; *On bloodletting against Erasistratos* 12, 76, 106; *On bloodletting against the Erasistrateans in Rome* 76; *On the causes of symptoms* 59, 68–70; *On difficult breathing* 47, 68, 153; *On the dissection of the uterus* 12; *On the secrets of women* 12; *On simple medicines* 150; *On therapeutics, to Glaucon* 77

Galenic medicine 6–7, 12, 26, 29, 35, 36, 52, 53, 58, 59, 68–70, 71, 73, 79, 83, 94, 100, 101, 108, 109, 116, 118, 126, 132, 140, 153; see also humoral medicine; non-naturals

gall-bladder 69

germ theory 113

ghosts 47, 50, 96, 153

Gove, Mary 98

Gowers, Sir William Richard 122, 131

Grafton, Anthony 46

grass 35–6, 39, 88, 81, 141, 152; in human diet 62

Green, Monica 151

green: analogies for 31–2; and menstruation 37; and sexuality 35; as envious 35, 38; and fear 39; as unripe 34–5, 62; as youthful 34, 40, 135; colour of skin 21; stools 112; see also grass

green sickness: earliest uses of label 19–20, 43

Greene, Robert 20–1

Gregory, James 129

Grmek, Mirko 65

Gruner, Christian 49

Guggenheim, Karl 15

Gynaeciorum compilation 35, 57, 126, 148–9, 151

gynaecology 1, 44, 103, 158; Hippocratic gynaecology, 11, 43–4, 49, 51–3, 66, 99, 107

Habershon, Samuel Osborne 3, 97, 124–5

haematology: see blood testing

haemoglobin 122, 123

hair 5, 31, 90, 160

Halban, Josef 73

Hall, Granville Stanley 66, 68, 88,135, 136, 138

Hamilton, James 91, 110, 111, 113

Hanawalt, Barbara 86

Hansen, Axel 60–1, 146

Hanson, Ann Ellis 75

Haraway, Donna 117

harem 136–7, 141

Harvey, Gabriel 46

Harvey, William 68, 69

headache 3, 21, 60, 108

heart 15, 38, 39, 46, 47, 48, 50, 69, 96–7, 99, 106, 121, 156; displacement of 117; tremor 78; see also palpitation

Heath, Clark; see Patek, Arthur

herbals 26, 27, 29; see also drug treatment

Herophilos 11, 73

Hesiod 62, 155

Hestia 54

Heywood, Thomas 95

hibernation 65

Hildegard of Bingen 36, 39

Hippocrates, 5, 10–11, 53, 61, 83; *Airs,waters, places* 155; *Aphorisms* 23, 88, 149; *Coan prognoses* 60, 61; *Diseases of women*, 11, 12, 49, 51, 52, 75–6; *Epidemics* 11, 52, 60, 75, 76, 107; *On ancient medicine*, 63, 65; *On the disease of virgins* 43–4, 47, 48, 49–53, 58–60, 62, 66, 70, 74, 79, 83, 84, 85, 88, 94–7, 99, 100, 103,

106, 109,140; *On generation/Nature of the child* 11, 70, 84, 99, 100, 109; *On the nature of man*149; *On the sacred disease* 50; *On superfetation* 75; *On the use of liquids* 24; *Prorrhetics* 60, 61; *Weeks*, 60

Hippocratic corpus: Latin translations, 45–6, 49, 51, 74, 94, 152–3 see *also* Calvi, Cornarius

Hirsch, August 136, 155

Hobby, Elaine 144, 148, 150, 157, 160

Hollick, Frederick 6, 15, 87

homeopathy 19, 28, 91, 113, 133, 134

hospital: rise of 117–8, 128; records 14

housework 129, 130, 138

Hudson, Robert 33–4, 59, 102, 117, 125

humoral medicine 6–7, 12, 22–3, 69, 78, 79, 83, 86, 99, 125, 149

humours: unconcocted 47, 68, 78

Humphreys, Margaret 2

hydropathy 125, 133–4; see *also* baths

hymen 51, 54, 55–6, 57–8, 80, 89, 124, 154

hysteria 7–8, 15, 93, 145, 148; male 146

iatrogenic disease 79, 125, 160

idleness 64, 66, 103, 139

imagination: dangerous effects of 41, 100, 136; maternal 64

imperialism 63, 81–2,140

innate heat 23, 69

insomnia 36, 97–8, 106

intelligence 49

Ireland 81, 157

iron: deficiency 33, 102, 104, 116, 160; use in treatment 125, 127–8, 131, 137

irritable bowel syndrome 139; see *also* constipation, diarrhoea

Irwin, Eleanor 39

Jacobi, Mary Putnam 137, 161

Jardine, Lisa 46

jaundice 22, 24–5, 33, 107; black 25; green 23, 24–8, 60, 107; white 144, 149

jealousy 38, 92

Joan of Arc 55

John Chrysostom 55, 58, 154

Johnson, Edward 30, 144, 150

Johnson, Walter 24, 30, 104, 119,144, 146, 148, 150

Johnston, John 118, 144

Jones, Ernest Lloyd 16, 90, 123–4

Joubert, Laurent 56, 80, 98, 146–7, 154–5

Kelly, Kathleen Coyne 154

Kitson, Jane 21–2, 25, 150

Klairmont-Lingo, Alison 157

Kneipp, Sebastian 125, 144

labia 124

laboratory 5, 10, 116–24, 141

Laennec, Réné-Théophile-Hyacinthe 120

Lane, William Arbuthnot 114, 115

Lange, Johannes 4–5, 6, 13, 18–19, 29, 30, 36, 37, 43–8, 54, 57–8, 61–2, 67, 68, 69, 70, 73–4, 79, 83, 94–7, 100, 105–6, 107, 139–40

Langham, William 27–8, 97, 126

lassitude 14, 72, 92, 96, 108, 130

lavender 127

Le Clerc, Daniel 44

lead poisoning 15

leeches 124, 154

leisure 37, 70, 103, 129

Leoniceno, Niccolò 61

leprosy 65

letter format, in medicine 7, 45; see *also* Lange

letters, women's 21

Lettsom, John Coakley 105, 114, 160

Liébault, Jean 32, 44, 53, 128, 152

life cycle 84–6, 108, 128, 158

literacy 23

Littré, Emile 12, 59, 60, 74, 147

liver 8, 46, 69–70, 82, 98, 107–12, 116, 126, 132; role in blood production 21, 47, 68–9, 97

Livy 46, 64

ps-Longinus 38, 39, 40, 151

Longus 39, 97–8

Loraux, Nicole 51

Lorkyn, Thomas 148–9

Loudon, Irvine 1, 15, 34, 35, 44, 51, 144, 148, 150

Loughlin, Marie 56

love: sensations of 39; unrequited 36, 40, 92, 95

love fever 19, 47, 53, 144
love sickness 4, 36–40, 67, 97–8, 108, 118, 136, 140, 151
Lucretius 39, 64–5, 95
lungs 24, 76, 116
lust 37, 41–2, 85, 86, 96, 103–4, 108, 136
luxury 63, 64, 65, 98–9, 139

MacDonald, Michael 29, 86
Maclean, Ian 1, 44
McMurtrie, Henry 130
madness 47, 50, 86, 92, 153, 159
magnetism 125
Mamillia 20–1, 35, 39, 42
Margaret, Countess of Cumberland 21, 158
marjoram 28
marriage 4, 48, 55, 138; age at 5, 20–1, 41, 46, 49, 50, 51, 57–8, 81, 83, 84–5, 87–8, 91, 92, 102, 106, 118; and nymphomania 41; and virginity 54–5, 86, 100; as therapy 48, 50, 58, 74, 77, 79–83, 84, 106, 107, 109, 110, 111, 124, 127, 138, 140; risks of 75, 78
Martinez, David 97
masturbation 41–2, 82, 90, 105, 145, 146
Maubray, John 3, 16, 33, 56, 97, 104–5, 153, 154
meat: avoidance of 46, 95, 100–2, 113, 127; in treatment of disease 101, 131
melancholy 92, 96
menarche, 4, 6, 10, 12, 21, 22, 23, 40, 49, 50, 53, 56, 70, 82, 84, 88, 100–1, 102, 103, 108–9, 110–11, 113, 123–4, 141; age at 51, 73, 77–8, 81, 84–5, 103, 109, 130, 133; and cities 91, 103; danger of 66, 88, 92, 137; preparation for 90
menopause 111
menstrual blood, nature of 73, 99, 109
menstruation 102, 108, 113, 126, 135, 156; and masculinisation 15; and pain 56, 57, 138, 156; diverted 23–4, 26, 27, 52, 76; fermentation theory of, 71–2; function of 9–10, 68, 72–3, 136, 156; Galenic model 68–70, 71; plethora theory of, 23, 72, 103, 108–9; role in health

11–12, 1[...]
154; vica[...]
Mercado, L[...]
145, 15[...]
Mercuriale[...]
154
Mezière, V[...]
microscop[...]
milk 23, '[...]
mint 28
miscarriage 107, 161
Mitchell, Silas Weir 130
mithridatum 25, 26, 126
monsters 63–4
Monte, Giambattista da 44, 78, 109, 152
Montpellier 19, 82, 88, 146
moon 128
Morantz-Sanchez, Regina 135, 138
mugwort 112, 127
Muscio 57

Napier, Richard 19, 22, 29–30, 86, 144
neohumoralism 82
nervous system 42, 67–8, 69, 82, 92, 120, 133
neurasthenia 15, 117
Nicolson, Malcolm 120
Nightingale, Florence 134
non-naturals 113, 129
nosebleeds 24, 52
novels 8, 41, 90, 133, 148, 152
numbness 50, 97
nuns 101
Nutton, Vivian 71, 147, 152
nymphomania 40–2, 88

oatmeal 104, 105, 112
observation 5, 13, 16, 32, 33–4, 122–3
obstructions 26, 28, 48, 50–1, 74, 78, 97, 126, 127, 132, 160; as possible pregnancy, 9–10, 107, 132; of channels entering womb 15, 26, 58, 69–70, 97, 103, 104, 106, 109, 126, 127
Oldham, Henry 24
Olive, Antoine 34, 88–90, 92, 98, 129
Oliver, James 125
onions, as remedy 25, 26–8, 30–1
orientalism 136–7
Ovid 37, 38, 140, 151
ovulation, 10, 72–3, 91

r William 21–2
s 97; and *chloros* 37; and fear 39;
and love sickness 37, 38, 46, 57,
97–8; and menstruation 58, 72, 76,
110, 127, 137; and nymphomania
37, 41; and pica 60, 106, 132; as
attractive 104–5; as key symptom
22, 30, 77, 80, 150; as sign of
pregnancy 9, 10; as sign of virginity
58; in Anna 30, 46, 58, 78; of blood
21, 123; of hair 31
palpitations 14, 48, 92, 100, 106, 108
Pandora 62, 64, 90, 155
Paré, Ambroise 58, 65, 106
parents of sufferer: *see* family
Paris Medical Faculty 34, 88, 146
parthenos, meaning of 49, 51, 54
Paster, Gail Kern 22, 76, 91, 154
Patek, Arthur and Heath, Clark 91,
117, 145, 146
patent remedies 128, 131–3
patient/doctor relationship 6–7, 8–9,
44, 107, 117–8, 119–20
Pechey, John 31, 128
penis 65, 84; bleeding 76, 149
pepper 25, 28, 98, 105
Phillips, Kim 87
phlegm: *see* humoral medicine
pica 10, 14, 16, 60, 61, 97, 98, 103–7,
108, 110, 159–60; and normal
menstruation 98; in pregnancy and
greensickness 106–7, 132
Pierce, Robert 8, 133
Pinault, Jody Rubin 57
plague 34; *see also* Athenian plague
plethora: *see* menstruation, plethora
theory of
Pliny 63, 65, 66, 155
Plutarch: *Dialogue on love* 73; *Life of
Demetrios* 38; on new diseases 63–5;
On the virtues of women 95
pneuma 48, 69, 79
poisoning, as model for green sickness
26
Pomata, Gianna 73, 75
Pontano, Giovanni 95
portal vein 69
Potter, Ursula 35
pregnancy 9, 10, 21, 44, 50, 51, 57, 73,
83, 88, 98, 106, 119, 154, 156, 159;
dangers of 57; overlap with chlorosis
9, 15, 107, 111, 146–7; signs of

106; tests for 133; therapeutic effects
of 48, 114; *see also* obstructions; pica
Priessnitz, Vincenz 134
Prometheus 62
prostitution 82, 154
Protestantism 4, 61, 140, 145
proverbs 4, 128, 145, 151, 158
ptomaines 113, 160
puberty 13, 22, 48, 83–90, 91, 101,
103, 129, 137–8; age at 51, 57, 60,
77, 89, 129; as vulnerable time 40,
47, 66, 83–8, 90, 92, 102, 108–9,
124, 137–8; growth spurt 102;
idealisation of 72, 87, 88–90;
premature 41, 82, 89
puberty gap 85, 87–8, 140
pulse 3, 14, 48, 69, 92, 118–21, 138

quantification: of menstrual loss 72;
surveys of sufferers 91, 130; *see also*
blood testing, pulse, stethoscope
quickening 9

Raciborski, Adam 6, 10, 41, 73, 81, 82,
84–5, 91, 101, 102, 107, 114, 118,
123, 129, 130, 144, 158, 159
Ranchin, François 53, 82, 118, 153
Ravenna 45, 51, 153
Rebello, Pedro 103–4
recipe collections 1, 27, 127, 160
red plants, use in treatment 28, 126,
150
Reece, Richard 124–5
rest cure 124, 130–1, 138
retention, distinguished from
suppression 9, 108
Reynolds, John 72
Rhodes, Peter 63
riding: dangers of 131; as therapy 129
Rigler, Lorenz 136
ripeness, imagery of 20–1, 35, 42, 47,
49, 50, 77–8, 80, 82, 104, 105; *see
also* fruit; green, as unripe
Rocher, Gregory de 80
Roe, Shirley 121
Rosenberg, Charles 2
Rosin, Heinrich 81–2
Rousseau, George 41, 152
Rousseau, Jean-Jacques 88–9, 91, 92,
135
Ruddock, Edward Harris 91, 113

rue 28, 126, 127
Rue, Ambroise 6, 87, 107
Rufus of Ephesus 100–1
Rutherford, John 67–8, 112, 119, 125, 160

sacred disease 50
sage 28
Salih, Sarah 56
Sappho 37–40, 140, 141, 151–2
Sawyer, Ronald 19, 25
Schenck von Grafenberg, Joannes 30
Schleiner, Winfried 145
Schultz, James 85
Schurig, Martin 4
Schwarz, Emil 59
seed, female 11, 12, 26, 53, 57, 64, 70, 72, 89, 101, 106, 147
self-denial 55
semen 23, 51, 56, 64, 79, 84, 89, 99, 136
Seneca 65
Sennert, Daniel 96, 119, 127, 139, 145, 154, 157, 158, 159–60
senses, role in medicine 88, 118, 122; see also observation, pulse, stethoscope
servants, domestic 72, 87, 91, 92, 131
sex: as cure for condition 4, 35, 37, 48, 74–5, 79–80, 82, 108, 110, 115, 127, 151; and imagery of war 80; in Eden 56
Shakespeare: Henry IV, Part 2 20; Love's Labour's Lost 37; Romeo and Juliet 35, 80, 148, 150
shame 44, 127
Sharp, Jane 9, 16, 19, 40, 56, 58, 75, 77, 82, 96, 98, 101, 106–7, 108, 119, 126, 127, 129, 144, 154, 157
Showalter, Elaine 8
Siddall, A. Clair 34, 125
Sissa, Giulia 54
skin 23, 24, 58–9
of sufferer, 33, 92
skin disease 33
Skrabanek, Petr 145
Slack, Paul 4
solitude 9, 92
Soranos 56–7, 85, 147
sperm: see semen
spices 98, 103, 105, 127, 133
spleen 2, 25, 69, 126, 132
Starobinski, 59, 60, 104

steel, as drug 127–8; see iron
Stengel 19, 31, 59, 104
Stephanus 53, 75
sterility 48, 83, 132, 138
stethoscope 120–1, 138
Stockman, Ralph 31, 91, 102, 113–4
stomach 29, 69, 78, 104, 107, 132, 150
Storch, Johannes Pelagius 23, 32–3, 72
Strange, Julie-Marie 128, 146, 159, 161
Sudell, Nicholas 31, 79, 112, 127
suicide 50, 59, 66, 95–6, 127
surgeons 32, 111, 151
sweat 27; menstruation through 24, 27
sweating: as symptom 38, 71, 106; as therapy 125, 129, 134
swelling 61, 94, 106, 132, 159; of feet 72, 96–7, 108
Sydenham, Thomas 14, 31, 61, 96, 118, 127, 147–8, 156
syphilis: sixteenth-century 13, 61; nineteenth-century 81, 121

Tait, Lawson 6, 16, 147
Tanner, John 3, 16, 80, 92, 118, 126
Tardy, Claude 53, 109
Taylor, Frederick 9, 123, 124, 131
tea 90, 105
technology, challenges to 120–3
Temkin, Owsei 144, 147
theriac 26, 150
Theriot, Nancy 146
Thucydides 63, 95
Tilt, Edward 11, 30, 124
timing of treatment 128
town and country 89, 90–2, 103, 105; see also countrywomen
Trabuc, C.-C. Marius 88, 104, 107, 110, 125, 129, 130
Trotula 35–6, 37, 40, 67, 70, 98, 140, 151, 154
Trousseau, Armand 6, 16, 30, 120, 121, 125, 157
tuberculosis, 121, 125, 144; see also consumption
Turner, Daniel 4, 32–3, 72, 107, 127

ulcer: gastric 15, 24; peptic 117
urine 28, 69, 125; and ovulation 73; examination of 45, 133; obstruction of flow 28, 97; pale, in chlorosis 31; virgin's 56, 154
uterine fury 53, 96

vagina 56, 58, *124*
van Foreest, Pieter 77, 127
van Helmont, Joan Baptista 62, 72
Vandereycken, Walter 102
vanity 28, 66, 92, 100, 105, 114, 115, 123
Varandal, Jean 19, 28, 31, 32, 40, 43, 60, 95–6, 105, 128, 136, 139, 144
vena cava 47, 69
venereal disease 133, 154; *see also* syphilis
ventilation 90, 91, 131, 133
Vesalius, Andreas 70
Vesta 54
vinegar 28, 98, 105, 134
Virgin Mary 54
virginity 4, 16, 28, 44, 49–51, 79, 80, 85, 89, 99, 124, 127; active 54, 81; definitions 53–6; diet appropriate to 95, 100–1; disguising loss of 53, 154; and imagery of conquest 80; passive 54; perpetual 57; restoration of 89; risks of 29, 57, 81, 93, 109, 115; of the soul 55, 58, 158; *see also* defloration
virginity tests 53, 56
voice 56, 62, 92, 154
vomiting 16, 92, 125, 127; morning sickness 106
von Noorden, Karl 81, 82, 92, 107, 131, 141

Wack, Mary 37, 40
Wailoo, Keith 117–8, 123
Ward, Gordon 15, 33, 117, 119, 123, 128

water 134; *see* baths
weakness 22, 108, 123; of digestion 112, 114; *see also* women, as weaker sex
Wear, Andrew 147, 148
white fever 2, 14, 19, 27, 47, 53, 119, 127, 139–40, 144
Whorton, James 113
widows 9, 28, 96, 132
Wiesner, Merry 87
Willis, Thomas 72
Wiltshire, Alfred 157
womb 2, 4, 15, 32, 44, 76, 98, 107, 108, 161; anatomy of 11, 12, 47, 68; and digestion 47, 99; and hysteria 7, 15; as cause of menstrual disorders 59, 68, 72, 109; as seat of disease 26, 44, 98, 109; closure of 53, 58, 99; expulsive faculty 78, 109; gravid 114; in virgins 15, 50, 69, 81, 84, 90, 115, 132; lining of 72; suffocation of 46, 53, 78, 106; vessels of 94, 99, 106, 109, 129; wandering 11, 83; weakness of 91, 103, 83, 109; *see also* uterine fury
women 103; as colder sex 95; as weaker sex 8, 50, 72, 88, 96, 105, 114, 119, 122, 129; in medical profession 118, 134–8, 151; role in food preparation 101; healers 132–3; work for 87; *see also* servants, domestic
Wood-Allen, Mary 105, 114, 130, 160

x-rays 117
ps-Xenophon 129, 159, 160

Yealland, Lewis 8
yellow bile: *see* humoral medicine

Lightning Source UK Ltd.
Milton Keynes UK
UKOW06f0619180915

258859UK00002B/28/P